RENEWAL
IN PSYCHIATRY

THE SERIES IN CLINICAL AND COMMUNITY PSYCHOLOGY

CONSULTING EDITORS:

CHARLES D. SPIELBERGER and IRWIN G. SARASON

Averill	• Patterns of Psychological Thought: Readings in Historical and Contemporary Texts
Becker	• Depression: Theory and Research
Brehm	• The Application of Social Psychology to Clinical Practice
Cattell and Dreger	• Handbook of Modern Personality Theory
Endler and Magnusson	• Interactional Psychology and Personality
Friedman and Katz	• The Psychology of Depression: Contemporary Theory and Research
Kissen	• From Group Dynamics to Group Psychoanalysis: Therapeutic Applications of Group Dynamic Understanding
Klopfer and Reed	• Problems in Psychotherapy: An Eclectic Approach
Manschreck and Kleinman	• Renewal in Psychiatry: A Critical Rational Perspective
Reitan and Davison	• Clinical Neuropsychology: Current Status and Applications
Spielberger and Diaz-Guerrero	• Cross-Cultural Anxiety
Spielberger and Sarason	• Stress and Anxiety, volume 1
Sarason and Spielberger	• Stress and Anxiety, volume 2
Sarason and Spielberger	• Stress and Anxiety, volume 3
Spielberger and Sarason	• Stress and Anxiety, volume 4
Ulmer	• On the Development of a Token Economy Mental Hospital Treatment Program

IN PREPARATION

Bermant, Kelman, and Warwick	• The Ethics of Social Intervention
Cohen and Mirsky	• Biology and Psychopathology
Iscoe, Bloom, and Spielberger	• Community Psychology in Transition
Janisse	• Pupillometry: The Psychology of the Pupillary Response
London	• Strategies of Personality Research
Olweus	• Aggression in the Schools

RENEWAL
IN PSYCHIATRY
A Critical Rational Perspective

with a foreword by Leon Eisenberg, M.D.

EDITED BY Theo C. Manschreck
Department of Psychiatry, Harvard Medical School;
Massachusetts General Hospital; and Department of
Psychology and Social Relations, Harvard University

Arthur M. Kleinman
Division of Social and Cross-Cultural Psychiatry,
Department of Psychiatry and Behavioral Sciences,
University of Washington School of Medicine, Seattle

HEMISPHERE PUBLISHING
CORPORATION
Washington   London

A HALSTED PRESS BOOK
JOHN WILEY & SONS
New York   London   Sydney   Toronto

Hemisphere Publishing Corporation
1025 Vermont Ave., N.W., Washington, D.C. 20005

Distributed solely by Halsted Press, a Division of John Wiley & Sons, Inc., New York.

1 2 3 4 5 6 7 8 9 0   D O D O   7 8 3 2 1 0 9 8 7

Library of Congress Cataloging in Publication Data

Main entry under title:

Renewal in psychiatry.

  (The Series in Clinical and community psychology)
  Bibliography: p.
  Includes index.
  1. Psychiatry—Philosophy.   I. Eisenberg, Leon, 1922- . II. Manschreck, Theo C.   III. Kleinman, Arthur.
RC437.5.C74   616.8'9'001   77-1244
ISBN 0-470-99108-9

Printed in the United States of America

DEDICATION

This volume honors Leon Eisenberg, our teacher and mentor. During his years as Chief, Department of Psychiatry, Massachusetts General Hospital, and later as Chairman, Executive Committee, Department of Psychiatry, Harvard Medical School, he has been the model for us of critical rationality in psychiatry. He has made us understand that a critical and rational approach to psychiatry must be anchored in a sensitive appreciation of the profoundly human experience of the clinical world and an indissoluble commitment to social justice as much as in serious scholarship and creative research. And he has fostered our differing inquiries into and critiques of psychiatry.

The chapters in this volume are pale reflections of the powerful and challenging vision he has transmitted to us of what psychiatric science should be.

Contents

Contributors

Jack Altman, Ph.D. Visiting Professor of Psychology, Institut National de la Recherche Scientifique-Santé, Université du Québec, Hôpital St. Jean-De-Dieu, Montreal.

David M. Bear, M.D. Research Associate, National Institue of Neurological Diseases, Blindness, and Stroke, National Institutes of Health, Bethesda, Maryland.

William R. Beardslee, M.D. Research Fellow, Department of Psychiatry, Harvard Medical School, Children's Hospital Medical Center.

Felton Earls, M.D. Assistant Professor, Department of Psychiatry, Harvard Medical School, Children's Hospital Medical Center.

Jeffrey Gilbert, M.D.[1] Assistant Professor, Department of Psychiatry, Harvard Medical School, Massachusetts General Hospital.

Gordon P. Harper, M.D. Research Fellow, Department of Psychiatry, Harvard Medical School, Children's Hospital Medical Center.

Arthur M. Kleinman, M.D., M.A.[2] Clinical Instructor, Department of Psychiatry, Harvard Medical School, Massachusetts General Hospital; and Lecturer, Department of Anthropology, Harvard University.

Anastasia Kucharski, M.D., M.A. Clinical Fellow, Department of Psychiatry, Harvard Medical School, Massachusetts General Hospital.

Theo C. Manschreck, M.D., M.P.H. Instructor, Department of Psychiatry, Harvard Medical School; Massachusetts General Hospital; and Department of Psychology and Social Relations, Harvard University.

Peter Mansky, M.D. Assistant Professor, Department of Psychiatry, University of Kentucky College of Medicine.

---

[1] Jeffrey Gilbert participated in the seminar, but did not contribute a chapter.
[2] Arthur Kleinman is currently Associate Professor of Psychiatry, Division of Social and Cross-Cultural Psychiatry, Department of Psychiatry and Behavioral Sciences, University of Washington School of Medicine, Seattle.

Michael Murphy, M.D., M.P.H.[3] Clinical Instructor, Department of Psychiatry, Harvard Medical School, Massachusetts General Hospital; and doctoral candidate, Harvard School of Public Health.

Timothy M. Rivinus, M.D. Clinical Fellow, Department of Psychiatry, Harvard Medical School, Massachusetts Mental Health Center.

Miriam Sonn, R.N., Ph.D. Psychiatric Nurse, Massachusetts General Hospital; and Department of Sociology, Brandeis University.

[3] Michael Murphy participated in the seminar, but did not contribute a chapter.

Foreword

THE PSYCHIATRIST'S DILEMMA

Leon Eisenberg, M.D.
Maude and Lillian Presley Professor of Psychiatry
Harvard Medical School

Why is it that for psychiatry there is a particularly urgent need for critical rationality, as so passionately and persuasively argued by Theo Manschreck and Arthur Kleinman in the opening chapter of this book? All of medicine, and not psychiatry alone, is under attack (Illich, 1975).

General discontent with medical care characterizes our era (Fuchs, 1974). Doctoring costs too much; and for all the cost, it has only marginal effects on mortality (McKeown, 1966). It's hard to get; and when it's to be had, it is too impersonal (Korsch et al., 1968). It's not the physician's power to affect the course of virulent diseases that is in question, but his or her relevance to the management of the day-to-day ills and the changes of aging that plague an increasing proportion of our population (McDermott, 1974). Yet it is for these that psychiatry, of all the medical specialists, has the most to say. Nonetheless, the aura of potency that emanates from surgical wizardry, "magic bullet" drugs, and the precision of the laboratory confers on surgeons and internists a scientific respectability denied to psychiatrists.

Our critics, and there are many, might highlight the flaws in our theories and the limitations on our practices as evidence of our need for critical rationality. Without denying those flaws and limits, I will focus on a very different reason—one that is at first glance paradoxical: the regularity with which our patients respond favorably to our interventions (a consequence of the extraordinary interpersonal sensitivity of one human being to another). The problem, as I see it, is not that psychiatrists sometimes fail in their efforts to influence patients, but that they so often succeed or, at least, appear to.

This may seem an outrageous claim. While some of our critics may begrudgingly acknowledge the utility of antipsychotic and antidepressant drugs, those familiar with the extensive literature on the evaluation of psychotherapy will point to the Scotch verdict of *not proven* in the majority of studies that have attempted to demonstrate the superiority of one method of treatment over another (Luborsky et al., 1975; Sloane et al., 1975). However, the very same data, looked at from the standpoint of outcome (and independent of the theory on which the treatment rests), are in remarkable agreement in reporting high levels of improvement (in the range of 80 percent), whether this be assessed by the patient's report of his or her own symptoms or by criteria based on role performance (Frank, 1965; Meltzoff and Kornreich, 1970; Weissman et al., 1974). It is customary to dismiss these benefits because they are "nonspecific" and bear little relationship to the theory of treatment on which they are predicated. Nonspecific they may well be, if specific refers to those aspects of technique that preoccupy therapists of one or another "school," but lack of specificity must not blind us to the near universal frequency with which benefit is claimed by the patient. Benefit, in the final analysis, is the aim of any medical intervention.

I make the point, not to argue that we rest content with an outcome that we do not understand and that may well be unrelated to the medical training of the psychiatrist, but to stress that what is a bonus for the sufferer is in fact an occupational hazard for the doctor. Just because we do so well, simply by "being" with the patient, whatever else goes on during the consultation, we are highly vulnerable to the error of ascribing the observed effectiveness to irrelevant epiphenomena in the psychotherapeutic process. Doing well, in this sense, invites the hubris of crediting ourselves with greater understanding than we have (Eisenberg, 1975).

Patients, in an all too human and unending effort to reduce the chaos that threatens to overwhelm them, attempt to impose meaning upon puzzling and enigmatic events. At times, they generate hypotheses that we, from the perspective that distance and disinterest permit, can help them dismiss. But the problem only begins there. If they are persuaded to abandon spurious ideas, they remain in urgent need of new meanings to relate old events and are more than ready to accept our efforts to provide them. Worse, from the standpoint of testing the validity of tentative hypotheses (and all the better for the reduction of anxiety), the new explanations are promptly incorporated into their belief systems. By acting upon them as if they were true, they make them, in a certain sense, true (that is, true for them). Thus, an idea put forth by the psychiatrist as a preliminary formulation, once it is assimilated by the patient, is so influential in altering the patient's behavior that it is only the skeptic (or critical rationalist) who will not mistake the social consequences of a psychodynamic interpretation for proof of its validity (Whitehorn, 1947).

CASE 1   Angela was a 19-year-old college sophomore when she came to see me with the complaint: "My mind doesn't function properly." She went on to report that other people's minds went into hers. Listening to others speak became "malignant" because she became a "receptacle" for chaotic ideas. Her symptoms, she stated, had been "building up for a long time." The immediate consultation had been prompted by a sharp decline in her ability to complete her college work. She had gone to the family doctor a month earlier "hoping it was something physical." She was distressed when he attributed her symptoms to "nerves" and referred her to me. She didn't believe it could be insanity because "my attitude isn't warped; I'm simply nonexistent as a person. It's the most miserable thing. I don't want to live if it doesn't clear up."

Over the next several years as I saw her weekly (this was before psychotropic drugs were available), her long-standing thought disturbance, confusion, and lack of pleasure in life underwent periodic exacerbations: radio waves penetrated her mind; she had visions that no one else could share; vague and distant voices seemed to be calling to her. These irruptions were accompanied by overwhelming anxiety expressed in the plea: "I must be going crazy. Am I going crazy? Tell me I'm not crazy."

Rarely was she able to report life events that might account for her acute distress. Her uncanny experiences were, however, "interpretable" as metaphors expressing aspects of her history and her current life space. Whenever I was able to offer an "interpretation" that, to her view, connected her bizarre mental symptoms to more understandable and ordinary human feelings, she would be visibly relieved. In subsequent interviews, she would refer to these interpretations as part of her new "understanding" of herself.

For example, on one occasion, she reported a radio message ordering her to kill her father. I "explained" that she, and not some foreign source, was the originator of the message and that it was "nothing more" than a dramatic expression of her own life experience in which her mother, herself schizophrenic, had made repeated attempts on her husband's life. Angela was angry with her father; yet she loved and needed him. By transferring the responsibility for the death wishes to the radio, she minimized her guilt and expressed her resistance to the act. (We never faced the dilemma of just who the "she" was who controlled this mental legerdemain.) It was up to the two of us together in treatment. I reiterated, to find ways for her ideas and feelings to be expressed directly in order to avoid the substitutive and symbolic alternatives that so distressed her. This "rational" explanation seemed to reassure the patient that she wasn't crazy or out of control and that she no longer needed to fear being impelled to carry out a command she dreaded fulfilling.

I was not then, nor am I now, at all confident that I understood the causes of her inner chaos. What I tried to provide was a coherent structure of meaning that made sense of her life history and of what she revealed to me about her own feelings. When these interpretations of her symptoms as metaphors succeeded in providing a matrix to make the strange and uncanny a part of the known and the familiar, there was a noticeable diminution of her anxiety. It is entirely possible that very different structures of meaning might have had the same beneficent result for the patient. However, I did not feel I had the right to conduct an experiment by deliberately offering interpretations constructed to be "false," simply to determine whether they, too, might be effective. The restraint stemmed not from any conviction that what I thought to be true was necessarily more therapeutic than some arbitrary alternative, but from my feeling that I had an ethical obligation not to tell the patient something I could not believe myself.

Did I make a difference? The patient was sure I did. I? I think I did. I believe she would have killed herself if she had become convinced she was "crazy." For her, the word "crazy" had many meanings, highly idiosyncratic. Between us, we negotiated a position that enabled her to fend off that self-definition. She remained out of the hospital; there was good reason to believe that hospitalization would have been a destructive experience for her. I doubt that she could have avoided it without some help from a "travel guide." Palliation, in chronic illness, is not a trivial good.

How did it end? She left town, still lonely and confused, to take a job. My only follow-up was a wedding announcement a year later. I know no more. Even if I did, it is not clear that additional information on the trajectory of her illness would shed any light on the meanings of the transactions between us.

If the Scylla of Delphic interpretation is patients' readiness to believe the doctor when psychic chaos threatens, its Charybdis is patients' insistence on presenting a more or less plausible psychogenic "cause" for somatic symptoms. What patients believe to be the source of the problem, so long as they have any hypotheses at all, will shape the history they present. Human consciousness is organized in such a fashion as to comprehend, or attempt to comprehend, behavior as though it be the result of one's own decisions. One says: "I hit him," and not: "My arm hit him," at least until the arm's performance is so foreign to the self that it cannot be forced into the framework of volition. Consider the following vignette:

CASE 2 Frank, a 25-year-old writer, was in search of psychotherapy "because" his decision to write his autobiography had led to such an intense inner preoccupation that he experienced alarming episodes of withdrawal from contact with his immediate environment. While driving, he might go into a reverie so compelling that to "bring myself back to reality," he found it necessary to execute a motor act such as shaking his head or stepping on the accelerator, "to jolt myself out of it." He went on to describe himself as unhappy, discontented with his life, and obsessed with reconstructing his past and dreaming of his future. In his opinion, it was unhealthy self-examination that had brought him to this pass and it was psychotherapy that he needed.

As part of the evaluation, I referred him to a clinical psychologist. My colleague reported that in the course of testing, the patient "threw his head sidewise and backward in ticlike fashion, with his jaws opening and closing rhythmically. His face was flushed and covered with sweat. After some seconds, he reassured me that he did this to restore his concentration." The psychologist described a number of evidences of psychopathology in his performance on the projective tests. The episode of head movement was attributed to "inhibition of hostility." The diagnostic formulation read: "This patient is attempting to protect himself by withdrawal and constriction, a process which is now beginning to show symptoms of a developing schizophrenia."

I had not been alert enough to recognize the clinical syndrome from the history Frank provided at our initial meeting. With the description of the specific episodes, I arranged for an electro-encephalogram, which revealed slow spikes in both temporal areas. On the basis of the overt behavior and the EEG findings, I made the diagnosis of temporal lobe epilepsy (a diagnosis Frank was most reluctant to accept) and prescribed diphenylhydantoin. Within a week of taking the medication, the patient reported the cessation of the episodes that had been the immediate reason for his seeking help. A very short time thereafter, he returned to New York in pursuit of a job offer. It had not been "he" who clenched his jaw to clear his mind; it was a jaw that clenched out of "his" control under the command of an irritable brain focus; it was a mind that blurred and refocused in such subtle fashion and brief interval as to enable the inner and outer events to be reintegrated into consciousness as acts of intention.

I was fortunate enough to see him a year later when he was passing through town and "dropped by" to bring me up to date.

His in-laws had refused to believe he had epilepsy and insisted that he stop taking the drug, a demand he complied with the more readily because of his own ambivalence. When medication was discontinued, the episodes recurred. This led to repeat examination and to reinstitution of the same treatment, followed by remission of symptoms. However, he had remained dissatisfied with himself and with his life; he was about to divorce his wife, an immature and histrionic woman who had attempted to commit suicide (for both of them) by turning on the gas when he was already asleep. Nothing about him supported the earlier suggestion that he was schizophrenic. However, he reported multiple neurotic symptoms. Treatment of the temporal lobe epilepsy had ended his psychomotor seizures but had had little effect on his psychological malfunction. He was encouraged to pursue his intent to seek psychotherapy.

Then, pity the practicing physician—and weep for the psychiatrist! Whatever complexities beset philosophers when they attempt to tease out the essential elements of a theory of causality and to explicate the logic of statistical inference, they do not have patients waiting upon them whose care must be based upon decisions that reek of imputed causal connections. The treating physician works in a context in which both he or she and the patient are bound together in a matrix of etiological hypotheses, frequently contradictory, often unsubstantiated, and much of the time with evidence inadequate for deciding on the relative merits of the alternatives. Worst of all, a significant component of the physician's therapeutic potency is his or her ability to make the patient feel the doctor "understands."

The most powerful test of truth in the scientific method is the susceptibility of predictions based on theory to disconfirmation by empirical evidence. Thus, international attention was focused on the study of the 1913 solar eclipse because the phenomena to be observed would provide a critical test for the theory of relativity. There was no reason to fear that the prediction would generate its own confirmation. Although the theory guided the specific observations that needed to be made, it could not affect the phenomena to be recorded. The heavens continue to spin on in their course and light continues to stream into space without regard to theories of field and force generated by scientists in their effort to comprehend the universe. When the first radio astronomers recorded unexpected celestial X-rays, there was no suspicion that radiation had not always existed nor that it would not continue to exist, whether or not astronomers have instruments to sample it.

Social and behavioral theorists face an altogether different problem in this respect. When the manpower economist, Carrter (1971), predicted a surplus of scientists for the subsequent decade by projecting the current numbers in training and anticipating trends in the job market, he was afflicted with the curse of Cassandra. Only if people did *not* believe him would his dire maledictions come to pass. For, if he were believed by students and their faculty advisors, fewer students would enter or be admitted to graduate training and the predicted surplus might be abated or even turned into an actual deficit. As the sociologist W. I. Thomas (Thomas and Thomas, 1928) pointed out almost forty years ago, "If men define situations as real, they are real in their consequences." This proposition provides major problems in the evaluation of general theory in social science; it is compounded as a source of knotty difficulties for formulating and testing theory and practice in psychiatry.

I am tempted to go further, but my assignment is to write a foreword, not a chapter. I shall content myself with having outlined, as a supplement to the arguments brought forth by my colleagues, additional reasons why critical rationality is essential to the development of psychiatry as a scientific discipline (Freedman, 1973).

It remains only to admit to my uncommon pride when Arthur and Theo informed me that they and their colleagues intended to dedicate this volume to me as their teacher. According to Erikson (1959) generativity, the crucial maturational process in the middle years of life, is "concern in establishing and guiding the next generation." Whether I have met that challenge adequately for either my biological or my intellectual offspring, I cannot judge; but I can attest to the very real satisfaction that the "next generation" has bestowed on this one by acknowledging a debt I would like to believe to be warranted. Having read the text and having seen for myself how far the writers have gone beyond what I could have written, I am all the more moved. One was, of course, at least momentarily disconcerted to note that one title considered for this volume was *Feet of Clay*, with some degree of reassurance being offered by the subtitle: *Quests and Inquiries into Critical Rationality in the Fields of Psychiatry*. Lest I fall into the psychiatric venal sin of overinterpretation, just having warned against it, I will accept the editors' assurance that it is psychiatry, and not the dedicatee, that suffers from that ominous syndrome *pedes argillaci*!

It remains a matter of considerable uncertainty—in the absence of definitive data—to speculate just how far graduate education influences the productivity of students in contrast to the role played by the gifts, the motivation, and the industry the individual student brings to his or her educational experience. I can perhaps take some credit for having, with the aid of my associates, selected so well. More than that, and unabashedly, I do take pride in the breadth and the depth of the interests reflected in the disparate chapters in this volume. The diversity speaks well for the academic environment in the Department of Psychiatry at the Massachusetts General Hospital, which has, as one of its hoped-for goals, the fostering of individual creativity. There can be no more persuasive demonstration that such a goal *is* attainable than the contributions assembled in this book.

REFERENCES

Carrter, A. M. 1971. Scientific manpower for 1970-1985. Science 172:132-140.

Eisenberg, L. 1975. The ethics of intervention: acting amidst ambiguity. Journal of Child Psychology and Psychiatry and Allied Disciplines 16:93-104.

Erikson, E. H. 1959. Identity and the Life Cycle. New York: International Universities Press.

Frank, J. D. 1965. Persuasion and Healing: A Comparative Study of Psychotherapy. Baltimore: Johns Hopkins Press.

Freedman, A. M. 1973. Critical psychiatry: a new and necessary school. Hospital and Community Psychiatry 24:819-824.

Fuchs, V. 1974. Who Shall Live? New York: Basic Books.

Illich, I. 1975. Medical Nemesis: The Expropriation of Health. London: Calder and Boyars.

Korsch, B., E. Gozzi, and V. Francis. 1968. Gaps in doctor-patient communication. Pediatrics 42:855-871.

Luborsky, L., B. Singer, and L. Luborsky. 1975. Comparative studies of psychotherapies: is it true that "everyone has won and all must have prizes"? Archives of General Psychiatry 32:995-1008.

McDermott, W. 1974. General medical care: identification and analysis of alternative approaches. Johns Hopkins Medical Journal 135:292-321.

McKeown, T. 1966. Medicine in Modern Society. New York: Hafner.

Meltzoff, J., and M. Kornreich. 1970. Research in Psychotherapy. New York: Atherton Press.

Sloane, H. B., F. R. Staples, A. H. Cristol, N. J. Yorkston, and K. Whipple. 1975. Psychotherapy Versus Behavior Therapy. Cambridge: Harvard University Press.

Thomas, W. I., and D. S. Thomas. 1928. The Child in America: Behavior Problems and Programs. New York: Knopf, p. 572.

Weissman, M. M., G. L. Klerman, E. S. Paykel, B. Prusoff, and B. Hanson. 1974. Treatment effects on the social adjustment of depressed patients. Archives of General Psychiatry 30:771-778.

Whitehorn, J. C. 1947. The concepts of "meaning" and "cause" in psychodynamics. American Journal of Psychiatry 104:289-292.

Preface

This book is the result of the joint labor of the contributors and the editors. The chapters in the volume are the product of a monthly seminar convened to examine the role of critical reasoning in psychiatric theory, research, practice, and education. Many of us look upon that experience as one of the most important we have had in both psychiatry and our general intellectual development.

Throughout the seminar and in the preparation of this volume, the editors received cooperation, support, and encouragement from the other contributors. The book belongs to all of us. But changes and errors relating to editing, and the ideas expressed in the Introduction are solely the editors' responsibility. Special thanks are due those contributors (and their families) who hosted seminar sessions, which frequently ran late into the night. Also, we wish to thank Suzanne Ryan for her typing assistance.

The editors send forth this volume with the hope that it will provoke critical thinking in the fields of psychiatry. At a time when much about psychiatry is being questioned and rethought, we seek to examine and criticize certain of its properties and to give illustrations of avenues that critical reasoning can follow toward the elaboration of psychiatric science. We have tried to be faithful to the spirit of intellectual commitment, rigorous inquiry, and enthusiasm that so brightly filled our seminar meetings and that we seek to transmit to our readers. We hold that critical rational discourse should characterize psychiatric practice, teaching, and research. Regardless of the limitations of this volume, if we have succeeded in sharing this vision, we have accomplished much of what we set out to do.

Theo C. Manschreck
Arthur M. Kleinman

CHAPTER 1

INTRODUCTION

Theo C. Manschreck, M.D.
Arthur M. Kleinman, M.D.

Several years ago, a group of young psychiatrists, a psychiatric nurse trained in sociology, and a research psychologist met in a seminar organized by the editors and decided to produce this book. The variety of chapters contained in this volume reflects their diverse interests in psychiatry. Despite the wide range of clinical and research subjects, their purpose is narrowly focused: to emphasize and decry the current deficit of critical rationality in psychiatry. Critical rationality means commitment to rational evaluation and derivation of knowledge. It encompasses the critical scrutiny of prevalent beliefs and practices; and it refers to the use of explicit values and rigorous methods, clear concepts and argument, precision in thinking, and supportive evidence to help us harness the creativity of imagination and intuition in the discovery of new knowledge. It promotes exacting standards for the process of inquiry, regardless of its object; and it is self-critical. It therefore qualifies as an indispensable standard governing clinical discourse, teaching, and research.

The means of accomplishing our purpose was to prepare a serious document to represent the spirit of the seminar and to honor an individual whose achievements as a teacher of psychiatry and mentor to several of us exemplify the best in critical rationality. That person is Leon Eisenberg, who currently holds the Maude and Lillian Presley Professorship of Psychiatry and heads the Department of Psychiatry at the Harvard Medical School, while playing a major leadership role in American psychiatry.

This introduction will serve as an overview of the context in which this book was written. First, we will examine background issues that influenced its genesis. Second, we will propose a critique of the present state of psychiatric thinking. Third, we will indicate the nature of critical rationality in psychiatry, and how critical rationality might remedy some of the present deficiencies in psychiatry. We will also discuss the implications of critical rationality for research, teaching, and practice in psychiatry. Finally, we will relate the chapters contained in this volume to the issue of critical rationality.

GENESIS OF THE BOOK

This enterprise began in 1972. At that time, the editors had just started psychiatric training and were becoming increasingly aware of important deficiencies in the fields of psychiatry. Coming from strong backgrounds in clinical medicine, we naturally focused initially on the widespread lack of interest in descriptive and diagnostic clarity in the clinical evaluation of patients. Almost without exception, psychiatric clinicians treat the diagnostic process as little more than an onerous chore. Later, we became alarmed by the realization that even the tenets of psychotherapy, for instance, are generally accepted and taught most uncritically. What seems more important than whether a patient improves is whether the trainee comprehends the case "correctly" or, more accurately, can offer a rhetorically convincing formulation in the name of one or another great classical theorist. Still later, we recognized how ubiquitous within psychiatry the practices of uncritical thinking and inattention to methodological issues are. Critical items in terminology, which everyone uses, are never clearly defined; curiously, the impact of research strategies and results arouses little interest. Finally, our awareness centered on the unfortunate conclusion that although psychiatry has the widest of interests in the broad understanding of human science, its practice is to isolate itself from the richness of contributions from other, relevant disciplines. Despite rapid and challenging advances in psychology, social anthropology, epidemiology, and the biological sciences, there exists no tradition for systematically incorporating these advances into the mainstream of psychiatric thinking and clinical practice and, perhaps more fundamentally, into the curriculum of psychiatric residents.

We were aware of these deficiencies in psychiatry and discussed them on numerous occasions. We saw little hope for reform and decided that at least in our own training and professional experiences, we would seek to maintain a high awareness of the need for critical thinking in dealing with human behavior and the many theories that seek to explain it. Another decision that we entertained was that at some point we would write a radical critique of psychiatry and emphasize these issues. As time passed and our initial experiences were corroborated again and again, our resolve grew stronger to carry out our plans.

In contrast to the experiences of many young psychiatrists, our training, under Ross Baldessarini, Leon Eisenberg, Thomas Hackett, Seymour Kety, Gerald Klerman, and Aaron Lazare, to mention a few, was excellent. We were neither wheedled nor proselytized into *believing* anything. This aspect of training was unlike that afforded other young psychiatrists in many American institutions, where there exists more of an apprenticeship than an academic training program, more indoctrination than intellectually open teaching, more professionalization into a trade than maturation into a scientific discipline. For this opportunity, which allowed us to avoid such indoctrination, we were particularly thankful, for this freedom gave us the basis on which to question carefully and relentlessly the obscurantism of psychiatric thinking. This adaptation suited us initially, but our growing level of disenchantment with all the fields of psychiatry led us to further decisions. One potentially successful approach to dealing with the inadequacy of critical thinking, which seemed so pervasive, was to begin to develop understandings in different areas of clinical psychiatry on our own. Then we could begin to share this kind of enterprise with one another and strengthen our resolve to continue to argue for a more rational psychiatry. The specific means of accomplishing this end was to create a seminar. In such a seminar, we envisioned the potential for the exchange of ideas, for support in searching out new areas of knowledge, a commonly embraced standard of reason, and respect for empirical knowledge and critical attitudes. This form was to be complemented by a content relevant to the interests and expertise of the individuals who would join us.

We then asked colleagues in training and some who had recently finished who shared these aspirations to meet regularly for the purpose of realizing these aims. Several preliminary meetings were held to discuss how we could best put our intentions into practice and examine their implications. We decided that each participant would independently, or in collaboration with a fellow participant, develop a critical understanding of a particular area of his or her choice and then present that understanding to the others in a seminar format. Each such study was to be carefully charted with a high degree of scholarly precision, and a serious respect for the standards of rigorous rational argument, logic, empirical evidence, and clarity, as opposed to innuendo, scholasticism, prevalent beliefs, and tradition, which seem to characterize the weaknesses of the psychiatric tradition we were reacting against. The purpose of the meetings, then, was threefold: first, to hear the progress of a member's thinking and judgment in a particular subject with which he or she had intimate involvement; second, to rigorously criticize, comment on, question, and contribute to the ideas of the speaker; third, and perhaps most important, to appreciate the common experience of rational discourse on a psychiatric subject as the norm, as a means of strengthening our individual preparedness to move further into our specialized interests and psychiatry in general. We hoped these efforts would have a salutary effect on each of us. The seminar met monthly in the homes of the members. Each meeting was devoted to two concise presentations, with at least an hour of discussion for each. Then each of us took the comments from the discussions and incorporated them into formal papers, which became the basis for the individual chapters in this volume. Theo Manschreck and Arthur Kleinman then edited these. They also prepared the introduction to orient the reader to the aims of the seminar and book.

THE PRESENT STATE IN PSYCHIATRY

Psychiatry is still a relatively young specialty within medicine. Its subject matter has only gradually been defined; initially, it dealt almost exclusively with the institutionalized insane. In the late nineteenth century, through the influence of Bernheim, Charcot, and Freud, psychiatry turned its attention to the noninstitutionalized—the neurotic and the characterologically disturbed. Now, in the latter part of the twentieth century, it finds entrance into a plethora of areas of human activity—law, literature, politics, abortion, community diagnosis and treatment, economics, population problems, death, the quest for happiness in sex, work, and play, self-realization, transpersonal identity—in addition to all the more traditional concerns it has had in the past.

Yet, though the extent of its interests has grown, the empirical knowledge base in psychiatry has remained small in relation to that in other clinical areas in medicine, and has increased at a disappointing pace. Indeed, there have been important breakthroughs—revolutionary changes in strategies of providing psychiatric care catalyzed by psychopharmacological advances, increasing sophistication in psychotherapy research, painstaking efforts in social and clinical epidemiology, the emergence of psychiatric consultation as a practical approach to problems in general clinical care, to name a few. But the daily lot of insightful psychiatric clinicians is to realize that although they know some things well, they proceed in their work essentially ignorant of vast areas of relevant human behavior. Hence, commentary abounds in the psychiatric literature on the drift away from medicine, the need for retrenchment, the quest for integration of disparate kinds of knowledge from eclecticism to pluralism to syncretism, the importance of clinical and experimental methodology, and the common experience of bewilderment among psychiatric residents. The reasons for this state of affairs have been commented upon in many ways. One of the most common responses is to see in contemporary psychiatry an identity crisis with implications for training and the direction psychiatry will take in the future (Torrey, 1975; Schwarz, 1974). This response comes from those psychiatrists who see themselves primarily as physicians. Their major concern is the expansion of psychiatric roles outside the traditional clinic setting. They see the limitations of psychiatric knowledge and expertise as fundamental reasons not to enter areas where, because of politics, enthusiasm, and perceived social need, psychiatry has overextended itself. These psychiatrists view medicine as the wellspring of psychiatric method and style and deplore recent trends that denigrate the traditional psychiatric interest in mental illness. Seymour Kety (1974) of the Massachusetts General Hospital has stated that

> psychiatry is an identity crisis precisely because it is not especially qualified to handle ... community, national and international affairs, poverty, politics and criminality. In each of these areas, we have responsibilities as citizens and human beings; we have yet to demonstrate any special competence as psychiatrists.

Or, as Sir Aubrey Lewis (1967) has stated succinctly, "The pretentions of some psychiatrists are extreme." Those who teach psychiatric residents from this vantage point often encourage tough-mindedness and skepticism in their students.

A second perspective on the contemporary psychiatric situation is that what is occurring is not an identity crisis, but rather a "developmental phase" of less worrisome proportions. The expansion of psychiatric responsibilities, so the argument goes, represents an opportunity, not a threat. Psychiatrists in this camp tend to be less medically oriented. They deemphasize the "disease concept," biological approaches to etiology, and somatic treatments. With the deemphasis is a corresponding increased interest in psychosocial aspects of psychiatry, "functional" etiology, and psychotherapy. Not surprisingly, they view involvement in areas beyond mental illness, such as politics, community development, and problems in living, as entirely appropriate for psychiatrists. There is an air of confidence and certainty among those who share this perspective, which is transmitted as a powerful influence to psychiatric residents, who face the uncertainties of clinical work.

We wish to offer a third perspective, initially noting criticisms of the first two. The first, we feel, is correct in its concern for emphasizing that psychiatry has drifted too far afield. However, there is a more far-reaching criticism than this that also applies directly to medicine. We might label this perspective the semicritical position in psychiatry. Thus, encouraging retrenchment and checking the expansion of psychiatric responsibilities, though important, are not all that is required to solve the crisis. The more serious critique of psychiatry's present trends has to do with the general lack of critical rationality in the monitoring of knowledge development and use. Psychiatry falls prey to this criticism more readily than medicine, not because medicine is innocent, but because the deficiency is more apparent in our chaotic field. This deficiency reflects a lack of concern for the role of knowledge in psychiatry—particularly how it is derived, how it is evaluated, translated, criticized, communicated, taught, and to what use it is put. In psychiatry, and in most fields in medicine for that matter, this subject is rarely addressed. No one desires to deal with "dry" philosophical issues that these questions raise; yet, precisely because there is a crisis in psychiatry, testing its rapid growth and responsibility against a relatively limited demonstrated competence, there is a need to examine these theoretical issues in depth. Questions concerning knowledge penetrate to the core of psychiatry's deficiencies.

In medicine, similar problems regarding knowledge have led to criticisms of overspecialization, the loss of the whole patient from the doctor's view, the disavowal of responsibility in relating to patients for the purposes of explanation, education, and other "nonorganic, nontechnological" aspects of patient care. The fact is that important strides in research and understanding in social and cultural anthropology, psychology, economics, and sociology hold the promise of being able to improve medical care success and to rigorously define what happens beyond biology to patients, if these advances can be translated into clinically relevant models. The rather obvious importance of these contributions is not generally reflected in medical care or medical training programs. Clearly, medicine and psychiatry have both been too caught up in specialized paradigms, the narrowly conceived organ approach of clinical medicine, and the broadly conceived deviance approach of psychiatry. Medicine has been loath to venture beyond its biological borders, and many of those who hold the semicritical position in psychiatry have accepted this posture as well.

The second perspective is more frightening. Implicit in its adulation of traditional models of psychiatric intervention is an assumption of certitude, almost Truth, concerning its formulations. There is among psychiatrists who hold this perspective a view that psychiatry has already been to the mountain and that the sacred tablets contain all that it is really crucial to know. Thus, there appears what to other scientists and professionals must seem an incredible sense of confidence in approaching new problems of enormous magnitude, such as politics, crime, and social change. Armed with traditional teachings, many psychiatrists blithely accept the role of expert and involve themselves, ill equipped by every other standard, in extremely complex questions beyond mental illness. The situation would be patently ludicrous if it were not for the widespread acceptance of this perspective, the general appeal of its certainty in a field full of suffering and anxiety-provoking unknowns, and the marked hubris that accompanies it. Critics of psychiatry continually examine this attitude and judge correctly that it represents a major failing, which has been encouraged by our society in the past and even at present.

To summarize, the first perspective, which we have labeled the semicritical position, assumes that psychiatry is all right within the methodological and biological context of medicine; it fails to see the limitations of the medical model in clinical medicine in its approach to questions of all forms of health care and illness behavior and, thus, does not push its critique far enough. There is safety in the rigid concepts of medicine. However, medicine is a narrowly conceived basis on which to examine and understand all forms of health and human behavior; and the medical models seems to lock psychiatry into a paradigm already discovered as too limited by medicine itself, and certainly too limited when applied to psychiatric issues. The second position, which we call the hubris position, assumes present psychiatric knowledge has some close approximation to truth, and, worse, that that truth can be applied to an enormous range of problems, internal and external to psychiatry. We see this position as very dangerous, for it rests on a base of certainty—at this point, mostly unverified—that allows it to delve into every area of human enterprise with a presumptiveness that threatens to undermine the whole field.

To understand how these two perspectives are maintained and how they manage to polarize the fields of psychiatry, we must consider psychiatry in the context of comtemporary society. At present, there are several different societal thrusts toward psychiatry. One is a radical critique of the entire profession that ends in rejecting part or all of it. This radical critique is associated with Szasz (1961), Torrey (1974), Laing (1967), and the so-called Counterculture, with its passion for psychiatric romanticism, encounter, and primal scream. While it raises some important questions, this critique vitiates itself in negativism and theoretical poverty, and throws the baby out with the bathwater.

Another and contrary orientation abroad is the folk mystique about psychiatry and psychiatrists (still present, though less powerful than in the past, thankfully); namely, that they are specially powerful in unlocking the secrets of the mind and healing social ills as well as personal ones. Finally, there seems to be a growing uncertainty in the United States and Europe about the uses and relevance of psychiatry in the future; in part, this is a response to psychiatry's disastrous ventures into wide areas of life; in part, it mimics the radical critique and psychiatry's showman image in the press; in part, it is based on misunderstanding and ignorance—but overall it is a reflection of the ambivalence, identity crisis, and widespread dissension in contemporary psychiatry.

Let us consider an alternative viewpoint. There is, in fact, nothing wrong with going about one's work in psychiatry with a special interest in psychotherapy, psychopathology, disease, or even crime and social change. The problem is that each of these separate areas of psychiatric endeavor has developed on the basis of a few insights and narrowly conceived frames of reference. Each area has had, it seems, its own set of rules, its own terminology, its own depth of knowledge, and usually a tremendous theoretical overgrowth that often has outdistanced its empirical basis. Communication with psychiatrists focused elsewhere has been difficult. Thus, we have the "special" psychiatries: the psychoanalytical, the psychopharmacological, the social and community psychiatries. Despite the diversity of these areas, Enoch Callaway, a distinguished psychiatrist, has pointed to one feature they have in common, "intellectual tunnel-vision" (Callaway, 1975). Each of the special psychiatries tends to develop an approach to things that excludes other approaches. Because of the temper of the times and the push for oversimplification and tunnel vision, the valid basis of each special psychiatry—its empirical findings and the rules that work within it—becomes obscured. Psychiatry, Callaway concludes, is an undisciplined discipline; and it will be unable to capitalize on potential payoffs in collaborative research unless it "tidies up the mess left by its snake oil salesmen," and ends the divisions engendered by advocates of special psychiatric techniques. The special psychiatries have sold themselves too well and now are struggling to fulfill their promises. The legacy of already broken promises seriously impedes psychiatry's scientific development and tarnishes its image among the rational disciplines concerned with the human sciences.

The view from the third perspective that we are presenting is that there is a crisis in psychiatry. It might well be labeled an identity crisis; however, the crisis is more fundamental than identity, although it certainly concerns identity. The present state clearly suggests that, increasingly, psychiatry has developed multiple partial identities through the variety of subspecialized areas into which it has entered. Yet, equally clear is the lack of a general identity for the field as a whole. Some might wish to keep this general identity linked to medicine; some feel it is available currently in the body of clinical and theoretical experience derivative from Freud and Meyer. Others, perhaps, do not care.

We feel there is a desperate need to define a general identity in psychiatry—an identity that would be a reasonable basis on which to reexamine the specialized endeavors within psychiatry, to determine their appropriateness. Such a definition, we believe, would benefit the teaching and learning of psychiatry. To define identity certainly requires that we understand what is currently lacking in the general identity of the field. The lack of a general identity in psychiatry has at least three features. The first is the lack of a common language and set of procedures for clinicians and researchers in the recognition and description of psychopathology and in diagnosis. The second is the lack of common methods for critically evaluating clinical and research ideas and new information that come into psychiatry from different areas and vitalize its growth. This lack extends also to methods for translating relevant ideas and information into clinical teaching and practice. The third is the lack of common values regarding the nature of our enterprise, which would be likely to describe what kind of knowledge we need and for what kind of purposes.

The unifying attribute of these features is the lack of a common discipline for approaching all questions in psychiatry. That is to say that the measures, principles, and values by which we may approach problems and examine ideas are neither clear nor consistent, much less explicit, throughout the fields of psychiatry. We feel these standards should derive from and develop through the workings of critical rationality. Later in this chapter, we will carefully define this term and discuss its meaning. In the rest of this section, we will consider several major traditions within psychiatry in an attempt to isolate and emphasize the reasons psychiatry has lost or never had an identity.

Let us examine, then, more closely the fields of psychiatry in order to discover the roots and consequences of this crisis. The purpose of this examination will be to disclose how each of three particular traditions within psychiatry has dealt with questions of knowledge and has itself contributed to a lack of general identity.

The clinical tradition, for the sake of clarity in our discussion, will subsume the psychotherapeutic and diagnostic traditions within psychiatry. In reviewing the biological tradition, we will be focusing on research into diseases and the impact of psychopharmacology. In reviewing the social and cultural tradition in psychiatry, we will attend to major influences only. We do not intend, nor feel it necessary, to exhaust the scope of activity within these traditions. Only the most outstanding and representative aspects of these traditions will be considered. We are looking at the main foci and their most influential factors.

The Clinical Tradition

At the dawn of this century, a group of independent investigators led our emerging profession—Freud, Kraepelin, and Meyer. Each examined clinical questions with a researcher's eye, biased by his own theoretical position. Each contributed magnificently to psychiatry. Much of their work influences the present as well. Until recently, Freud, particularly, and Meyer have had dominant influence in clinical training and practice in the United States.

Two crucial consequences for psychotherapy and diagnosis followed from this intellectual and historical influence on American psychiatry. The first was the fact that the teaching of psychiatry came to mean the teaching of Freudian and Meyerian ideas. Clinical and theoretical psychiatry, thus, became largely congruent in its scope, methods, and assumptions with the views of these important men. The second consequence was the relative absence, until recently, of Kraepelinian teaching in general, and particularly of Kraepelin's views on diagnosis and disease in psychiatry. As we hope to demonstrate, these two consequences were not independent but very much related.

The Freudian and Meyerian tradition   Imagine, if you will, the difficulties facing the practitioner at the beginning of this century, when confronted with "hysteria." What was one to do? Apart from excellent descriptions, no effective treatment was available, nor was much known about this particular clinical problem. Because of his own frustrations in treatment, Freud traveled to Paris to learn of Charcot's work. Out of his studies, Freud developed the brilliant closed system of psychodynamic theory, a pioneering, comprehensive attempt to explain behavior that linked motivation, unconscious experience, and emotional development. From the theory, a crucial additional feature developed, a treatment called psychoanalysis, which was consistent with it. This potent and somewhat mysterious art was practiced by the guild of talented individuals who surrounded and were trained by Freud. Hysteria, particularly, could be conceptualized and its treatment derived through the understanding of psychic mechanisms taken directly from the theory. The electrifying qualities of the theory and the mystique of the treatment led rather rapidly to its acceptance and use. The anxiety of treating conditions like hysteria was partially allayed.

Several factors contributed to the feeling of certainty among those who believed Freud's ideas. His unorthodox views created a sense of embattlement, enhancing unity and morale. The internal consistency and clarity of his model of behavior and a theoretical language that could be shared added substantially to the confidence of those who espoused it. Since all behavior fell within reach of its explanatory powers, the theory moved well beyond the fragmented picture of nineteenth-century psychological life—associationism, introspection, and faculty psychology—which preceded it, and offered a relatively universal explanatory system for all human behavior. Further, it was closely associated with a treatment modality in an age where specific therapy for conditions like hysteria was largely absent.

One unhappy feature of the growth of the psychoanalytic movement in psychiatry has been the absence of a significant research tradition in the clinical sphere. This is particularly noteworthy in view of the experimental quality of the initial investigations Freud and his followers engaged in. Whereas psychological and social scientific, as well as biological, research in fields related to psychiatry have experienced mushroom growth in methodology development, techniques of measurement, and the power of demonstration, there has been relatively little to distinguish the development of psychoanalytic research beyond the classical case description and the production of brilliant hypotheses, many of which are incorporated untested into the body of "clinical knowledge" passed on to psychiatric residents, often as if they were rules governing human behavior. Relatively few of these hypotheses have been given controlled, experimental verification. And there seems to be no interest in altering this situation. As Holzman (1970) commented:

> The question remains as to when ultimate experimental validation of psychoanalytic formulations should occur. The author of this book agrees that psychoanalytic formulation should be subjected to experimental or other empirical validations but favors a different timing than that demanded by strict operational or positivistic approach. To guard against nipping preliminary exploration in the bud, there must be a period in which curiosity and inquiry into the unique and novel are fostered while the results of natural observations are awaited and then formalized.

How long, indeed?

Without a research tradition and a research community organized to verify the hypotheses of psychoanalytic theory, the movement took several directions. There was conflict within the Freudian camp, and the fragmentation that resulted led to the establishment of closely related theories as promulgated in the writings and schools of Alfred Adler and Carl Jung, for example. Outside of this classical tradition, Adolf Meyer proposed brilliant and related ideas to account for the aberrations of mental experience and to develop his own variety of clinical interventions. That work expanded with the development of the interpersonalist school of Harry Stack Sullivan, the first truly American form of psychiatry.

In the United States, Freud and Meyer, through their ideas and the traditions they established, have had the most significant impact on clinical training in psychiatry over the years. Yet the combination of brilliant hypotheses and the absence of a research tradition eventually led to increased skepticism. Challenged by new ideas and viewpoints contrary to prevalent belief, the focused clinical tradition in American psychiatry through the fifties became a divergent, chaotic assortment of narrowly conceived, interventionist views—Gestalt therapy, encounter therapy, existential therapy, psychodynamic therapy, client-centered therapy all developed. It is interesting that none of these schools has established a firm and creditable research tradition.

What is disturbing about these developments is the persistent absence of critical methodology and thinking, self-examination, and research rigor within these clinical traditions, which have fostered polemics and closed bodies of theory in place of open, dispassionate criticism and rational integration. Psychotherapy research, for instance, has struggled with poor support and virtually none of its main tenets effectively introduced and accepted in clinical training programs. As Eisenberg (1973) has commented:

> Most neurotic patients will report themselves improved following outpatient psychotherapy of almost any stripe. The very multiplicity of apparently successful schools of therapy betokens a lack of specificity, which raises questions about the adequacy of the theories upon which each is based. Further, psychotherapy, no less than drug therapy, has a potential for toxicity that is far from trifling. If it can produce change, then it is to be expected that it will sometimes yield further psychic disequilibirum, rather than the desired re-equilibration, when imprudently applied. It too can promote dependency, consume disproportionate amounts of personal effort and become a way of life for the patient. There is no better index of this problem than the veritable explosion of "sensitivity," "transaction," and "encounter" groups with their share of chronic attenders, a phenomenon which says more about the loneliness of contemporary men and women than it does about the effective management of personal distress and alienation. What stands out is how miniscule is the investment in research in contrast to the resources committed to the doing of psychotherapy. This balance must be redressed if present ignorance is to be remedied.

The main developments in knowledge in this tradition have been the elaboration of hypotheses and the redefinition of theoretical ideas. These have determined what are appropriate "data," and these data have in turn been used to justify theory, following the classical direction of self-fulfilling prophecies. The traditions developed by Freud and Meyer have, however, had an important humanizing effect on medicine in general. Rather than merely categorizing the difficulties that patients present, under the influence of this tradition, practitioners have learned to listen and to try to understand the suffering of their patients, and have treated personal biography as an essential aspect of sickness.

But practical knowledge has not grown significantly. Nor has much been done to create a common standard for developing knowledge within this clinical tradition. One reason, then, for the lack of attention to standards and the enlargement of practical knowledge in clinical psychiatry has been complacency—a complacency that is supported by the mythology of the present capacities of our understanding. Another influence that currently stifles the passion for critical approaches to knowledge derives from a more sophisticated but equally troublesome mythology. Many psychiatrists believe that though we clearly do not fully understand psychiatric anomalies, we do possess, at least, a valid theory and optimal treatment—if we are able to use it effectively. The key word is effective; for in order to achieve effective treatment, according to this view, one must believe in its efficacy. A corollary view registers dismay at attempts to inform residents, for instance, about our lack of understanding of the process or effectiveness of psychotherapy. After all, if one reduces the residents' confidence by revealing certain "inadequacies," one will necessarily interfere with their ability to be effective. This tragic stance toward knowledge about psychotherapy undermines psychiatry. As Leon Eisenberg (1973) stated:

> There is no area more central to medical research than the exploration of this potent therapeutic modality so that we can prescribe it with specificity, in such a fashion as to enhance personal growth, in such dosage as to be proportionate to need. Dismay at the state of the art justifies no derogation of its value. To the contrary, it is precisely psychotherapy that holds great promise of major benefit to medical care, once we have learned to control its power.

Psychiatrists who approach clinical psychiatry and, in particular, psychotherapy, from narrow, traditional viewpoints, also strongly dislike skepticism about psychiatric knowledge. They fear the potential despair that threatens to engulf those who question. That despair, they argue, will result inevitably in nihilism, both diagnostic and therapeutic. Many who believe this consider themselves great humanists and liberals; they see criticisms like this one as reactionary and antihumanistic. But let us be quite clear: their view espouses at its core authoritarian teaching and wishes to exclude open access to knowledge. Thus, it detracts from learning and discovery and can have no place in an open discipline anchored in the scientific tradition. The lack of development of cogent standards crucial to psychiatry's identity is an inevitable consequence.

The thrust of the preceding ideas is a not-too-subtle endorsement of obscurantism and unquestioning and obsequious learning. The clear impact is to foster suspicion for new ideas, methodological concerns, and rationality—in short, it is anti-intellectualism. Those who feel most threatened rationalize the poverty of psychiatric knowledge in a very uncritical manner and propose no possibilities for real improvement. They promote a turning away from inquiry. They offer a model for psychiatric residents that is stifling and that has closed minds, rather than opened them. This viewpoint in clinical psychiatry has led us astray. Lacking a significant research tradition, it has turned to obscurantism, authoritarian teaching, and has closed off inquiry, with ruinous results. Dogma prevails. As Akiskal and McKinney (1973) point out:

> Extremists from this camp have generated an anti-intellectual climate which has even permeated academic circles. To the extent its proponents have assumed anti-methodologic postures they represent a serious hindrance to the scientific development of psychiatry. They rely mainly on ill-defined, non-standardized, and somewhat mystical techniques. . . .

The formation of numerous psychotherapies has only alienated psychiatrists further. What little there is in the way of critical rationality in this tradition has been ignored.

The Kraepelinian tradition Before the turn of the twentieth century, Emil Kraepelin extended Karl Kahlbaum's contribution that psychiatric illnesses should be considered as longitudinal units by adding etiology as a key feature of their definition. Out of these efforts came the notion of disease entity in psychiatry. Etiology, in Kraepelin's view, was to be understood through the investigation of biological aspects of these "entities." He proceeded to examine all manner of psychopathological changes associated with diseases of established etiology—infection, trauma, tumor, etc.—and he proposed a classification scheme for those psychiatric entities that could not be assigned a known cause. Manic depressive insanity and dementia praecox thus entered the vocabulary of clinical psychiatry. The tradition generated by Kraepelin's remarkable contributions lived on, particularly in Central Europe and Scandinavia. His work became a standard for clarity in the description of psychopathology. Research into natural history, genetics, and the treatment of psychiatric entities flourished.

Although Freud did not explicitly attack Kraepelin's views, Freud's concepts of etiology were linked to developmental and not biological factors in the group of illnesses he studied. With an approach to etiology similar to Freud's, Meyer felt inspired to attack Kraepelinian views himself and even went so far as to counter Kraepelin's classificatory schema according to his own preconceptions; hence, he gave us such terms as schizophrenic reaction and manic depressive reaction.

Kraepelin propounded a brilliant approach to psychiatric illness; however, he, like Freud and Meyer, must be criticized for his lack of openness to alternative views. Kraepelin clearly linked himself to the increasingly sophisticated clinical medicine of his day and, thus, to its methods, assumptions, and limitations. The search for biological causes became a passionate enterprise.

Before we attempt to resolve this clash over etiology, let us note that both viewpoints preconceive the kinds of causes that should be considered. In fact, for both viewpoints etiological concepts are ideal, that is, not demonstrable in concrete terms, even today. In the face of limited knowledge, such preconceptions tend to become rigid, unmodifiable, and, consequently, harmful. It is perhaps a historical quirk that Freudian and Meyerian views came to dominate American psychiatry. But regardless of why they did, the impact of their dominance resulted in the deemphasis, decrying, and, more commonly, the ignoring of the Kraepelinian position.

What influence may be traced from the lack of acceptance of Kraepelin's views in American psychiatry? Perhaps the strongest influence has been in diagnosis. Put simply, the importance of description and diagnosis shrinks to the extent one believes that the key determinant of psychopathology is development. Diagnosis in the United States has been in disarray for years. The American Psychiatric Association officially sanctioned a formal scheme of diagnosis in the *Diagnostic and Statistical Manual* of 1952. This committee-derived product reflected the diversity of views on the scene at that time. Thus, there were classical Freudian neuroses, Meyerian reactions, and even Kraepelinian diseases as diagnostic groupings.

Over the last thirty or so years, studies of diagnosis have demonstrated frequently the drawbacks of nosology and the unreliability of psychiatric ratings of psychopathology. It is also clear that part of these difficulties is attributable to orientation and training, often through the workings of implicit preconceptions of Freudian- and Meyerian-trained psychiatrists that bias their observations. If psychiatric disturbances are, in fact, merely the consequences of an interplay between experience and constitution, and the key clinical issue resides in the specifics of that interplay, then each illness is unique except for common patterns of development and the understanding derived from looking at the form of the illness—its presenting features, its course, its complications, etc., are not nearly so crucial as unraveling the historical web that has caught the individual in his or her present situation. Freudian and Meyerian views have been attacked justifiably—their preconceptions are challenged by the effectiveness of somatic interventions. Again, in the face of little knowledge, much has been assumed and little verified.

We can be hopeful in the knowledge that attempts are under way to improve on diagnostic performance. Yet, until psychiatrists accept the critical attitude of examining carefully their own preconceptions

and of developing accommodations to new knowledge, these difficulties will persist. Tragically, the effect of preconception in psychiatry has been to perpetuate tunnel vision.

Although the general picture of clinical psychiatry appears gloomy,
there are reasons for optimism. As mentioned, research in psychopathology holds real promise for breakthroughs in the development
of a common language and standardized clinical procedures (see, for
example, Cooper et al., 1972; Feighner et al., 1972; Wing et al.,
1967). Multidisciplinary attempts to study the interaction between
physician and patient from initial encounter through the clinical
evaluation and the negotiations that appear crucial to effecting
patient satisfaction and compliance with treatment interventions also
signal a commitment to understanding how to provide optimal care
(see, for example, references to Chapter 3 in this book, and Lazare,
1973, 1975). The investigations carried on under the banners
of ego psychology and coping and adaptation continue to provide
rich results for advancing our knowledge of human behavior (see, for
example, Hartmann, 1958; Lazarus, 1966). Learning theory, with its
offspring behavior therapy, shows increasing applicability for a range
of clinical problems (see, for example, Bandura 1969; Wolpe, 1973).

One very promising development in clinical psychiatry is the
emerging discipline of psychiatric consultation, or liaison medicine.
Perhaps because it has clear links to the pragmatic goals of clinical
medicine, and because it draws on multiple distinct bodies of
knowledge to accomplish its tasks, consultative psychiatry challenges
the older approaches of clinical psychiatry with a clear-cut and
organized requirement for knowledge. What will be the foundations
for knowledge in this clinical field? Certainly, the clinical psychiatric
traditions just discussed offer an inadequate basis for working in this
area. This field illustrates the great need for the critical use of new
sources of knowledge: communication theory, medical sociology and
anthropology, and medical and neurological aspects of psychiatry, to
name a few (Lipowski, 1973). Consultative psychiatry represents a
promising arena for critical rationality in that here the need for a
constructive, practical, and synthesizing stance toward knowledge is
quite clear. We are hopeful that as this field of psychiatry elaborates
a distinct epistemological framework (one that should be integrative),
that framework will have a positive influence on the growth and
organization of knowledge in clinical psychiatry generally.

The Biological Tradition

The biological tradition has remained tied to psychiatry mainly
through the efforts of Kraepelin. Kraepelin proposed in 1892 that
psychiatric diseases should have identifiable cerebral pathology and

biological etiology. However, this ideal has seldom been attained in investigation. The psychoses associated with niacin deficiency and syphillis represent two such contributions. Yet the great majority of psychiatric illnesses have not fallen before the biological investigators. In fact, what search there has been for biological answers to the enigmas of psychiatric anomalies has been costly and generally unproductive. Cerebral pathological investigations, perhaps because of insensitive and imprecise technology, have had uncertain and usually negative results. One has been to denigrate the usefulness of biological approaches to psychopathology. As might be expected, this stance has been taken by many in the Freudian and Meyerian camp, but, interestingly enough, it has also characterized many biological researchers.

Many of the biological researchers investigate normal functioning instead of the psychopathology, believing that through an understanding of normality, we can begin to understand the processes that have not yielded to previous biological strategies. This particular approach deserves some emphasis. Research directed at normal mechanisms of function often provides little payoff for psychiatric interventions. Not that this is an inappropriate area of research; the question is, however, should psychiatrists spend time at such activities in their research endeavors when trained biochemists and neurophysiologists can perform these same tasks as well or better? Why not apply the tools of research to pertinent clinical questions? This wedding of clinical problems and research pragmatics seems essential in a field with far too few engaged in serious research (Brodie, 1973).

A further comment on this situation has to do with the imposing lack of theoretical development in biological psychiatry. There is, in fact, no organized theory of psychiatric disturbances from a biological perspective. There are, indeed, highly developed models, such as the catecholamine model of affective disorder and genetic models of schizophrenia; nevertheless, there are at this time no means by which such models may be adequately translated into an understanding of the diversity of psychiatric anomalies. One is struck by this imposing feature of biological psychiatry, which perhaps militates against the translation of relevant biological findings into clinical practice and teaching. The lack of a unifying theory appears to be due to significant skepticism about the value of theories in psychiatry; perhaps this ties in with an empiricist atheoretical tendency in the biomedical fields generally. No doubt, a lack of confidence in the theorizing that has gone on in the clinical tradition has supported skepticism. While no one would venture to say that an overall unifying theory of biological aspects of psychopathology should be proposed, there is strikingly little attempt even at mid-range theorizing in this area. The result is clear: a number of very important empirical results, a diversity of narrowly focused conceptual models, and little or no means of translating the findings from one model to another or from one area of psychopathology to another.

One may conclude that the present state of psychiatry, with respect to biological investigations, reflects the development of several very specific and useful treatment techniques (e.g., drugs, convulsive treatment, etc.) and models that have been exploited in an attempt to find specific mechanisms underlying various areas of psychopathology. At the same time, many psychiatrists engage in "basic" biological research largely unrelated to pertinent clinical issues. There is little theoretical unity to these important contributions or activities. Thus, it remains difficult to teach residents and psychiatrists who work in other fields within psychiatry about this basic subject matter.

The Sociocultural Tradition

The sociocultural tradition really represents several traditions and reflects in its numerous contemporary viewpoints different levels of theoretical development. Much of the older sociocultural tradition in American psychiatry derives from Adolf Meyer or, more accurately, from the efforts of his students, who pursued his ideas in research and clinical work. The social epidemiological investigations of Alexander and Dorothea Leighton and colleagues in Nova Scotia and Nigeria are singular accomplishments. These workers used Meyerian ideas to explore meaningful connections between the role of sociocultural factors and the prevalence of psychiatric symptomatology and impairment (Leighton, 1959; Leighton et al., 1963; Hughes et al., 1960; D. Leighton, 1967). It is striking that correlation of these same factors with specific psychiatric diagnoses was not a focus; this reminds us of the relative disinterest in the disease approach associated with Meyer.

Many programs of research have continued along these lines, branching into cross-cultural investigations as well. Theoretical development has been considerable and yet, in many ways, has remained quite isolated from major advances in sociocultural science outside of psychiatry. Furthermore, some of the best cross-cultural research in psychiatry has been done by anthropologists. Much of this work is largely unknown to general psychiatrists (see references in Chapter 3 in this volume). But a new tradition of social and cross-cultural psychiatry is emerging, with strong bonds to anthropology and sociology. Evidence of this newer movement may be found in the increasing numbers of psychiatrists with undergraduate and graduate degrees in these fields, as well as in the recent expansion of psychiatric contributions to social and cross-cultural research (see, for example, Fabrega, 1974; Levy, 1973; Kleinman et al., 1975; Yap, 1974). What is most interesting about the growth of this new stream of research and teaching in psychiatry is that frequently these are contributions as much to anthropology, social and cross-cultural studies, and health care research as they are to psychiatry, thus strengthening interdisciplinary bonds. Such work adds to the identity crisis in our field by making less clear the border between psychiatry and these disciplines. But this has had an enriching influence so far, even though we now require redefinition of what are appropriate problems and approaches for psychiatrists engaged in such inquiries. This development suggests that a too formal division of labor and problems among related disciplines is not desirable. And it raises a question we shall mention here and return to below: the relationship of psychiatry to the social sciences, which Edward Sapir, Yale anthropologist and linguist, once referred to as the question of what psychiatry could offer anthropology, a question that we shall turn on its head.

Perhaps the most potent stimulus to sociocultural work in psychiatry in the United States was the federal funding commitment to community mental health in the 1960s. Yet the results have been discouraging from the standpoint of a psychiatric identity. Although the areas of concern for investigations were clearly defined—social causes and correlates of psychiatric disorder, prevalence of psychiatric disorder, prevention, comprehensive services for large numbers of individuals with diverse social and cultural backgrounds—no unified theory or set of approaches characterized these efforts. Moreover, the volumes written to report on the activities of that era indicate that very little was done with rigor or method to match the problematic task or the level of support given. A number of empirical studies and a paucity of theoretical contributions were the main products. Whole practical fields developed, such as crisis intervention, in which a variety of concepts and clinical experience relating to specific patient problems, such as divorce, grief, abortion, and unemployment, were pulled together into a nebulous theoretical structure, organized by a special terminology, and then forged into a full-blown field within psychiatry. As Brodie and Sabshin (1973), two prominent psychiatrists who wrote on trends in psychiatric research during the sixties and early seventies, pointed out:

> One of the striking findings of this survey involves the paucity of papers on the social causes of psychiatric illness. Social psychiatric concepts had produced important formulations about etiology during the 1950's and by the beginning of the 1960's it appeared that we were on the verge of developing new constructs to account for social factors in psychopathology. Quite clearly, these constructs have not emerged between 1963 and 1972

and this void may represent a significant commentary on the past decade. One of the most important questions about this issue concerns the emphasis on the development of practical programs during the 1960's, rather than on theory-building. Papers on the delivery of mental health services represented a large component of the papers we categorized as non-research. It is conceivable that these efforts siphoned off potential research on social etiology.

At the same time that this financial largesse was available, American psychiatry nevertheless remained relatively isolated from the broad achievements and increasing sophistication of sociocultural research conducted by professional social scientists. Bridges between community psychiatry and social science have been difficult to build. The passions of territoriality and mutual suspicion have generated many barriers. The persistent hubris of dynamic theorizing has irked many social scientists, who directed their efforts initially to criticism and more recently, unfortunately, to downright avoidance of psychiatry. Further problems have arisen when, even after developing a liaison between the two disciplines (psychiatry and social science), their focus and even their languages seem to differ. The paradigms that can help us translate the useful concepts of both disciplines into meaningful ideas for successful collaboration are lacking. For example, the deviance model of labeling theory in sociology and the disease model in psychiatry could lead to comparative theoretical and research evaluations that would affect both and could produce an integration within an overarching framework. But, so far, this has not happened; and only polemics have resulted from the interaction of these incomparable (as now held) paradigms.

Now, with crumbling federal financial support and an increased demand for effective care coming from health consumers, the need for practical, efficient translation of socioscientific insights looms larger for psychiatry and medicine. Narrow-minded bickering and isolationism are ludicrous luxuries of the past.

Here we need to pose the more fundamental question raised by the newer stream of social and cross-cultural psychiatry mentioned above: What role might social science (anthropology, sociology, social psychology, language and communication research, etc.) play in psychiatry? First, social science would provide much needed scientific supports, not only for social and community psychiatry, but for psychiatry in general. Certainly, these fields contribute in essential ways to our understanding of the social and cultural context of disease; clinical interaction and communication between psychiatrist and patient; the workings of therapeutic milieus and psychiatric hospitals; the social outcome of treatment; the socialization of professional psychiatrists and their relation to other mental health professions; the social, organizational, and cultural influences on psychiatric practice; and other important questions as well. In particular, cross-cultural psychiatry, until very recently a small and isolated backwater in our field, already has begun to contribute to psychiatry in several promising ways. It has taken advantage of certain "natural" experiments—culture-bound disorders, traditional healing systems, diverse ethnic and cultural beliefs about mental disorders, the impact of social development (modernization) on psychiatric disorders and treatment practice—in order to raise fundamental questions about how we conceptualize, evaluate, and treat mental illness in our own society. In so doing, it has frequently used psychiatric problems and approaches to examine basic issues in clinical care generally, running from the family context of care to the impact of cultural beliefs on symptoms and treatment interventions and outcomes (Fabrega, 1974). Furthermore, by 1980 when more than three-fourths of the world's population will be non-Western, only a sophisticated cross-cultural approach to psychiatry will prevent the imposition of Western European and American psychiatric models (and biases) on non-Western populations and encourage construction of a comparative, truly international, scientific psychiatry applicable in all cultures (see Yap, 1974).

The future may hold the prospect of social and cross-cultural psychiatry acting as a bridge for bringing relevant components of social science into psychiatry and medicine; for providing useful knowledge of nontechnological clinical care with scientific support; and for encouraging integrative cross-disciplinary research on problems that fall between psychiatry and social science. Thereby, this field may enable psychiatry to have an influence on social science. The emergence of medical anthropology and reemergence of culture and personality research on a sounder footing may indicate early examples of such an influence. But in order to accomplish these possibilities, this field needs to follow a critical rational direction that liberates it from the hold of old and unproductive disciplinary biases, unuseful approaches, and irrelevant and unimportant questions. Lacking such direction, the field most likely will wither, contribute neither to academic nor clinical psychiatry, and not have a potentially valuable relationship with social science. Perhaps no other field of psychiatry faces such uncertainty as to the outcome of its exciting challenges. Will we move beyond the superficiality and abuses of community psychiatry? Critical rationality is essential for the construction of new theory, teaching paradigms, and research on clinical strategies in social and cross-cultural psychiatry. A critical rational approach could spell the difference between the successes of a new tradition and failures of an old one in this inchoate, but essential, field of psychiatry.

THE NATURE OF CRITICAL RATIONALITY

The present state in psychiatry may be analogous to late
nineteenth-century psychology, which William James (1892) described
as

> a string of facts; a little gossip and wrangle about opinions; a little
> classification and generalization on the mere descriptive level; a strong
> prejudice that we have states of mind, and that our brain conditions
> them . . . this is no science; it is only the hope of science.

We agree that much is amiss in psychiatry. We further agree that
contemporary difficulties reflect a lack of general identity, or more
accurately a firm foundation, for psychiatry. However, we disagree
both with those who ignore this problem and with those who
attempt to solve it by calling for a return to the bosom of medicine.
We argue that neither of these responses holds real promise for
psychiatry. The former has pushed the fields of psychiatry almost to
anarchy; the latter would restrict the fields to the practical, but
narrowly conceived approaches of medicine.

We feel the fields of psychiatry have a loosely knit, fragmented
identity, exemplified by the "special psychiatries," and derived from
a fascinating and complex history, a firm linkage to medicine,
specific clinical interests and responsibilities, and specialized areas of
expertise. Growth has been characteristically undisciplined. On the
other hand, throughout the fields of psychiatry, we feel a broad
consensus could be formed as to what constitute the fundamental
features of psychiatry. First, psychiatry has a clear clinical purpose:
to provide the best care for patients who suffer from psychiatric
disturbance. Second, psychiatry must draw relevant knowledge from
multiple domains—for example, biological science and behavioral and
social sciences—in order to accomplish its purpose. Third, and
fundamental, psychiatry shares with medicine explicit values that
guide clinical and research interests, namely, the therapeutic imperative: to help, to prevent, to cure, to palliate, and not to harm (see
Chapter 2 for discussion of this issue).

These views certainly reflect the potential for a firm and unified
foundation or identity for the fields of psychiatry. As we have
surveyed the present state of psychiatry, however, it has become
abundantly clear that there exists little agreement among psychiatrists
as to how to put these features into actual practice. What
psychiatrists say and what they do seem too diffuse and diversified,
not to mention inconsistent, to hope for that. Furthermore, there are
major barriers to the realization of this consensus: (1) the fields of
psychiatry are undisciplined; they are not sufficiently self-critical,

receptive to new ideas and other visions, or rigorously methodical in their approaches to new kinds of knowledge; (2) the fields of psychiatry are not organized to systematically introduce, evaluate, and integrate emerging concepts and findings from other disciplines that could help accomplish their task.

Clearly, what is needed is some tool, a fine instrument, if you will, to enable psychiatrists to overcome these barriers. Indeed, a means by which to discipline these undisciplined fields and to organize the emerging knowledge of extrapsychiatric fields that will allow us finally and thankfully to lay aside the issue of identity crisis, which in the light of present debate appears unresolvable. In short, psychiatry, the undisciplined discipline, has grown feet of clay and requires a firm foundation on which to form an identity.

We therefore propose a constructive potential solution to these difficulties. It may appear deceptively simple: we suggest that all psychiatrists employ a critical stance toward knowledge, a stance that we call *critical rationality*. That stance we believe will enable psychiatry to discipline itself and to evaluate and integrate systematically knowledge throughout the fields of psychiatry. And it will aid psychiatry to understand and even grow in reaction to the withering effects of anti-intellectualism, irrationality, and antiscientific interests massing in our midst.

Throughout this introductory chapter, we have alluded to the importance of critical approaches to knowledge. We have used the term "critical rationality" to describe the essential aspects of that commitment (we disclaim any particular relationship between critical rationality as we use this term and critical theory, the ideology promulgated by members of the Frankfurt Institute for Social Research). What then is critical rationality? How can it serve psychiatry in a time of crisis?

In proposing the term "critical rationality" to describe this approach, we have obviously combined its two component concepts, criticism and rationality. We have done this for a specific purpose. We wish to emphasize that rationality alone is not a sufficient answer to overcome the barriers that prevent psychiatry from achieving unified identity. We also wish to stress that several different meanings for the term "criticism" can be linked strategically to the concept of rationality in order to construct a comprehensive approach fully responsive to psychiatry's present deficiencies. In the following pages, we will discuss first the concept of rationality and then the meanings of criticism relevant to it. We will next suggest several examples of how critical rationality may be put to use in psychiatry, then comment on the implications of its introduction.

There is nothing obscure implied by our use of the term "rationality." Rationality, naturally, refers to reason (we will use the two terms interchangeably), the product of centuries of Western philosophical and scientific tradition. It therefore implies certain rules and methods of inquiry; for instance, the standards of inductive and deductive logic and the scientific method. In addition, it fosters certain values and principles. These include clarity in the presentation of concepts, precision in thinking, and explicitness of argument and assumptions. Especially important for its use is the dialectical development of ideas through the careful scrutinizing procedures of questioning, debate, and reflection. This helps to disclose the limits and depth of our knowledge. These rational tools unblock the way for inquiry. As Abraham Kaplan (1964) has so wisely stated:

> Everything depends on the conduct of enquiry, on the way at which we arrive at our conclusions. Freedom from bias means having an open mind, not an empty one. At the heart of every bias is a prejudice. That is to say, a pre-judgment, a conclusion arrived at prior to the evidence and maintained independently of the evidence. It is true that what serves as evidence is a result of the process of interpretation—facts do *not* speak for themselves; nevertheless, facts must be given a hearing, or the scientific point to the process of interpretation is lost.

Perhaps it is obvious to think that rationality should undergird the workings of any organized approach to the discovery of knowledge. But psychiatry is a particular area of inquiry that differs fundamentally from psychology, biochemistry, and economics. In addition to pursuing actively the understandings and knowledge that originate in related areas, psychiatry must translate findings from its own inquiries and from other fields into applications useful for patient care. This is not necessarily true for the former fields. Because of this fact, the relationship between psychiatry and knowledge must assuredly differ from that in other disciplines, but must be similar to that found in other applied sciences, including medicine. This raises a crucial question. How can rationality—this nonspecific instrument— serve as a guide with respect to the issue of developing meaningful, practical, and applicable knowledge in psychiatry? We believe an indication of the answer to this question lies in Whitehead's brilliant contributions to the understanding of the nature of the relationship between theory and practice of reason. Reason, after all, has a substantial history in Western culture. The lessons from this history significantly illuminate aspects of the present state in psychiatry.

Whitehead (1929) argues that it is useful to think of rationality as having two separable functions. One is speculative, or theoretical, and the other is practical. Speculative, or theoretical, reason has the function of piercing to the general behind the specific, of transcending particular methods, to what Whitehead calls "the flight after the unattainable." Before the Greeks, this function of reason was anticipated in the intuitive imagination reflected in ancient, inspirational religious activity. The Greeks, however, discovered the significant secret that speculative reason was itself subject to orderly method. That unique secret was the apprehension of how to be bound by method, even as it was transcended. The Greeks, thus, invented the logic of discovery—the broadest form of logic. The experiences of centuries have given us the criteria that Whitehead (1929) points out should be the basis for assessment of any particular belief. They are:

1. Conformity with intuitive experience
2. Clarity of propositional content
3. Internal Logical consistency
4. External Logical consistency
5. Status of a *Logical* scheme with:
   a. widespread conformity to experience
   b. no discordance with experience
   c. coherence among its categoreal notions
   d. methodologic consequences

These criteria are not easy to apply. The medievalists stressed deduction, often carelessly ignoring criticism of premises presumed to accord with experience. Moderns have stressed induction, assuming that looking at experience is a straightforward operation—but being careful to admit only observations that conform to experience. Speculative reason searches for complete understanding; it is evident in the urge for theorizing in psychiatry. Its proper satisfaction is elucidation.

The practical function of reason is to discover method and clarify methodology; as Whitehead illustrates, practical reason befits the fox, speculative reason, the gods. Thus, practical reason refers to the careful exploration of method with a view to fulfilling an immediate purpose. It eschews speculation in the pursuit of practice. Kaplan (1964) points out this practical function of reason with respect to methodology:

> The aim of methodology [the study of methods], then, is to describe and analyze these methods [procedures such as forming concepts and hypotheses, making observations and measurements, performing experiments, building models and theories, providing explanations and making predictions], throwing light on their limitations and resources, clarifying their presuppositions and consequences, relating their potentialities to the twilight zone at the frontiers of knowledge. It is to venture generalizations from the success of particular techniques, suggesting new applications, and to unfold the specific bearings of logical and metaphysical principles on concrete problems, suggesting new formulations.

The two functions of reason, though separable, are intimately connected; they thrive on each other. Speculative reason must be harnessed by its practical counterpart. Whitehead (1929) states:

> The supreme verification of the speculative flight is that it issues in the establishment of a practical technique for well-tested ends, and that the speculative system maintains itself as the elucidation of that technique. In this way there is the progress from thought to practice, and regress from practice to the same thought. This interplay of thought and practice is the supreme authority. It is a test by which the charlatanism of speculation is restrained.

There is, however, a problem. The problem for rationality in general, and for rationality in psychiatry in particular, is that these two functions of reason have troublesome natures in the hands of its users. They have a tendency to stagnate because of dogmatism. They lack discipline.

The satisfaction that derives from the workings of a particular method stifles innovation. Current practice, because it appears to work, becomes the sole focus of intellectual activity. Consider in the present state of psychiatry the importance of the catecholamine model in biological psychiatry. In the United States, this powerful and practical method has virtually monopolized the efforts of numerous biological researchers. Similar, but less stifling, perhaps, has been the effect of crisis intervention "theory" on social psychiatry. Isolated from logically related disciplines of social science, that field has seized on this diffuse "theoretical" structure as a means of ordering multiple observations, diverse clinical problems, and social needs in order to achieve the appearance of a formidable body of knowledge. In clinical psychiatry, the advocates of various psycho-therapies spend much energy claiming sole possession of the means of therapeutic success, despite the consistent demonstration that most forms of psychotherapy can be effective. Specialized interests militate against support and/or organization of methical attempts to disclose the salient variables of favorable therapeutic outcome. Practical reason tends to stagnate in self-satisfaction; a powerful model begins to dominate thinking. It shapes our notion of what constitutes evidence. Instead of testing hypotheses, it tends to search only for evidence to corroborate them. Powerful methods embody themselves in institutions and professional organizations that have special interests; the discovery of knowledge assumes a secondary role. Kaplan (1964) illustrates:

> By pressing methodological norms too far, we may inhibit the bold and imaginative adventures of ideas. The irony is that methodology itself may make for conformism—conformity to its own favorite reconstructions—and

a conformity even less productive than one at least imitating scientific colleagues.

There is, as Whitehead (1929) comments,

> an active interest restraining curiosity within the scope of method. Any defect of that interest arouses an emotional resentment. Empiricism vanishes.

Speculative reason tends to stagnate when it does not result in practical applications, techniques, and methods. In psychiatry, in the early twentieth century, the push for complete understanding led to a premature closure of thinking, oversimplification, and isolationism in both the Freudian (and Meyerian) and Kraepelinian camps. Unverified hypotheses replaced knowledge and became dogma. In some cases, research slowed almost to a standstill. Residents were taught to be uncritical, to accept the tenets of dominant ideology.

Stagnation becomes evident when a particular methodology no longer deals with main issues. Minor questions dominate debate. Obscurantism becomes prevalent, suspicion of new ideas increases, and authority is invoked as an ultimate arbiter. As Whitehead (1929) complains:

> Obscurantism is rooted in human nature more deeply than any particular subject of interest. It is just as strong among the men of science as among the clergy and among professional men and business men as among other classes. Obscurantism is a refusal to speculate freely on the limitations of traditional methods. It is more than that: it is the negation of the importance of such speculation, the insistence on incidental dangers.

Whitehead thus orients us to answer the question we posed earlier: How can rationality serve as a guide with respect to the issue of developing meaningful, practical, and applicable knowledge in psychiatry? His contribution is to lay before us an analysis of what the natural history of reason is in the hands of its users. He does this by clarifying the dialectical relationship between the two functions of reason: theory and practice. Theory (speculation), for which the Greeks invented the logic of discovery, helps create practical techniques; these techniques in turn serve to restrain imagination and theorizing by keeping them wedded to real issues and practical problems.

Reason, then, is a tool; as a tool, it promotes certain values and is productive and consequential only insofar as it is skillfully and thoughtfully applied. It can be employed to lead to new understandings, or it can promote obscurantism. Similarly, reason in psychiatry can only be effective if it is used skillfully and thoughtfully. Our argument is that psychiatrists have been and continue to be undisciplined in their use of reason. As a result, disunity prevails, and new knowledge enters the fields of psychiatry with considerable difficulty. Theorizing in psychiatry must be related to relevant problems. Practical techniques must be examined constantly and not be allowed to monopolize efforts. Obscurantism may then be avoided. But how is this dialectical tension to be maintained in psychiatry?

It is here that the notion of *criticism* comes to play a significant role in forming the approach we propose. First, "critical" refers to and emphasizes the reflexive character of rationality. That is, critical rationality constantly orients us to the evaluation of methodology, including its own. In order to prevent stagnation, those who profess the use of rationality must scrutinize themselves critically to disclose the limitation and potential of their thinking. For example, psychoanalysis is a rational theory; however, there have been few attempts among its devotees to commit themselves to a critical stance toward it. The result has been inbred stagnation and unrestrained speculation. Had there been an attempt to critically evaluate this theoretical structure, psychiatry might now be the benefactor of a far more productive clinical tradition.

Second, criticism underlines and means the constructive quality of rationality: the thoroughgoing motivation to see the merits and faults of viewpoints, of new ideas as well as established ones. In this sense, much of the interest that generated this seminar and volume came from a critical stance toward psychiatric clinical practice. Our resulting disenchantment led us to organize efforts to develop new understandings and to reform thinking on numerous issues from a systematically critical and rational point of view. In a related sense, the term criticism also points to the importance of negation as a tool for evaluating ideas; in science, verification and falsifiability are essential criteria for acceptable statements concerning knowledge. To be able to verify statements requires evidence, e.g., observations. To falsify statements requires that we be able to articulate in advance what events, were they to take place, would falsify our predictions (Hanson, 1971; Popper, 1968). These notions form part of the spirit of what is critical in rationality.

Third, criticism means what Polanyi and Prosch (1975) refers to as the analysis of tacit (or personal) knowledge. That is, examining the tacit subsidiaries we make use of to move *from* pieces of unintegrated (and usually unexamined) knowledge *to* more or less explicit knowledge focused on a problem. Much of the time, this integration is *ad hoc* and unanalyzed. Although this may be less of a problem in research, it is virtually characteristic of clinical reasoning. A critical rationality in psychiatry, in this instance, would make the study of clinical judgment a major avenue of research, and would use the study of clinical judgment as a pedagogic vehicle for teaching future clinicians (Feinstein, 1967; Lazare, 1973).

Fourth, critical refers to the normative element within rationality. We would promote awareness of the purposes and ends that constitute the consequences of rational scientific endeavor. In his famous work *The Eclipse of Reason*, Max Horkheimer (1947) laments the evolution of rationality in the West insofar as interest in means, and ignorance and disavowal of responsibility for ends, have become an essential feature. By calling for an explicit awareness of such failings, our approach can perhaps avoid the naive exuberance that accompanies the introduction (and often goes on long after that) of new treatments, particularly new psychotherapies. Furthermore, such an awareness can orient psychiatrists to the social and political implications of their work. Psychosurgery for prisoners, the excessive use of civil commitment procedures, the abortion problem, labeling of people as psychiatrically ill for social and political reasons—all call for a critical rational appraisal.

Whitehead (1924) proposed a constructive way in which theory and practice work in dialectical tension. He was wise to note, then, that reason (rationality) is only a tool. People may use it skillfully, if unthoughtfully; and it can promote stagnation. In psychiatry, we must also be aware that rationality is only a tool. Present rationality tends to promote obscurantism and stagnation in psychiatry. In order to prevent both, we have proposed the joining of criticism to the notion of rationality. Through the workings of a *critical* rationality, then, we may hope to maintain an appropriate dialectical tension between the two necessary and useful aspects of psychiatry—theory and practice—and consequently et the fields of psychiatry moving again.

Critical rationality, therefore, represents a stance toward knowledge and issues in which knowledge and values intersect. It is a tool that, if put to appropriate use, can go far to discipline the fields of psychiatry and help them overcome isolationism, both inside and outside psychiatry. The implications, if such an instrument could be used throughout psychiatry, would be considerable. Perhaps it would be useful to illustrate some of the possible applications that a critical rational approach might generate.

One obvious example of the usefulness of a critical rational approach in psychiatry relates to training. We would argue that such an approach has multiple ramifications as to how to organize teaching and what to teach psychiatric residents. In that a critical rational approach represents a useful and basic instrument for the fields of psychiatry, we would propose at the outset that it be made a fundamental teaching approach of the entire training program. Let us consider how a critical rational approach might influence the development of a basic curriculum for psychiatry residents and structure the process of training.

First, we will suggest comparisons between the traditional approach and the one we propose. Then, we will look at two subject areas as examples.

The traditional approach to psychiatric training has the following characteristics: (1) There is a lack of explicit, general goals for training. Are young psychiatrists to be trained to become biological researchers, psychotherapists, or administrative psychiatrists? What constitutes the "core curriculum" (a favorite phrase) for residents? There is no consensus on these matters. Hence, we have training tracks, generalist programs, and what is paraded before residents as eclecticism. (2) Methodical, rigorous, and critical approaches to knowledge in psychiatry are deemphasized. (3) The great bulk of teaching time is focused on supervision—usually of psychotherapy (most often, some variant of current dynamic theory, but also behavior therapy). Relatively little time is devoted to in-depth exploration of relevant disciplines, for example, neurosciences, psychology, medical aspects of psychiatry. Thus, traditional training has the character more of apprenticeship than of disciplined scholarship. (4) As a result of both unclear goals and a relative disinterest in rigorous approaches to knowledge domains, there is a pronounced tendency to rely, year after year, on an unimaginative curriculum dominated by the traditional filler: dynamic psychology, long-term psychotherapy, crisis intervention, social and community psychiatry, and so forth.

As an alternative, a critical rational approach to the issues of training would have the following characteristics: (1) the formation of explicit goals for training:

a. to introduce a variety of relevant subject areas.

b. to develop a critical attitude toward the evaluation of information.

c. to achieve an in-depth understanding of the subject areas, in order to recognize the limits and potentials of the knowledge and disciplines presented.

d. to foster the development of integrative approaches, utilizing intradisciplinary and interdisciplinary contributions in concepts and methods.

(2) Instead of a deemphasis of method, there would be a clear commitment to teach residents a critical rational approach, both explicit (by stating the ground rules for rational discourse in the presentation of patients and ideas, and by stating the goals sought and methods used) and implicit (by having teachers employ the tool

routinely). (3) Instead of an apprenticeship, the model for teaching would be to use as many techniques as needed (including supervision) to promote gradually the increasing independence of the residents through disciplined scholarship, by helping them to develop thorough, in-depth understandings in order to increase their confidence in their ability to know their limits, to know what to do in order to answer a specific question outside of their expertise, and to know the means by which to increase competence in a specific area of interest. And (4), instead of traditional subjects, this curriculum would attempt to deal carefully with a variety of disciplines deemed basic to psychiatry's needs and taught from the standpoint of their relevance to specific issues in psychiatry. These disciplines might include biomedical subjects (the neurosciences, epidemiology, genetics, psychopharmacology), behavioral sciences (cognitive, developmental, and personality psychology, learning theory, psychopathology, psychophysiology), social sciences (medical sociology and anthropology, social psychology), communication sciences, and humanities (ethics, philosophy of science, logic, history of psychiatric ideas and institutions).

Let us elaborate these suggestions for a general curriculum with respect to two specific examples. First, we will consider the training of residents in the area of psychotherapy. The teaching in this area would be organized to conform to the explicit general goals outlined above. Initially, residents would be introduced to the relevant aspects of directly related, basic subject areas: linguistics, communication theory, social psychology, social and anthropological studies of the healing relationship, learning theory, psychodynamic theory of transference, and so on. The various psychotherapy schools could be presented systematically, with attention to the scientific bases of each. Then, residents could develop on the basis of this and prior experience critical approaches to psychotherapy itself. Much of this development would come from a critical reading of the literature, determining assumptions and deficiencies of various studies, appraising arguments, and, perhaps most pertinent, critically examining the residents' own experiences in providing psychotherapy to patients. Residents could begin to achieve a profound understanding by learning the significant areas of established knowledge, the key questions generating research, and, perhaps most important, what is not known. A detailed examination of the literature on psychotherapy research of all persuasions from analytic therapy to techniques of behavior control (e.g., propaganda, brainwashing) would be useful for these purposes. Attempts might be made to generate general conclusions from this large literature, noting how effective each of the various psychotherapeutic modalities is and what appears to be effective about them generally. Among the lessons and limitations: Psychotherapy works, but we do not know how. Some general attributes of successful treatment are known; theory may contribute little to efficacy.

Finally, residents could be taught first, then asked to develop later, integrative approaches to understanding psychotherapy. From within the established fields of psychiatry, residents could learn how to apply techniques such as behavioral therapy, hypnosis, or psychodynamic therapy to individual or group psychotherapy. Residents might wish to compare the relative assumptions and efficacies of psychoanalytic and behavioral techniques, noting their strong similarities and underlining their differences. Knowledge of social psychology and sociocultural factors relevant to the doctor-patient relationship might form the basis for more effective interventions in social therapeutic milieu treatment, the so-called therapeutic milieu, which is frequently the basis for inpatient treatment in psychiatry. Study of the sociocultural and psychological features of doctor-patient relations from the perspectives of medical anthropology and cognitive and social psychology might lead to increased comprehension of the factors promoting or detracting from patient compliance and satisfaction. Or, as Lazare (1976) has recently done, residents might turn to studies of diplomacy, labor relations, and collective bargaining to draw important information and concepts to help learn about the process of negotiating treatment plans with patients.

A second example of how a critical rational approach might elaborate a teaching program could be the subject of schizophrenia. Again, the goals would be those outlined above. First, residents would be introduced to the relevant subject areas. These could include: the history of the psychiatric concepts of schizophrenia, psychosis, disease; the classic contributions of Kahlbaum, Kraepelin, and Bleuler; the psychologies of schizophrenia (Jungian and other dynamic theories, learning theories, cognitive theories); the biological aspects of schizophrenia (genetics, neuropsychology, biochemistry, psychopharmacology, and model psychoses—including drug-induced psychoses, temporal lobe epilepsy, and other known causes of psychotic disease); the social aspects of schizophrenia (labeling theory and studies of deviance, the "social breakdown syndrome," and institutional influence on behavior); recent and contemporary approaches to the study of diagnosis and outcome (the World Health Organization International Pilot Study of schizophrenia, the Schneiderian, Langfeldtian, American Psychiatric Association, and Washington University approaches to syndromal diagnosis); contemporary treatment (psychopharmacology, psychotherapeutic techniques, Schizophrenics Anonymous, and behavior modification, e.g., token economies); and efforts at prevention (epidemiology, genetic counseling, high-risk group study and surveillance).

Second, residents would, through critical encounter with these subjects, begin to develop increasing sophistication regarding the usefulness and limitations of the diagnosis of schizophrenia; these experiences would be augmented with frequent case presentations, patient interviews before groups of residents, and regular reports by residents of required follow-up and management of patients. Third, as a result, a critical approach would gradually characterize the efforts of residents in this area. Instead of providing oversimplified formulas for approaching schizophrenia, the effort would be to indicate the complexities of the subject, the limits of present knowledge, and the understanding achieved through working with the basic conceptual problems in the field and criticizing one's own approach as well as the approaches of others, based on actual applications. In this way, the residents could function as doctors while working out their understandings of these problems.

Fourth, there would be an emphasis on creating integrated approaches to our understanding of schizophrenia. For example, one might wish to pursue understandings related to the concept of schizophrenia from an interdisciplinary standpoint: To what extent— and supply a description—do patients who receive the diagnosis of schizophrenia (according to research criteria developed by several groups) have cognitive impairments in attention, language function, and perception; also, are there other neurological disturbances (such as fine coordination, two-point discrimination, stereognosis, and graphesthesia); and is there in these same patients evidence of certain biochemical changes (e.g., platelet MAO enzyme; see Murphy and Wyatt, 1972)? Further integrations could be devised by learning to employ factor analyses of various dimensional aspects of these disturbances. For example, residents could learn to separate logically the social, psychological, and biological experiences of schizophrenic patients in order to integrate these dimensions within an epidemiological framework of risk factors or a medical framework proposing specific pathogenic mechanisms—both of which could be tested either on populations of patients or in individuals through intensive and in-depth case studies. Through such exercises, residents could develop quite sophisticated understandings of the subject; moreover, they could gain an appreciation of methods now, or potentially, available that may help to answer present unknowns in this mystifying area.

Within the fields of psychiatry, an obvious need to which a critical approach might also speak is the development of effective means for overcoming disciplinary barriers to ensure the flow of relevant knowledge into psychiatry. An important example here is an elaboration of a mechanism for systematic translation, application, and evaluation of knowledge *from* other fields *to* psychiatry. Such an elaboration might conform to the following translational paradigm (following and extending Nida, 1974): (1) elicitation of new knowledge from another field; (2) its analysis in terms of that field; (3) its translation from the concepts of that field into relevant models in the language of a particular field of psychiatry; (4) its reconstruction in terms of related concepts in that psychiatric field and in other fields of psychiatry; and (5) feedback based on evaluating the results of its actual application to particular problems in psychiatry, which will change that knowledge for this specific field of psychiatry, psychiatry generally, and the extrapsychiatric discipline from which it is derived. In the same way, such a translational paradigm might be a means of systematically translating among the different fields of knowledge in psychiatry, and thus of generating a framework for integrating those now quite separate systems of psychiatric knowledge, that is, the "special psychiatries." Here, then, are uses to which a critical rational approach to theory and psychiatry could be profitably applied.

Perhaps an example would make this specific instance of a critical approach clear. Suppose we wish to take the concept of the sick role from medical sociology and bring it to bear on psychiatric illness following the arguments used by Kleinman in Chapter 3. We are arguing that, for the most part, such transfer is done unsystematically on an *ad hoc* basis. In the model presented above, we present a framework—the product of a critical rational approach—that can be applied systematically to that process. That model calls for analyzing what the sick role concept means in sociological parlance, and then translating the meaning into a specific conceptual domain in psychiatry, such as psychopathological concepts about illness, or social psychiatric concepts of course of illness and its determinants, or a cross-cultural psychiatric concept of cultural patterning of illness and societal responses to it. This means, in part, defining the sick role concept in psychiatric terminology. This step would be followed by reconstructing our theory of illness with this concept. We would then apply the concept to a particular problem, such as one commonly encountered in consultation psychiatry: hypochondriasis with secondary gain or malingering. The results of our application would be evaluated with regard to validity and benefit (heuristic or clinical) when compared with existing concepts. Finally, this evaluation based on a specific application would feed back to refine this interdisciplinary conceptual transfer and show what needed to be clarified or elaborated in order to make the sick role concept useful. Feedback might also include some input into medical sociology, which might affect how this concept is defined and used there. Abuse of the sick role as a concept then might be used as a means of integrating a number of categories in psychopathology, ranging from hysteria to malingering, which could be applied in psychiatric consultation to specific clinical problems, as Kleinman argues in Chapter 3.

Along the lines of this translational paradigm, for example, communication theory models of dyadic communication might be transferred into studies of psychiatric doctor-patient interactions. The same kind of approach might be used for biological concepts as well.

Another example of critical rationality applied to psychiatry might be the rigorous elaboration of an analytic dichotomy between *disease* and *illness*, in which the concept of disease stands for a primary malfunctioning of the biological and/or psychological processes, and the concept of illness stands for secondary psychosocial and cultural reactions to disease. Using this dichotomy, we might review the diagnostic categories to see where these conceptual distinctions would be beneficial in thinking about and treating psychiatric disorders. We know that acute disease can occur in the absence of illness (e.g., acute intoxications). Chronic disease, on the other hand, is always accompanied by illness, which usually provides the major issues for clinical management. Indeed, illness may be fulminant when disease grows quiescent. Perhaps malingering, alcoholism, drug abuse, and homosexuality could be regarded as illnesses in the absence of disease. The value of the distinction is that it bears on a major issue in clinical care: scientific technology usually treats disease, not illness; communication and "caring" aspects of doctor-patient relationships usually treat illness, rather than disease. Psychotherapy can affect disease, but its primary impact is on illness. Most dissatisfaction with modern health care indicates ineffective or absent treatment of illness. This critical elaboration of a useful dichotomy suggests models for responding to problems in primary psychiatric care (lack of compliance, patient dissatisfaction, medical-legal actions) as much as in primary medical care. We might argue from this perspective that psychiatric consultation often is asked to augment medical care devoted entirely to disease by treating illness. Limits of space do not allow us to demonstrate how this model can be applied to actual cases, but it should be obvious that this is an analytic distinction potentially entailing powerful clinical consequences. For example, should the treatment of disease/illness be separated into two distinct clinical functions of two distinct health professional roles (e.g., doctor and nurse; or general medical doctor and psychiatrist); or should an attempt be made to reunify these traditionally integrative functions in the role of the doctor? This is a problem for a critical rational approach in psychiatry that needs to be elaborated fully, following the steps of our translational model, and that could be tested as a framework for integrating biological, behavioral, and social concepts into psychopathology and psychiatric treatment (for further notes on the illness/disease argument, see Eisenberg, 1976).

Implications and Conclusions

The implications that follow from a critical rational approach as evidenced in the examples discussed include the *spirited and directed attack on key clinical problems* through new clarifications, a more precise *sorting out of the issues*, and the *building of interdisciplinary bridges*. Certainly, also, we can more readily understand the usefulness of theorizing, which is crucial to the development of knowledge, particularly for the purpose of finding unity in diversified areas of investigation. There is a need, then, for a less substantial theorizing (we would suggest a mid-range theorizing) that does not try to provide a framework for all facts and needs, but pulls together various empirical findings and aids in integrating them with systematic observations from other disciplines. As in the examples above, this translational purpose and integrative function for mid-range theory provides a standard toward which investigations from many diverse areas in psychiatry can move. The result will be a greater unity of psychiatric knowledge, without a loss of any particular approach.

A further implication of a critical rational approach in psychiatry is a *new humility* generated from an awareness of the limitations about present psychiatric knowledge. Some examples: Psychotherapy works, but we do not understand how; though we are able to distinguish schizophrenia from other disturbances in many cases, at this time we neither have the capacity nor the methods to halt the natural course of this process, nor to predict (even with genetic knowledge) accurately those who will experience this serious disturbance in their lives. Our understanding of hysteria, though perhaps extended by Freud, still is remarkably poor; we are unable to treat hysteria, much less to define it clearly. A host of related and currently obscure issues reside in the notions of psychogenic psychosis, "borderline character," and "culture-bound disorders." As these disturbances are thought to be very prevalent, it behooves us to understand them.

This humility is coupled, however, with a clear-headedness. The despair of nihilism only threatens those who cannot face reality. Humility only puts us in context; it does not prevent us from increasing our effectiveness as psychiatrists. A critical rational approach indicates where we may profitably proceed, since such an approach is grounded in responding to psychiatric problems by being relevant, practical, and effective.

The implication of a critical rational approach with respect to the issue of identity in psychiatry is singularly important. We feel that the identity crisis in psychiatry cannot be solved by present approaches. Psychiatry must transform its feet of clay by disciplining itself; the issue of identity may then dissolve.

To summarize, critical rationality is an approach with special features. It encompasses the dialectical functions of reason—practical and theoretical—which have come to us in highly developed form after centuries of experience. But psychiatry, we hold, requires a more explicit and self-conscious approach than mere reason; after all, most psychiatrists feel they are exceptionally rational. The problem is that the fields of psychiatry lack discipline and a firm foundation and may stagnate if they are not pulled together in a productive manner. Critical rationality becomes a powerful instrument for psychiatry, because it can help overcome the barriers that promote disunity inside and outside the fields of psychiatry. The purpose of combining criticism with rationality is to attempt to provide explicit reference to certain needs. These include a need for a unified approach to knowledge; a need for rigorous self-discipline in that approach (the reflexive character of methodology); a need for an approach that can develop means for introducing new concepts into research, teaching, and practice; a need to increase our awareness of the manner in which we think and act in our work (the analysis of tacit or personal knowledge) as well as our awareness (the normative context) of the far-reaching consequences of what we do throughout the fields of psychiatry; and a need to recognize that though we must, because we are doctors, act (apply that knowledge in therapeutic interventions), we tend to rationalize our actions afterward rather than understand first in order to act effectively.

Ultimately, it will be each psychiatrist who, in seeking to use a critical rational approach, will either succeed or fail. The chapters of this volume represent substantial attempts to deal critically and rationally with significant issues in different fields of psychiatry. We believe that this approach can bring about renewal in psychiatry.

CHAPTERS

As we introduce the specific chapters of this book, several points should be made. First, the participants in the seminar wrote their chapters after receiving constructive and critical encouragement for their ideas and their field of psychiatry from all participants. In this sense, each of us shared in the creation of the entire book. Second, critical rationality was an explicit approach for the process of developing and writing on each topic, down to the final editing. That stance meant that among the many points we have already discussed, traditional authority would not serve as the final word on an issue. Third, the variety of areas dealt with is an indication of the relevance of critical rationality to the fields of psychiatry. This diversity might, under usual circumstances, mask the crucial commitment to rational approaches to knowledge development represented here. It should be clear that although the content of each chapter is important, the significance of the work as a whole is in its documentation of a crucial experience of dealing with knowledge together in different fields of psychiatry in a rational manner.

We have, therefore, divided the chapters into three parts according to the type of knowledge issue for psychiatry with which each dealt. In observing the chapter titles within each part, one immediately notices that there is a variety of topics; but the key is that each chapter considers a particularly and widely important kind of question within its specialized frame of reference. Thus, in the first part, Issues That Require Clarification and Reconceptualization in the Fields of Psychiatry, the chapters deal with specific problems that have confounded psychiatry for some time. However, the intent is not to rehash concepts or merely to review these problems. It is rather to approach issues through a critical evaluation and rational process of analysis in order to clarify and find new solutions.

Theo Manschreck, a psychiatrist with interests in cognition and general psychopathology, has written a chapter on acute psychosis. He proposes a reasonable and yet far-reaching change in the way we diagnose and organize our understanding of this significant psychiatric problem.

Arthur Kleinman, a psychiatrist who investigates the healing relationship cross-culturally, and who is specially trained in social science, has written a chapter on sociocultural science contributions to understanding psychopathology. He introduces a new approach to the vexing questions of how to conceptualize, how to utilize therapeutically, and how to teach the powerful sociocultural influences in psychiatry.

Peter Mansky and Jack Altman have written a chapter on drug dependence in which they draw together concepts and research findings from pharmacology and psychology to forge a new model for understanding this troublesome phenomenon. The model has implications for prevention, treatment, and research. Mansky is a psychiatrist with an extensive background in opiate pharmacology research and a strong interest in psychopathology. Altman is a research psychologist who has designed and collaborated on inter-disciplinary approaches to the study of drug dependence.

In their chapter, Timothy Rivinus and Gordon Harper have attempted to integrate recent reformulations in the field of adult psychosomatics with understandings derived from the study of development and familial influences on children, to develop a comprehensive view of illness in children. This view will, they feel, supply a basis for conceptualizing illness multidimensionally at all ages. They illustrate the usefulness of their approach with clinical observations from a psychosomatic inpatient unit of a children's hospital. Rivinus is a child psychiatrist and researcher in this area. Harper is a child psychiatrist and pediatrician with special interests in developmental psychology.

The second part of the book, Issues That Determine the Frontiers and Limits of the Fields of Psychiatry, has two quite distinct chapters. This part is devoted to a consideration of certain issues under examination in psychiatry and other disciplines. Thus, these chapters carefully analyze the possibility for translation of various concepts and tools into and out of psychiatry. David Bear, a psychiatrist, has written a pioneering essay on temporal lobe epilepsy, a problem he has worked on for several years. He extends our views on the importance of this particular neurological disease for psychiatry by indicating its potential as a model for understanding such diverse functions as emotion, language, and learning, as well as for gaining insights into personality disorder and schizophrenia. Anastasia Kucharski, a psychiatrist who has pursued advanced studies in history, discusses psychohistory and the rationality of psychiatric ventures into historical explanation. In an era when psychohistory is fashionable, her argument demands attention.

The third part of the book, Issues That Provide Novel and Significant Perspectives in the Fields of Psychiatry, reflects the power and applicability that a critical rational approach can lend to new and intuitive insights. By themselves, such insights stir our imagination, but fail to effect important advances. By harnessing them, critical rationality expands their effectiveness for psychiatry. Miriam Sonn, a nurse and sociologist, draws from her experiences in psychiatric nursing important observations regarding the nature of being a psychiatric patient. This enlightening inside viewpoint, which brings to this subject an approach from phenomenological sociology, represents a virtually untapped source of knowledge within psychiatry. Equally novel in its focus is Felton Earls' chapter on the relationship of fathers and psychopathology. Earls, a child psychiatrist, has done a service to rational exchange on this topic by highlighting past achievements and proposing new directions for effecting useful interventions in the study of this issue. Harper, in a second chapter, proposes a new look at the general problem of what kind of relationships are important from the developmental perspective by investigating where child development takes place, as opposed to with whom it takes place. William Beardslee, a child psychiatrist and veteran of the 1960s civil rights struggles, has contributed a chapter based on his experiences of tracking down civil rights activists who have remained in the South a decade after the movement peaked. He has looked at the present life styles of these men and women and contrasted them with their courageous pasts; and he clarifies the issues relevant to the general psychosocial adaptation and coping that such singular events in life demand.

REFERENCES

Akiskal, H. S., and W. McKinney, Jr. 1973. Psychiatry and pseudopsychiatry. Archives of General Psychiatry 28:367–372.

American Psychiatric Association (APA). 1952. Committee on Nomenclature and Statistics.

Bandura, A. 1969. Principles of Behavior Modification. New York: Holt, Rinehart and Winston.

Brodie, H. K., and M. Sabshin. 1973. An overview of trends in psychiatric research: 1963–1972. American Journal of Psychiatry 130: 1309–1318.

Callaway, E. 1975. Psychiatry today. Western Journal of Medicine 122:349–354.

Cooper, J. E., R. E. Kendell, B. J. Gurland, L. Sharpe, J. R. Copeland, and R. Simon. 1972. Psychiatric Diagnosis in New York and London. London: Oxford University Press.

Diagnostic and Statistical Manual of Mental Disorders-(DSM-I). Washington, D.C.: American Psychiatric Association.

Eisenberg, L. 1973. The future of psychiatry. Lancet 11:1371–1375.

_____. 1976. Delineation of clinical conditions: conceptual models of "physical" and "mental" disorders. In Ciba Symposium No. 44: Research and Medical Practice: Their Interaction. Amsterdam: Elsevier Excerpta Medica North Holland, pp. 3–23.

Fabrega, H. 1974. Disease and Social Behavior. Cambridge, Mass.: MIT Press.

Feighner, J. P., E. Robins, S. B. Guze, R. Woodruff, G. Winokur, and R. Munoz. 1972. Diagnostic criteria for use in psychiatric research. Archives of General Psychiatry 26:57–63.

Feinstein, A. R. 1967. Clinical Judgement. Huntington, N.Y.: R. E. Kreiger.

Hanson, N. R., 1971. Observation and Explanation: A Guide to the Philosophy of Science. New York: Harper & Row.

Hartmann, H. 1958. Ego Psychology and the Problem of Adaptation. New York: International Universities Press.

Holzman, P. S. 1970. Psychoanalysis and psychopathology. New York: McGraw-Hill.

Horkheimer, M. 1947. Eclipse of Reason, New York: Seabury Press.

Hughes, C. C., M. A. Trembley, R. N. Rapaport, and A. H. Leighton. 1960. People of Cove and Woodlot: Communities from the Viewpoint of Social Psychology. New York: Basic Books.

James, W. 1892. Psychology, Briefer Course. New York: Holt.

Kaplan, A. 1964. The Conduct of Inquiry. Scranton, Pa.: Chandler.

Kety, S. S. 1974. From rationalization to reason. American Journal of Psychiatry 131:957–963.

Kleinman, A., P. Kunstadter, E. Alexander, and J. L. Gale. 1975. Medicine in Chinese Cultures: Comparative Studies of Health Care in Chinese and Other Societies. Bethesda, Md.: Fogarty International Center, National Institutes of Health.

Laing, R. D. 1967. The Politics of Experience. New York: Pantheon.

Lazare, A. 1973. Hidden conceptual models in clinical psychiatry. New England Journal of Medicine 288:345-351.

———. 1975. Patient requests in a walk-in clinic. Comprehensive Psychiatry 16:467-477.

———. 1976. Personal communication.

Lazare, A., F. Cohen, A. Jacobson, M. Williams, R. Mignone, and S. Zisook. 1972. The walk-in patient as a "customer": a key dimension in evaluation and treatment. American Journal of Orthopsychiatry 42:872-883.

Lazarus, R. S. 1966. Psychological Stress and the Coping Process. New York: McGraw-Hill.

Leighton, A. 1959. My Name is Legion. Foundations for a Theory of Man in Relation to Culture. New York: Basic Books.

———. 1967. Is Social Environment a Cause of Psychiatric Disorder? Psychiatric Research Report 22, American Psychiatric Association.

Leighton, A., T. A. Lambo, C. C. Hughes, A. H. Leighton, J. Murphy, and D. B. Macklin. 1963. Psychiatric Disorder Among the Yoruba. Ithaca, N.Y.: Cornell University Press.

Leighton, D., J. S. Harding, D. B. Macklin, A. M. MacMillan, and A. H. Leighton. 1967. The Character of Danger: Psychiatric Symptoms in Selected Communities. New York: Basic Books.

Levy, R. 1973. Tahitians: Mind and Experience in the Society Islands. Chicago: University of Chicago Press.

Lewis, A. 1967. The State of Psychiatry. New York: Science House.

Lipowski, Z. J. 1973. Psychosomatic medicine in a changing society: some current trends in theory and research. Comprehensive Psychiatry 14:203-215.

Murphy, D., and R. Wyatt. 1972. Reduced monoamine oxidase activity in blood platelets from schizophrenic patients. Nature 238:225-226.

Nida, E. 1974. Toward a Science of Translating. Leiden, Holland: Brill Press.

Polyani, M. and H. Prosch. 1975. Meaning. Chicago: University of Chicago Press.

Popper, K. 1968. The Logic of Scientific Discovery. New York: Harper & Row.

Schwartz, R. 1974. Psychiatry's drift away from medicine. American Journal of Psychiatry 131:129-134.

Szasz, T. S. 1961. The Myth of Mental Illness. New York: Harper & Row.

Torrey, E. F. 1975. The Death of Psychiatry. Baltimore: Penguin Books.

Whitehead, A. N. 1924. The Function of Reason. Boston: Beacon Press.

Wing, J. K., J. L. Birley, J. E. Cooper, P. Graham, and A. Isaccs. 1967. Reliability of a procedure for measuring and classifying the "present psychiatric state." British Journal of Psychiatry 113:499-515.

Wolpe, J. 1973. The Practice of Behavior Therapy. New York: Pergamon Press.

Yap, P. M. 1974. Comparative Psychiatry. Toronto: University of Toronto Press.

PART I

ISSUES THAT REQUIRE CLARIFICATION AND RECONCEPTUALIZATION IN THE FIELDS OF PSYCHIATRY

ACUTE PSYCHOSIS
Attempts at Clarification

Theo C. Manschreck, M.D.

INTRODUCTION

One of the most puzzling and curious practices of psychiatric clinicians is the unthoughtful diagnosis of states of acute psychosis. I find the practice puzzling because acute psychosis is one of the most complex diagnostic problems. I find it curious because the facility with which the diagnosis is usually made belies the complexity. From my own observations, such peremptory diagnosis may have several unfortunate consequences:

1. The diagnosis is frequently wrong, even when the clinical condition is clearly a psychiatric disturbance.
2. As a result, proper treatment and/or management of the patient may be delayed or never achieved; costs consequently mount, and suffering is increased.
3. Particularly when the incorrect diagnosis is schizophrenia, the resulting stigmatization and self-deprecation of the patient and family may be profound.
4. By glossing over the importance of making distinctions and of precisely identifying the clinical presentation, psychiatric thinking remains muddled; and our colleagues in other medical disciplines may justifiably consider us intuitionists, malcontents, and diagnostic nihilists.
5. As commented on by Baldessarini (1975), our capacities to test numerous hypotheses relevant to etiology and treatment of a variety of psychoses have been negatively influenced by "a lack of descriptive and differential diagnostic rigor in psychiatry, particularly in America."

While there has been some change in diagnostic practice in the United States (Baldessarini, 1970), influenced in large part by the development of increasingly effective somatic treatments (phenothiazines, tricyclics, lithium carbonate, and so on), the great majority of patients who present clinically with acute psychosis are rapidly labeled schizophrenic. Several cases seen in the last few years at the Massachusetts General Hospital will illustrate these points.

CASE 1   Mrs. S. B., a 47-year-old divorced Italian woman, part-time seamstress, presented with a three-week history of suspicion and subsequent open expression to family that they were trying to poison her. Stopped eating, withdrew from family contact, isolated herself; except for intermittent outbursts of anger, became virtually mute. Family concern led to psychiatric consultation.

Previous personality   Introverted, quiet, no known psychiatric disorder.

Mental state   Mute, except for expression of delusional material of persecutory quality, no evidence of hallucinations, "waxy flexibility."

Physical state   Evidence of recent weight loss.

Diagnostic impression   "Acute schizophrenia."

Treatment and course   Initially placed on low doses of phenothiazines, followed with trials of antidepressants, psychotherapy. Discharged with some improvement.

Subsequent course   Readmitted three months and again six months after discharge with complete relapse into presenting symptomatology. On exam, found to be underweight again and manifesting profound psychomotor slowing. Treated at second admission with eight ECT treatments leading to some improvement and discharge. At third admission, she was treated initially with high doses of chlorpromazine, which led to remission of delusional thinking. For the first time, her condition was viewed as an affective psychosis, and she was started on doxepin 250 mg daily, with subsequent reversal of weight loss and maintenance of remission until two years later when symptoms recurred following four months off medication. This relapse responded rapidly to reinstatement of medication.

CASE 2   Mr. D. F., a 20-year-old white male, unemployed. Presented to my service with diagnosis of acute schizophrenia, in transfer from an out-of-state psychiatric hospital. While visiting his mother, previously labeled schizophrenic, who lived separated from the rest of the family, this patient had experienced increasing disorganization of thinking over several weeks, leading to frenetic door-to-door salesmanship, interspersed with proclamations to people on the street that he was the Messiah, and his mother, the Virgin Mary.

Previous history Hospitalization one year previously with diagnosis of acute schizophrenia, based largely on grandiose delusions and "bizarre" behavior involving patient and a neighborhood statue of the Virgin Mary. He was found by police lying in the arms of the statue. He had been treated with chlorpromazine in high doses and discharged improved within a month, only to lapse into severe depression one month later.

Mental state Verbose, rapid speech with flight of ideas. Delusions of being Jesus Christ. No formal thought disorder.

Physical exam No abnormalities discovered.

Treatment and course Responded well to haloperidol and lithium carbonate (900 mg daily). For the first time, the diagnosis of manic depressive psychosis was entertained.

Subsequent course Psychosis developed six months after discharge, following discontinuation of medications. Patient refused to take lithium subsequently, did well for six months, then experienced minor relapse not requiring hospitalization. This he treated successfully with haloperidol; he decided then to begin lithium regularly. Functioning well in group psychotherapy setting since then.

CASE 3 Mrs. D. J., a 37-year-old white woman, employed intermittently, and mother of a retarded 2-year-old son. Presented in acute crisis related to personal losses and threat of loss of son to state children's agency.

Previous personality and history Judged previously to be "schizoid" or "inadequate personality" during state hospital admission for overdose of diazepam. Given the diagnosis "acute schizophrenia," for reasons of "flattened affect, poverty of thought production."

Mental state Tremulous, tearful woman. Speech usually slowed, with occasional push of speech. Thinking: slow progression, occasionally pressured, and self-possessed, without formal or content disorder. No evidence of suicidal ideation or hallucination.

Physical state Without weight loss; mild diaphoresis, increased pulse, respiratory rate.

Treatment and course Further investigations into intellectual functioning led to finding that the patient operated with a borderline retarded IQ. Historical information from family, school, and work records revealed consistently poor performance. Patient was felt to be suffering from acute anxiety symptoms related to specific precipitating events. She was treated with diazepam and supportive psychotherapy and discharged in several weeks.

Subsequent course No evidence of psychotic symptoms or signs for more than three years. There was one episode of personal crisis that resulted in a mild overdose of diazepam.

Note that in each case the diagnosis of acute psychosis was schizophrenia, and this decision was later shown to be wrong. In Case 3, for instance, there was even poor documentation for the impression of acute psychosis. As a result, treatment that led eventually to successful control of symptoms was delayed. Obviously, these patients received less than optimal care, costs were consequently high, and suffering—both personal and familial—was unduly prolonged. The quality of clinical thinking that concluded with the initial diagnosis of schizophrenia is appalling. Clearly, also, such lack of rigor undermines the potential for successful research on important etiologic and therapeutic questions. These and similar experiences lead inevitably to distrust and at best skepticism for clinical psychiatric diagnosis.

Indeed, there is a great deal of evidence beyond personal experience to reinforce this skepticism. Baldessarini's study (1970) of the changes in diagnostic practice in affective disorder shows vividly the shifting sand quality of diagnostic bedrock in our field. His findings strongly suggest that the availability of new and effective forms of treatment may bias the observer in the difficult problem of differential diagnosis. The frequencies of schizophrenic versus affective psychosis from 1944 to 1968, as diagnosed in a university psychiatric clinic, revealed abrupt increases in the rate of schizophrenic diagnosis in the beginning of the phenothiazine treatment era and a sharp increase in the rate of affective psychosis diagnosis in the subsequent era of lithium treatment. Furthermore, as one group of diagnoses increased, the other decreased.

In 1959, Pasamanick and his co-workers reported a little-publicized study of diagnostic practice in three comparable wards in a university teaching hospital. Despite closely matched populations of patients, the study revealed very different diagnostic statistics on these wards. The study shows that differences in diagnostic assignment reflected clinician bias, which differed according to the school of psychiatric theory to which the clinician belonged. Analytically trained psychiatrists tended to diagnose fewer cases of schizophrenia and more characterological and psychoneurotic cases. More organically oriented psychiatrists tended toward the reverse. Were diagnoses of no real importance, such findings would not be worth mentioning except perhaps in a pedantic debate, but the fact is that the diagnoses had significant consequences. They were related to length of hospitalization, type of treatment afforded the patient, including drugs, convulsive treatment, and psychotherapy. Clearly, diagnosis has profound implications. And as Pasamanick emphasizes, "Despite protestations that their point of reference is always the individual patient, clinicians in fact may be so committed to a particular psychiatric school of thought that the patient's diagnosis and treatment [are] largely predetermined" (Pasamanick et al., 1959).

A series of promising and significant contributions to the study of diagnosis in psychiatry has resulted from collaborative American-British (New York-London) diagnostic projects (Professional Staff, 1974; Sandifer et al., 1969). These studies have shed light on diagnostic practice and have helped isolate the reasons for differences across the Atlantic. Their findings strongly suggest that training, definition for psychopathological phenomena, the threshold for the recognition of psychopathology, and the concepts of various disorders in psychiatry—all have influence in this problematic area (Cooper et al. 1972).

Rosenhan's now famous experiment (1973a) in which he and several others obtained admission to twelve different psychiatric hospitals by feigning a history of auditory hallucination while otherwise behaving normally points to similar diagnostic shortcomings. Seven of eight experimental "pseudopatients" received the diagnosis "schizophrenia" both on admission and discharge. The fact that not one psychiatric diagnostician nor any managing psychiatrist appeared concerned enough to learn whether the single-symptom complaint of hallucination possibly reflected a reversible and treatable organic disease is, frankly, embarrassing. The fact that nine of the twelve hospitals, where these unfortunate events occurred, had approved psychiatric residency training programs is also disturbing (Rosenhan, 1973b).

The cases presented above, which are representative of many others, as well as the studies cited, indicate the kinds of difficulties that result from present practice. Yet psychiatry has been slow to recognize these difficulties and to combat them with specific interventions. Distrust and skepticism for diagnosis have been a reasonable result of past sins; the need for reform in accordance with rational and scientific approaches has become a clear mandate.

The kind of thinking that operates in the psychiatric diagnosis of acute psychosis—and particularly differential diagnosis—is, in fact, an appalling combination of "professional" folklore and carelessness. All of us, inside and outside of psychiatry, suffer from the results; clearly, something should be done to alter this situation. Yet the problems of diagnosis and differential diagnosis of acute psychosis are complex. Over the years, leading thinkers in clinical, research, and theoretical psychiatry have developed a variety of solutions, often contradictory ones, and consequently compounded the confusion. Thus, each generation of young psychiatrists inherits at best an amalgam of principles and conceptual approaches woefully inadequate to meet the task of distinguishing these most serious psychiatric disturbances.

This chapter is an attempt to provide a new perspective on this problem. I wish, first, to describe succinctly the general problems in the diagnosis of acute psychosis; second, to understand some of their origins; third, to break new ground with a clarification and modification of the concept of disease entity in psychiatry; and, finally, to suggest a set of proposals that provide a schema for approaching diagnosis and differential diagnosis anew. These proposals, I hope, will also serve as a logical starting point to indicate potential research needs.

GENERAL PROBLEMS IN THE DIAGNOSIS
OF ACUTE PSYCHOSIS

Problem 1 Acute psychosis in the absence of readily identifiable coarse brain disease tends to be diagnosed as schizophrenia. At the extreme, acute psychosis has become synonymous with acute schizophrenia and psychotic symptoms and signs have become synonymous with schizophrenic ones.

This problem refers most particularly to the American experience, for which cases discussed in the introduction are illustrative. There has been "the tendency to label as 'schizophrenia' almost any serious mental or behavioral disorder with a fairly clear sensorium and lacking depression as the most striking feature" (Baldessarini, 1975). Indeed, in part, this practice must be attributed to the erroneous clinical impression that affective psychoses are relatively uncommon. But perhaps more central to the issue are the facts that although the *Diagnostic and Statistical Manual II* of the American Psychiatric Association (APA) lists other forms (but does not specify their characteristics), psychiatric practice in the United States recognizes only two kinds of psychotic disturbance in the so-called "functional" group of psychotic illnesses; and the criteria for their diagnosis are vague and too broadly defined. For example, the relevant description of schizophrenia:

295.4 Acute Schizophrenic Episode

This diagnosis does not apply to acute episodes of schizophrenic disorders described elsewhere. This condition is distinguished by the acute onset of schizophrenic symptoms, often associated with confusion, perplexity, ideas of reference, emotional turmoil, dreamlike dissociation, and excitement, depression and fear. The acute onset distinguishes this condition from simple schizophrenia. In time these patients may take on the characteristics of catatonic, hebephrenic, or paranoid schizophrenia, in which case their diagnosis should be changed accordingly. In many cases the patient recovers within weeks, but sometimes his disorganization becomes progressive. More frequently remission is followed by recurrence. (In DSM-I this condition was listed as "Schizophrenic, acute undifferentiated type.") (APA, 1968)

Other factors contributing to this problem would include the well-known effect that knowledge of effective treatment interventions has in biasing clinical diagnostic judgment, as discussed above. Toxic states, particularly secondary to alcohol and amphetamine, are frequently diagnosed as "acute schizophrenia." Patients suffering from these disturbances often cannot provide important historical information because of gross disorganization or confusion in thinking. In an effort to appear decisive, and guided by the experience that patients with similar symptoms have responded well to antipsychotic medications, clinicians may well make a premature diagnosis. Naturally, the results can be devastating.

Thus, in the extreme, this tendency to diagnose schizophrenia fosters clinical practice in which the concepts of acute psychosis and schizophrenia have become synonymous. Examples have been reported by Abrams et al. (1974), who noted that 50 percent of patients who satisfied research criteria for mania had received prior diagnoses of schizophrenia. These psychiatrists also conducted an investigation into forty-one cases of "paranoid schizophrenia" admitted to an acute treatment unit and found that two of these forty-one satisfied research criteria for schizophrenia, whereas half satisfied research criteria for mania. Certainly, the broad definition of schizophrenia tends to be reflected in and to support a rather inclusive use in diagnosis.

Problem 2 The practice of equating acute psychosis and acute schizophrenia obscures investigations of the former and confuses the "ontological" status of the latter (i.e., is schizophrenia a disease or a syndrome?)

Many psychiatrists consider acute psychosis a general classification of disturbances that subsumes a number of syndromes and diseases. An unfortunate aspect of the present difficulties is that acute psychosis, which, in fact, may be the outcome of a multiplicity of clinical disturbances, has increasingly been ignored as a specific object of research investigation. The readiness with which acute psychosis tends to be diagnosed as "acute schizophrenia" contributes to confusion and the lack of delineation of the entities within this category. This situation, of course, gives rise to questions about our ability to deal with several controversial issues. In European psychiatry, for instance, there is a tradition of distinguishing numerous acute psychoses, among them psychoses in which etiology is considered to be largely psychological, the so-called psychogenic psychoses. Cycloid psychosis represents another kind of disturbance subsumed under acute psychosis that many psychiatrists feel is a valid clinical entity (Fish, 1964; Fish, 1967; Perris, 1974). Another issue is the thorny problem of distinguishing acute atypical mania presentations. Still another is the issue confronting clinicians who must distinguish psychoses associated with medical disease from other psychoses and must do so rather frequently. The diagnosis of patients who suffer from acute losses and develop persistent hallucinations provides a similar headache for practitioners. The use of the term "acute schizophrenia" exemplifies the obscurity that blankets our understanding of acute psychosis. An analogue from medicine would be the practice of labeling all clinical presentations with febrile signs and symptoms as measles. Measles would be the most heterogenous of diseases, and one can imagine the difficulties of providing effective treatment for this "disease" as well as distinguishing other entities if this "diagnosis" had become as unthoughtfully used as "acute schizophrenia."

Furthermore, critical questions arise regarding whether acute schizophrenia is a disease, a syndrome, or both. Originally posited as a disease by figures such as Kraepelin and Bleuler, the constellation of signs and symptoms, known as dementia praecox and later schizophrenia, is seen in other clinical entities with known etiology. By not defining clearly what does and does not constitute acute schizophrenia, and by not differentiating carefully those conditions that might mimic acute schizophrenia, clinical psychiatry obscures the question of what schizophrenia is. In short, carelessly diagnosing acute schizophrenia in cases of acute psychosis inevitably increases the variety of clinical pictures to which that term applies. This leads to hodge-podge groupings. And acute schizophrenia becomes a vaguer and vaguer concept. Psychiatrists for the most part would argue for a distinct grouping of schizophrenia, but actual practice undermines the likelihood of careful definition of that distinctiveness.

Paralleling the difficulties produced by the breadth of the concept of schizophrenia and the obscurity it bestows on the discovery and understanding of clinically similar conditions is the fundamental lack of agreement on what constitutes the more general concept of psychosis—how do we define this clinical term? One of the most unrewarding enterprises in psychiatry is to look for a common meaning for psychosis. The varieties of meanings that find use in clinical settings is legion and most disturbing. One hears colleagues claiming that patients "look psychotic" because of "bizarre behavior," that patients manifesting anxiety and/or extreme agitation are "acting psychotic." As confusing as these very unacceptable and vague interpretations is the labeling of the suicidal patient as psychotic, a practice still in vogue among some psychiatrists. These comments and labels are in fact nothing more than interpretations. They are interpretations based primarily on custom and the prevalent lack of descriptive precision in clinical observation. They allow clinicians to soft-pedal clarity, for the sake of appearing sophisticated. They help create a sense of knowledge, where in fact no such knowledge exists. Psychosis is an inferential concept; that is, one infers from clinical observation data that psychosis is present. Clearly, the data base for any inference will have tremendous bearing on its validity. In most cases, when one asks for the data base for such an inference, the answers are disappointing. Instead of an explicit inference, there is all too often an implicit or tacit use of knowledge. If, as psychiatrists, we hope to clarify the meanings of schizophrenia and psychosis and to develop valid knowledge about them, including the ability to answer the questions we have raised about acute psychosis, then present practice must cease and a more thoughtful approach must develop.

Problem 3 The diagnosis of acute or chronic schizophrenia tends to be very unreliable.

Though the definition and the use of the term "acute schizophrenia" are broad, there is a remarkable lack of agreement in its application to a given case. There are at least three reasons for this low reliability. First, there is the problem of theoretical orientation. Pasamanick et al.'s study (1959) strongly implied that the different diagnostic practices among psychiatrists arise not from different patient populations, but rather from the bias and orientation of the diagnosing physicians. Diagnosis, insofar as it rests on individual observation, is at core a subjective activity (Polanyi and Prosch, 1975). Yet there are ways to limit this subjectivity, as we will discuss.

A second reason is the psychiatric nomenclature. Ward et al.'s studies (1962) on psychiatric diagnosis showed that the reasons for the lack of reliability of diagnoses made by two psychiatrists rested 62.5 percent on the inadequacy of the nosology, in requiring impractically fine distinctions and providing unclear criteria. According to Spitzer et al. (1975a), this source of unreliability may be called a "criterion variance;" it is the largest source of unreliability.

Closely tied to these reasons is the third, namely, obscurantism. Diagnoses, after all, don't mean too much, so why bother? This feature of current psychiatric thinking derives, I feel, from the facile acceptance of certain axioms, such as psychosis represents a "normal response" to environmental stress. In some cases (compare below), this opinion may reflect what actually happens, but to generalize from it to all psychosis leads to neglect in the careful appreciation of clinical symptomatology. Why do some clinicians hold this view? They do so because the practical intervention for a given case is assumed to lie in the psychological realm through the achievement of the goals of insight, strengthening of useful defense mechanisms, and adaptation. If "functional psychosis" is merely poor adaptation, then the need for precise observations of the clinical picture is lessened and high standards for diagnosis and differential diagnosis are only of academic (i.e., pedantic) interest. The very fact that various treatments have become so undeniably successful in dealing with severe psychiatric disturbances destroys this argument. In the face of such practical advantages to dissecting clinical phenomena carefully, I find it unconscionable that psychiatrists have not moved beyond old teachings.

Problem 4 Given that the diagnosis of acute psychosis is itself problematic, in part because the concepts of schizophrenia and psychosis are vague, it follows that differential diagnosis has become a hopelessly complex exercise and a process without clear standards.

Precisely because the concepts of schizophrenia and psychosis are not clearly defined, their usefulness in diagnosis is seriously in question. When used to describe a patient's malady, they impart none of the usual pieces of information important to clinicians: (1) what to do in terms of treatment, (2) what complications the patient may expect, (3) what prognosis is likely. A psychiatrist would be acting irresponsibly if he or she attempted to develop treatment and inform about complications and prognosis solely on the basis of information such as: "The patient is psychotic," or "The patient is acutely schizophrenic." Consider an analogous situation in medicine. Confronted with the report of a diagnosis of myocardial infarction, an internist would first see the patient and then determine clinical treatment procedure. Interest would focus on degree of cardiac failure, concomitant disease, respiratory difficulty, presence of arrhythmia, and electrocardiographic changes. The difference between the situation in medicine and that in psychiatry is that the basis for saying a patient has a myocardial infarction (i.e., clinical presentation, confirmed by electrocardiography and enzyme studies) is much clearer than the basis for saying a patient has acute schizophrenia. The internist may then proceed more confidently than his psychiatric colleague to develop the relevant clinical formulation. The likelihood for error is greater in the second case, precisely because the data base from which the inference, schizophrenia, is drawn does not contain an independent validating criterion. For schizophrenia there is no such validating independent criterion, and the diagnosis must rely entirely on clinical, historical, and examination data. As the data are derived from individual observations, where there is a high potential for subjectivity, the likelihood of error is increased. Indeed, given the different theoretical schools in psychiatry, the data base may differ from clinician to clinician according to the theoretical conceptions used to determine what the facts are; diagnosis then becomes a self-fulfilling prophecy.

Clearly, if it is difficult to define the clinical presentation of psychiatric disturbance, the possibility of differential diagnosis diminishes. Differential diagnosis requires the clearest observations and knowledge. Without these, it will fail to be a viable component of clinical evaluation. How do clinicians, for example, distinguish the toxic deliria, mania, temporal lobe epilepsy, and schizophrenia? What standard or logical approach lies behind their diagnostic efforts? Since the diagnosis of acute psychosis is generally performed in a peremptory manner, these questions are often bypassed or not considered. The difficulties in the whole process of diagnosis, therefore, contribute to the meaninglessness of differential diagnosis.

There are several conclusions that can be drawn from the analysis of these problems. First, given that psychiatry is not a charlatan's field, it follows that the present state of affairs does not imply the presence of an evil conspiracy to obscure our understanding of acute psychosis, but rather is a consequence of psychiatry's past. The contemporary picture reflects profound traditional and historical influences. Psychiatry grew out of medicine, but with an object of interest not so clearly defined, namely, diseases of behavior. Second, there can be no doubt that these problems pose an unavoidable challenge to progress in the characterization of psychosis. Despite their imposing significance, no viable solutions have been put forward to resolve them fully. Third, one concludes that any approach to their solution involves three related areas of conceptualization in psychiatry: (1) disease entity, (2) psychosis, and (3) diagnosis. In the following sections, I will attempt to describe the historical attempt to grapple with these concepts and highlight contemporary approaches as well. By this means, I believe, another dimension in understanding the nature of the issues will become clear. Fourth, these problems point beyond themselves to a deeper issue, the relationship of psychiatry to medicine, and the meaning of this relationship to psychiatry in terms of values, methodology, and knowledge. In order to propose a solution to the general problems in the diagnosis of acute psychosis, we must address this implicit issue directly.

THE CONCEPT OF DISEASE ENTITY

In the history of psychiatry, disease entity has been an ideal concept that has undergirded a medical model structure for psychopathological investigation. It has been ideal in that few psychiatric disturbances have really fulfilled criteria for disease as developed in other branches of medicine. General paresis of the insane and the psychosis of pellagra we now understand to be a result of particular etiological factors, namely *treponema pallidum* and niacin deficiency, respectively. (Ironically, these disorders, which do fit the disease entity model, are now generally regarded as part of the venue of general medicine and neurology rather than psychiatry.) The nature of schizophrenia, anxiety neurosis, and psychopathy, however, alludes such clear etiological insights. The history of the use of this concept in psychiatry merits attention.

During the eighteenth and early nineteenth centuries, many medical investigators who focused on psychiatric maladies were part of a tradition in which almost all psychopathological entities achieved disease status. Thus, pyromania, delusion, and hallucination all received the designation disease. Prominent neurologists and physicians who might be called neuropsychiatrists today, opposed this view in the mid- to late nineteenth century. This group, among them Carl Wernicke, held that there was only one psychiatric illness, *Einheitspsychose*, or unitary psychosis. All psychiatric disturbances were considered manifestations of this unified disease entity, which began in young adult life with anxiety and depression, progressed to frank psychosis via "furor," and by life's end finally presented in dementia. All these manifestations, in fact, represented only one common disease. This view was the most prominent one when two German physicians presented their revolutionary concepts.

In 1874, Kahlbaum proclaimed that the basic unit of disease in psychiatry was the entire course of illness; the total pictures of psychiatric abnormality constitute distinct diseases. To this profound notion, Kraepelin joined the principle of etiology as the basis for systematic approaches to disease in psychiatry, a view of revolutionary importance in conceptualizing disease throughout medicine in the nineteenth century. Genuine disease entities, according to Kraepelin in 1892 (in Jaspers, 1963), had the following characteristics:

1. similar causes
2. similar basic psychological form
3. similar development and course
4. similar outcome
5. similar cerebral pathology

Kraepelin had thus defined psychiatric disease as more than simply brain disease, but had left it clearly linked to biological etiology. Kraepelin held that by investigation of outcome and the particular form of psychological disturbance in a disease, one could develop means for detection at an early stage. Of crucial significance was the clear mandate to consider the disease entity in its *longitudinal* course (Jaspers, 1963).

A different view was exemplified in the later work of Eugen Bleuler. Bleuler considered the basic units of psychiatric investigation to be constellations of signs and symptoms (symptom complexes or syndromes) which occurred as regular patterns among his patients. In schizophrenia, for example, Bleuler determined the symptom complex to consist of disturbed associations, autism, ambivalence, and incongruous emotional expression. He proceeded to study this complex in depth to discover its psychological nature. This approach, emphasizing *cross-sectional* features of psychiatric disturbance, clearly differed from Kraepelin's (Bleuler, 1950).

Kraepelin's and Bleuler's approaches are reflected in the different compositions of the dementia praecox and schizophrenia groups, respectively. Kraepelin conceived of the former with very narrowly defined criteria and with a poor outcome. Bleuler conceived of the latter through his investigations of psychological deficit, and tending to dismiss outcome as a criterion of definition, he found a group of patients with a different natural history from those of Kraepelin. In fact, Bleuler's groupings are very broad and reminiscent of *Einheitspsychose.*

Kraepelin's investigations resulted in the division into two groups of all those psychoses that could not be explained on the basis of demonstrable cerebral pathology. Thus came into being the concepts of manic depressive psychosis and dementia praecox. Since 1892, Kraepelin's approach has held a dominant influence in Europe. Yet, because there has been a lack of fulfillment of disease entity criteria, particularly in terms of etiology, there has also been a proliferation of other views, such as Bleuler's. Kraepelin's teachings held no particular practical advantage in terms of determining treatment, as specific treatment was not available. Without clear data to support the cerebral etiological criterion, other approaches to etiology could and did develop. Certainly, also, the clinical demand to fit a given case into one of the two categories raised troublesome issues; the fact is that it is often very difficult to distinguish between dementia praecox and manic depressive insanity.

On a more positive note, one could consider the Kraepelinian formulation of disease entity as the basic spur to a tremendous outpouring of research investigation. Clinicians undertook to follow cases and attempted to develop prognostic criteria in dementia praecox. These contributions had tremendous import in an age when knowledge of outcome laid the basis for almost all predictions regarding a given patient. To be able to forecast improvement, possible downhill course, or the likelihood of remission was a formidable triumph. Thus, in this sense, the notion of disease entity provided a valuable orientation for clinicians. The point is, however, that this notion, although powerful, did not unite all psychiatry.

Karl Jaspers (1963) argues that the opposition of the unitary psychosis view versus the discrete disease entities view remains largely unresolved. The latter view has been correct in so far as the idea of disease entities has led to fruitful investigations; yet the former is also correct in that no *real* disease entities à la Kraepelin have been elucidated. Even for general paresis of the insane, Jaspers holds, no consistent psychological form has been determined; furthermore, no one has yet diagnosed with certainty a known somatic disease using only psychological data. Jaspers states his own conviction that the fundamental groupings of Kraepelin have been different from prior classifications in that, with Kraepelin's notion of disease entity, these groupings have provided a useful and productive basis for promoting psychiatric investigation. Jasper's own view represents a harmonizing alternative to the unitary psychosis/disease entity dichotomy: Disease entity has proved to be a powerful concept in psychiatry, and it is not to be abandoned (see also Roth, 1963). It provides an economical, ideal separation of the vast array of psychiatric disturbances, and this is a valid orienting point for clinical work. However, when it becomes rigid, it fails to allow for the richness and complexity of clinical individuality that most clinicians see as the rule, rather than the exception. If this notion of clinical individuality were lost, the concept of disease entity could function to harm rather than to support meaningful clinical progress. We are still at the level of description in psychiatry, and, as Jaspers comments, we should suspend judgment on the question of disease as we carefully attend to collecting rich, unbiased clinical descriptions.

Nothing has dramatically altered the present situation in psychiatry. One can trace fairly clearly the influence of the discrete disease entity viewpoint among those psychiatrists who have held a strong medical orientation. The work of the Washington University group, for example, has had the goal of refinement—through studies of outcome, family transmission, and natural history—of the validity of clinical entities. The World Health Organization International Classification of Diseases (WHO, 1967) has organized an etiology-based classification of psychiatric disturbances. While no group still holds to a unitary psychosis viewpoint, except perhaps the followers of Karl Menninger (Menninger et al., 1963), its influence can be found in at least two places. First, there is the tradition in psychiatry that views psychiatric disturbance not as a disease, but as a reaction to events, characterized by a combination of biological, constitutional, and environmental determinants. This view, held by Adolf Meyer and his students, has had a tremendous impact on American psychiatry, particularly through the efforts of the interpersonalist school of Sullivan. Second, there is the view held by Hans Eysenck and others that psychiatry has two domains, the medical and the behavioral. The former domain includes medical diseases that manifest themselves as psychiatric disturbance; the latter domain includes all other behavior disorders and has as its proper basis psychology. The so-called functional psychoses and neuroses represent disorders of psychological functioning, not discrete disease entities. These disturbances exist on a continuum of severity with normal functioning and are not qualitatively distinguishable from normal. This dimensional view of psychiatric disturbance has prominent advocates who tend to argue that disease distinctions are consequently meaningless (see Strauss, 1973).

From my own reading of the present situation in psychiatry in America, I see widespread confusion concerning the concept of psychiatric disease. The language of clinical psychiatry belies this fact, with its lack of a commonly understood notion of what psychiatric disorder is. One hears the terms "reaction," "malfunctioning," "maladaptation," "disease," "disorder," etc., presumably all used to refer to the same object. Indeed, it is likely that not all that passes for psychiatric disturbance is in fact a disease entity; the problem is that except for the work of a few individuals, psychiatry refuses to deal with this issue explicitly. As a consequence, we continue to toil clinically with an imprecise notion of what a psychiatric disturbance (see section on Diagnosis) is. When we consider that our role is to diagnose and treat psychiatric disturbance, this fundamental shortcoming weakens our effectiveness. And it is a special burden for residents in psychiatric training.

THE CONCEPT OF PSYCHOSIS

The term "psychosis" is considered by many to be a psychiatric albatross. This criticism and concern arise from an understanding of the application of the term in medical and social situations and an appreciation of its many meanings. To the average person, psychosis is indicative of "craziness," "being out of touch," "insanity"; and it conveys a sense of foreboding, fear, mystery, and even frank danger. To the professional, the term appears to have some clinical usefulness, perhaps as a gross distinction about severity of psychiatric disturbance or impairment of social functioning, but it is rarely explicitly defined. Much discussion in the psychiatric literature centers on this concept, particularly in attempts to distinguish it from neurosis, to clarify the legal meaning of sanity, and to relate it to the concept of disease. But at present, we may accurately judge that the term "psychosis" reflects much confusion, and consequently is obscure in meaning.

The sources of this confusion, particularly in professional usage, not to mention the lay definitions, are several. Historically, the term has had numerous definitions; these definitions have reflected implicit theoretical views regarding the nature of what is being described. These thinly veiled, camouflaging, ontological biases contributed to the confusion. Another source of confusion lies in the general way in which terminology in a field changes.

The term "psychosis" was introduced in 1845 by Feuchterleben to refer to the psychological manifestations of mental disorder as opposed to the underlying neurological condition. The illness itself was still called a "neurosis," or nervous disease (Bowman and Rose, 1951). In this era, physicians believed that "mental" illnesses were really organic illnesses, i.e., neurological disorders. Thus, a disease entity viewpoint produced the term. The thrust of this view was directly parallel to clinical medicine, in that the important problems for clinical study were held to be the accumulation of descriptive data, physiological and psychological, about diseases and the development of classifications based on symptomatology. Emil Kraepelin, as discussed earlier, represented the culmination of this viewpoint.

Almost simultaneously, in the late nineteenth century, a somewhat different orientation in psychiatric thought arose, partly in response to the expansion of psychiatric practice to include non-insane sufferers from mental disorder. Prior to this time, the province of psychiatry was somewhat arbitrarily limited to the group of mental patients who were institutionalized. Now, ambulatory patients became a major focus of psychiatric practice. As a result, a legal and social distinction developed as a convenience to differentiate the insanities and the milder forms of disorder, or "psychoses" and "neuroses." Charcot and Bernheim in France influenced the acceptance of this distinction when they established the importance of "ideas" in the development of psychopathology. "Mental causes" became a preoccupying interest; and, as Bowman and Rose (1951) point out, the term "psychoneurosis" was first used in this period.

These attempts to apply scientific method to psychological data in order to work out some purely psychological theory for understanding and treating mental disturbances represented a movement to explain mental phenomena rather than to just describe them. The most influential figures in developing this orientation were Freud and later Meyer.

Freud and Meyer both believed in the importance of the contributions of heredity and constitution to the unfolding of mental illness. However, their emphasis in training and treatment was on the interaction of these influences and environment—the development, actually, of illness—rather than on *specific cause* of illness; this emphasis, they believed, correctly prepared psychiatrists to understand the nature and occurrence of *psychiatric symptoms*. As the basis for his classification, Freud relied on certain concepts about the theoretical structure of the human psyche; thus, for example, the defense neuropsychoses. Meyer proposed to classify reactions on the basis of the extent of involvement of the personality of the patient. Yet, each of these men clearly considered mental illness to be an adaptive response, and each took a developmental, rather than a specific etiological, approach.

In his last written work, *Outline of Psychoanalysis* (1949), Freud stated:

> The neuroses and psychoses are states in which disturbances in the functioning of the [psychical] apparatus come to expression. We have chosen the neuroses as the subject of our study because they alone seem to be accessible to the psychological methods of our approach . . . (One of our principal findings is that) neurosis (unlike infectious diseases, for instance,) has no specific determinants. It would be idle to seek in them for a pathogenic factor . . . . It is *quantitative disharmonies* that must be held responsible for the inadequacies and sufferings of neurotics. The determining cause of all the varying forms of human mental life are to be looked for in the interplay between inherited dispositions and accidental experiences.

Meyer based his classification on the notion that mental disturbances represent adaptive *reactions* of the psychobiological organism and that every such reaction is an understandable result of the psychological development of the individual up to the occurrence of the disturbance (Meyer, 1910).

These views are significantly different from Kraepelin's. The nineteenth-century medical concept of disease is much less evident. Disharmony involving environment and heredity, as reflected in development, forms the focus instead. Psychosis is seen as a "maladjustment at some stage in a psychobiological [Meyer] or psychological [Freud] developmental process" (Bowman and Rose, 1951).

Compounding the confusion generated by the different approaches to psychopathology is the set of difficulties to which all terminologic science tends to be prey. These problems, as Strömgren (1969) points out, create a guaranteed mess. They are: (1) the arbitrary choice of terms (e.g., Feuchterleben's use of psychosis); (2) the influence of common usage (e.g., lay concepts of "craziness"); (3) changes in meaning (e.g., from *Einheitspychose* to the divisions of psychosis by

Kraepelin to the schizophrenic reactions of Meyer); (4) broadening of usage (e.g., the practice of labelling certain amnestic syndromes as Korsakoff's psychosis).

Much of the contemporary confusion surrounding the concept psychosis, then, can be traced to differences reflected in theoretical orientations of those who use the term, and to the natural history of the term itself. But a great deal of the confusion can be traced to the lack of even good attempts to define it at all in the major textbooks. Most psychiatrists tend to refer to several notions as essential when trying to define psychosis: (1) some form of break with reality, (2) some encompassing disturbance of personality, affecting it in every sphere; and unlike neurosis, in which normal functioning continues outside of certain areas of conflict, (3) some disturbed and disordered behavior, and (4) the form of the symptoms (as distinct from the content) is not understandable in the light of information about the patient's previous personality and present circumstances.

Many of these criteria have been used to distinguish neurosis from psychosis. Depending on one's point of view—whether one is a discrete-disease-supporter (the all-or-none position) or the continuum-from-normal-supporter (the more-or-less position)—the term "psychosis" will mean something quite different, even if it is descriptively defined in a similar manner. The former group will usually see little or no connection between previous personality and present psychosis, and the latter will make every effort to see the development of psychosis from previous personality.

The all-or-none position is held by many medically oriented psychiatrists in the United States and Great Britain. The Washington University group is an example. The more-or-less position is held implicitly by many psychodynamically oriented psychiatrists and is a very explicit viewpoint among many psychologists. Those who hold the more-or-less position argue, as we will discuss later, that dimensional approaches to psychosis offer more fruitful rewards clinically and in research than discrete disease approaches (Claridge, 1972; Eysenck, 1956).

DIAGNOSIS

Diagnosis is a central issue in our attempt to find a way out of the problems posed by present-day clinical practice. Diagnosis is such a muddled problem in psychiatry that it will take some effort before we can clarify the issues, much less begin to forge a solution. The following is an attempt in that direction. I begin by defining diagnosis, distinguishing its properties, and suggesting how it may be analyzed for the purposes of research investigation. Then I develop an argument that the diagnostic problems reflected in our present inability to solve the problems of acute psychosis arise from two sources, the nosology itself and the process by which diagnoses are made. I next consider what appears to be required for a scientific practice of diagnosis in psychiatry—the standards we should strive for. Then I discuss contemporary attempts to solve these problems.

Diagnosis refers to:

1. a classification system or nosology
2. the process of deciding which nosological entity is appropriate for a given case
3. and the decision, opinion, or "label" resulting from that process

Probably because it tends to imply treatment and prognosis, the third usage receives the most clinical attention. However, it is the first two usages that are fundamental to our understanding of the diagnostic chaos in contemporary psychiatry. These two, classification and the process of class allocation, have been studied in a number of ways; the verdict of more than thirty years of research in psychiatric diagnosis is that there are embarrassing inadequacies in both that call all diagnostic endeavor into question.

For purposes of research, there are two logically distinct features of diagnosis: the nature of the diagnostic entity and the nature of observation and enumeration. These two features are closely related to the concepts of validity and reliability, respectively. These concepts might be seen as two fundamental properties of diagnosis. Validity refers to the conformity of the diagnosis with reality, or the facts. Reliability refers to the consistency with which patients are diagnosed. Obviously, validity is particularly tied to the classification scheme itself, and reliability is particularly tied to the process of class allocation. Noting this, one can readily envision the kind of research that ensues in attempts to investigate both features.

Having set the stage with the formal properties of diagnosis, we may now consider more carefully the role psychiatric diagnosis plays in the generation of the problems discussed in the introduction to this chapter. I believe this troublesome situation has two sources. The first is the inadequacy of the nosology itself, which arises from the multiple functions of nosology in psychiatry, the haphazard quality of its historical development, and the critical limitations of its most contemporary example, the *Diagnostic and Statistical Manual II* (APA, 1968). The second source is the inadequacy of the process of diagnosis itself, which arises from the nosology, the training, and the orientation of psychiatrists.

The Nosology

All classification systems have a variety of functions. This is particularly true of the classification system in psychiatry. Knowing these functions is useful in two ways. First, this knowledge distinguishes the variety of tasks we require of our nosology, and, second, it enables us to begin the process of improving the nosology by calling attention to inappropriate, contradictory, or unscientific functions. The following is a tentative list of functions:

1. to indicate etiology
2. to predicate rational treatment
3. to indicate prognosis, including complications, and to suggest pathogenesis
4. to aid communication, as a "shorthand" description of behavior for a specialized language
5. to influence social or legal decisions
6. to provide a basis for research investigations
7. to increase the confidence of professionals and the patient

Certainly, one can conceive that all these functions might play a role in the diagnostic scheme of any medical discipline. Yet, although this variety is present in other branches of medicine, in psychiatry it is especially important. The reasons for this are multiple, historical, and complex. Clearly, interest in behavior and its anomalies cannot be restricted to the medical domain; behavior—particularly disordered behavior—affects all aspects of social, cultural, and political life. Thus, it is not surprising that psychiatry might be called on in numerous apparently nonmedical circumstances to lend its expertise (e.g., prediction of violence, certification of sanity) and that its nosology might be enlisted as an aid or reference in them (and even as an instrument of social control). How well psychiatry can handle such assignments is another matter.

Panzetta (1974) suggests that there are three kinds of functions for psychiatric nosology, namely, descriptive, administrative, and interventional. I would add research (although Panzetta tends to include this function in the descriptive and interventional), giving us four kinds. Each of them has had and continues to have considerable influence on our nosology. An awareness of these influences will serve as a basis for elaborating our critique of the nosology.

In the eighteenth and nineteenth centuries, as well as our own, description led to the establishment of numerous psychiatric entities. For example, pyromania, catatonia, hebephrenia, and so forth, were at one time both description and diagnosis. The descriptive orientation in psychiatry also has led to the grouping of psychiatric symptoms into syndromes and, through the efforts of Kraepelin and

Kahlbaum, disease entities. In our own time, a survey of psychiatric nosology reveals the considerable importance description plays in the derivation of diagnostic categories such as the individual personality disorders, the neuroses, and the situational reactions. The performance of the descriptive functions of nosology is fundamental; it provides a basis for communication and study of behaviors of psychiatric interest.

The period of the Enlightenment saw the blossoming of the administrative functions of psychiatric nosology. Insanity, or the loss of reason, became a paramount concern. What is the nature of moral and legal responsibility in the insane sufferer? How should society respond to these people? These complicated questions have continued to be asked, and though the decisions about them have not been inherently diagnostic, they have clearly referred to diagnostic criteria. Today, the administrative functions of nosology are reflected in the issues of involuntary hospitalization, commitment, and even in the change of status of alcohol intoxication from public nuisance or crime to a medical and psychiatric disease.

Though the interventional functions of psychiatric nosology (to predicate treatment) are not well developed, they have experienced an explosive growth over the last few years. Interventional functions relate most clearly to medical concerns, to medicine's therapeutic imperative, the concern for decreasing suffering by prevention, cure, or palliation. Thus, it is not surprising that interventional functions are closely tied to etiological models of psychiatric disturbance. This is not to say that therapeutic interventions are not possible before etiological sophistication has developed in a field. We are increasingly aware of the powerful qualities of even "clearly useless" therapies in the process of providing help. Placebo effects are not to be underestimated. However, with the development of scientific medicine, particularly since Sydenham, has come increasing success in maximizing our therapeutic interventions, even when etiology has not been fully understood. Witness the success of smallpox vaccinations, digitalis preparations, and public health measures against unsanitary living conditions and impure water. What is certain is the fact that intervention, in order to be successful, relies on the scientific ordering of observations. Had the work of Kraepelin and Bleuler not preceded the observations of French researchers in the early 1950s, one might well wonder if the discovery of phenothiazines would have gone unnoticed in terms of its psychiatric intervention potential. We know, for instance, that meadow saffron, which contains colchicine, was used in the ninth century to treat gout; but this effective medicine was unfortunately discarded, probably because no one could adequately test its efficacy (Shapiro, 1959). Psychiatry requires preparation in order to capitalize on discovery and intuition.

The interventional functions of psychiatric nosology are not well developed. Even in general medicine, the diagnosis of appendicitis does not necessarily imply a particular intervention. Yet this diagnosis usually has more interventional consequences than the diagnoses of depression or obsessive neurosis, for example. This comparison suggests the primitive nature of psychiatric nosology. By and large, the interventions available to psychiatry in the eighteenth and nineteenth centuries were palliative: the preservation of physical health, a pleasant environment, a caring group of healers. In this century, we have witnessed the development of numerous treatments—dynamic psychotherapies, somatic treatments, and sociotherapies. The somatic therapies, in particular, have led to increasingly sophisticated interventions. And though the evidence may be somewhat contradictory (Bannister et al., 1964; Kreitman, 1961), diagnosis tends to imply certain treatments in psychiatry.

The research function of psychiatric nosology has long been present. From the first attempts to count cases of mental disturbances, nosological definitions have been the basis for studies comparing normal and disturbed populations. This function is quite useful and important. Research findings are the major challenging force to change nosology. Clear definitions of psychiatric disturbance, even if not entirely valid, are profitable starting points in research. Wrong definitions will be discovered, when tested against the findings of research. But our nosology's present imperfections limit our efforts to find the appropriate information efficiently.

The variety of psychiatric nosological functions has several consequences. First, there has been no consistent, systematic classification based on the needs of any one of these functions, although some attempts were made during the late nineteenth century. Many of these attempts were, in fact, taxonomies, or orderly classifications based on presumptive relationships among psychiatric disturbances. Their lack of utility, as well as their unwieldy complexity, aided their demise. Second, in some fashion and with greater or lesser emphasis, each of these functions has been perpetuated in the contemporary nosology, known as the *Diagnostic and Statistical Manual II* (APA, 1968).

Therefore, it is not startling that the history of nosology in psychiatry has not developed along clear scientific lines, but in response to etiological views, administrative needs, and theoretical concerns that often bias objectivity. Out of the apparent chaos of nineteenth-century nosology, Kraepelin shaped a system of classification based on his concept of disease entities and rooted immovably in an etiological frame of reference. Because of a primary interest in hospitalized patients, the nosology of characterological and neurotic disorders was relatively less well developed in Kraepelin's scheme.

Attempts to delineate these disorders arose largely from other traditions, such as those fostered by Freud and Meyer. In the United States, the 1952 edition of the *Diagnostic and Statistical Manual* (APA, 1952) reflected the influence of Kraepelin, Freud, Meyer, and the concerns of practitioners who in World War II had found a number of prevalent problems not represented in prior nosologies; psychophysiological reactions, traumatic neurosis, etc., thus became recognized officially. On the other hand, the diagnosis of psychogenic psychosis, particularly popular in Scandinavia, found little favor in the United States, because the view that *all* psychosis is in some sense psychogenic in origin has been a theoretical bias in our country.

The result of this historical development is a crisis in diagnosis. *DSM II*, a revision of the 1952 manual, has done little to improve matters. The derivation of nosology from so many traditions and with so many functional concerns has profound implications for the validity of that nosology. Logically, validity may be absent, present in different categories, found in multiple permutations; we simply have no basis in the nosology itself to make a judgment about its validity. Nevertheless, this manual is the official nosology of American psychiatrists. But there are other pertinent criticisms of *DMS II*.

Despite the fact that any nosology in psychiatry begins with an "arbitrary focus," as Panzetta (1974) points out, no such feature is explicit in *DMS II*:

> The important concept to recognize is that the nosologic process begins with a decision about how to define the most general sense of the term disease (or its semantic equivalent). . . . "Decision" is the operational term here. Decision means selecting from alternate possibilities. There is no absolute definition but rather a series of relatively congruent definitions depending on one's focus. . . .
>
> If one studies DSM II one realizes that nowhere is there a definition of "mental disorder," which is the general word used to label the group of disorders to be "nosologized." (Panzetta, 1974)

He concludes that "mental disorder" in *DSM II* comprises those behaviors that have traditionally been considered with that label. The result of this lack of conceptual focus is to produce a nosology that reflects many viewpoints on what constitutes mental disorder and give them each a place. This establishes a kind of empirical nosology, but one for which generalizations that might give order to its separate components are not forthcoming. What do these disorders have in common? As there is no definition, for example, in terms of social norms, psychological symptoms leading to individual pain, disease, etc., we are given no principle on which to judge whether new behaviors should fall within the same categories.

Another problem with *DSM II* received attention in Ward et al.'s study (1962) of the nomenclature, in which it was clear that fine distinctions between neurosis and personality disorder were difficult to make. The degree of anxiety, or its lack, ego syntonicity or ego alien quality of subjective experience of patients so labeled, and the pattern of the disorder seem to be ineffective points of differentiation. This feature of *DSM II* contrasts with the increasing denotative clarity of the specific neurosis or personality disorders. We must note:

> the increasing connotative obscurity as we generalize first to the level of differentiation between "neurosis and personality disorder," and even more [obscurity] as we generalize to the level of "mental disorder." (Panzetta, 1974)

Panzetta's analysis of the conceptual problems inherent in *DSM II* moves on to discuss the lack of "time framing" in this nosology. Acute or chronic, time of onset, mode of onset, transience or durability—these characteristics are for the most part not specified in *DSM II*. As a consequence of this deficit in specification, certain difficulties may arise. Panzetta (1974) points to Shephard's comparison of an initial survey of prevalence of childhood disorders with one taken later that disclosed that much of the behavioral disorder detected in the earlier survey was absent in the second.

DSM II operates from a reductionistic orientation toward human behavior. The seemingly inherent principle in each nosological category is to see that category as derived from "internal factors,"

> be they somatic, dynamic, or habitual. There is no place for a contextual or environmental factor to be seen as operative, except perhaps in the "transient situational disturbances." (Panzetta, 1974)

This latter factor is one of a variety that general systems theorists hold to be significant. Their theoretical stance derives from increasing sophistication in concepts of causality. The linear causality of nineteenth-century physical science has proved increasingly unhelpful in biological science. Biological events, the argument goes, must be conceptualized as being influenced at multiple levels of organization:

> It is no longer sufficient to explain cellular metabolism excessively in terms of intracellular and infracellular events. The context of the organism is as important as the component parts of the organism in understanding the behavior of the organism. (Panzetta, 1974)

In summary, we find significant parallels between the problems of *DSM II* and the problems of psychiatry itself. Specifically, *DSM II* has the following shortcomings:

1. the lack of a clear definition of what constitutes psychiatric disturbance
2. the lack of clear delimiting criteria to separate classes of disorder, such as neurosis and personality disorder
3. the lack of guidelines to determine which diagnosis applies in cases where clinical conditions suggest two different possibilities—which takes precedence? should the two be chosen together?
4. the lack of objective criteria for defining disturbance, including exclusive and inclusive criteria
5. the lack of single model conceptual rigor—e.g., we have mixed together disease, reaction, alcoholism
6. the lack of time framing in the definition of psychiatric disturbances
7. the tendency toward reductionism

At this juncture, the search for viable solutions consumes much interest. There are basically two approaches to a solution: (1) to abandon the old entirely, or (2) to improve the old with radical revision.

For abandonment Among the alternative approaches, if we abandon the old, is to develop a dimensional classification scheme. This type of classification, advocated by Eysenck (1970), Claridge (1972), and Strauss (1973), among others, is a powerful one; it rests on description and measurement, and represents more of a methodological approach than a model. Fundamentally, it is an attempt to identify patterns of behavior whose frequency and uniformity may provide a basis for scientific classification. Although no disease entity concept is implied or assumed, the requirement for clearly defined methods of measurement is.

As opposed to the typing of behavior disturbances, the dimensional approach seeks after the concept of dimension in behavior. Much of its work has been based on factor analytic techniques that have helped carve out a limited number of factors or dimensions that describe an individual's behavior. These include, in Eysenck's work (1970)—neuroticism, introversion, extraversion, and psychoticism. These factors represent continuous dimensions, which extend from normal to severely disturbed; there is no discontinuity in these dimensions to be readily identified as syndromes or diseases. Generally, all individuals have scores on neuroticism and psychoticism factors, further supporting the objection against discrete syndrome identification.

The dimensional approach derives much of its power from a negative assessment of the present adequacy of what may be described as a typological or categorical approach. Specifically, typological systems in psychiatry lack definitive validity to the extent that is common in other branches of medicine. That is, there are few independent sources of validation, such as lab tests, for type diagnoses. Second, there is no definitive evidence for the discontinuity of important psychiatric variables that would buttress the case for discrete groupings. Ratings on the dimensions of psychoticism tend to fall on a bell-shaped curve, for example. Third, there is no definitive evidence for groupings in the distribution of key variables to support a position for real types (Strauss, 1973).

Historically, measurement represents a distinct advance over mere classification. It is in the area of measurement that the power of the dimensional approach has its greatest influence. The ability to quantify promotes precision and research. The ability to single out variables contributing to psychiatric disturbance lends possibility to the search for effective therapy.

What assessment may be made of the dimensional approach?

1. It represents a powerful methodology, based on statistical techniques, that gives it the advantages of measurement, usually seen as representative of a distinct advance over mere classification.

2. It crystallizes the criticism of present-day psychiatric diagnostic practice by its contributions to the precise measurement of behavioral differences and the development of a more scientific classification scheme.

3. It accords with the common observation of continuity of behavioral differences and demonstrates them systematically.

4. It allows the quantitative interrelationships among variables to be precisely acknowledged. It asks, for instance, does a change in A lead to a change in B, rather than, does A cause B?

5. It avoids the necessity of arbitrarily fitting individuals into particular categories, by defining their disturbances precisely through key variables.

Upon more critical appraisal, however, we find that there are several features that tarnish the quality of this potential solution to our diagnostic difficulties.

1. It avoids the disease concept, but would be a potentially meaningless approach if it did not relate its findings to laws derived from the experimental study of behavior. Thus, the dimensional approach must have an implicit theoretical basis. Furthermore, any dimensional model is limited until it fits into a coherent theory of

behavior. Thus, the dimensional approach has, as its name suggests, a quantitative view of behavior differences, the more-or-less viewpoint. By not positing diseases, it does not escape into an agnostic position in the debate about disease because it makes its own ontologic claims.

2. It is reductionistic. By describing individuals on the basis of several psychological dimensions, it does not increase our understanding of the multiple levels of human behavioral organization.

3. Though it tries to place itself within a coherent behavior theory, it does so at the expense of disease concepts, which have aided medical progress. It gets rid of the disease concept and thus ignores one focus for the development of homogeneous groups of psychiatric disturbances. Attempts within the dimensional camp to retain the syndromal groupings by organizing concepts based on segments of various dimensions represent an interest in retaining these important concepts (cf. type factor approach below).

4. The dimensional approach has not yet given us the wherewithal to diagnose organic disturbances that manifest themselves in behavior.

5. The dimensional approach may never be as capable of describing new variables as the typological approach. An example of this notion is the concept of schizophrenia spectrum disorder, which offers one insightful means of ordering genetic inheritance data on schizophrenia. The dimensional approach fails to account for variations in psychopathology in blood relatives of schizophrenics (genetic spectrum concept), and this failure is crucial, since it suggests that the dimensional approach would neither predict nor likely discover such a pattern.

6. By failing to categorize into discrete types, or diseases, the dimensional approach also fails to fulfill what seems to be an important psychological need to achieve a sense of mastery and knowledge, which accompany the bestowal of a name.

7. It is impractical (and perhaps even antitherapeutic, in a medical sense) in that it fails to suggest treatment. Here, it shows its essentially nonmedical origins and purposes.

8. Reasonably successful attempts to validate traditional groupings by statistical techniques and the failure to usefully integrate all symptomatic findings in dimensional assessments as described by Maxwell and others are further reasons why the dimensional view is less effective (Everitt et al., 1971; Maxwell, 1972).

It should also be noted that the statistical approach is not limited to the production of dimensional analyses of behavior. The *type factor* approach utilizes factor analytic techniques as well; it accepts, however, the groupings of psychiatric nosology, then attempts to discover subgroups within them. In doing so, it preserves the advantages of precise measurement, but falls prey to the attack that proceeds against that nosology. Its major difficulty is that it is cumbersome.

For revision One of the most industrious efforts for revision comes from the Washington University Department of Psychiatry. Through careful review of the literature and the initiation of numerous studies designed to determine correlates of syndromal groupings, these investigators have sought to validate the existence of psychiatric entities. The ideal basis for this nosology is disease, in the medical sense. Instead of basing classification upon the "best clinical judgment and experience" of a committee and its consultants, which was the basis for *DSM II*, this group has used clinical description, family studies, and follow-up of the course of illness, to develop diagnostic criteria for fifteen psychiatric illnesses (Feighner et al., 1972). These illnesses represent a refinement of certain diagnostic categories in *DSM II*, based on systematically collected information and exclusive and inclusive criteria; numerous entities from that manual have not been included, however. This exclusion arises not from their lack of reality, but from their lack of validation at this stage. These fifteen groupings are not considered final but are open to revision. The standards for such revision are scientific evidence that demonstrate effectively distinctions among the groups tentatively validated, or the presence of new groupings. These efforts are in accord with the fundamental needs of nosology in clinical medicine (Moriyama, 1960).

In a large study on the psychobiology of depression, the "Feighner criteria" have formed the basis of an expanded version, the so-called *Research Diagnostic Criteria (RDC)* (Spitzer et al., 1975b), which includes a number of other categories and follows the same kind of guidelines as its parent form. While it is true that both sets of diagnostic criteria originated to meet research needs, that is, clear and distinct, homogeneous sample definitions, they have obvious clinical relevance. The original criteria are now used at a number of centers and have been published as a book (Woodruff et al., 1974). Furthermore, the Research Diagnostic Criteria promise to be a lasting contribution in the development of *DSM III* (Spitzer et al., 1975a).

The Process of Diagnosis

The process of deciding which nosological entity best fits a given case is complex. There are three stages in this process: (1) observation, (2) interpretation, and (3) class allocation.

Observation refers to the part of the diagnostic process in which skilled selective perception occurs. It is skilled in that its quality depends on personal experience, expectation, and purpose. It is selective, like all perception, and depends on the vigilance of the observer. Because perception is not total, but focused mainly as a function of factors in the observer, observers operate from their peculiarly subjective standpoints (using tacit or personal knowledge), and when they deal with complex phenomena, the likelihood of disagreement increases.

Interpretation is the translation of the data of observation into the constructs of psychopathology (depersonalization, anxiety, obsession, compulsion, and the like). Central to its operation are clear definitions for such constructs and accurate observation.

Class allocation is the fitting of observed and interpreted data to classes of disease. Rarely, if ever, in actual practice can there be an ideal fit; usually, the fit is within an acceptable range of variance from the standard.

Clearly, there is room for error or other variations in each of these stages. For example, observers may vary in many ways, such as in orientation, training, value attributed to the diagnostic process; hence, their observations may vary. Error may result from plain ignorance. And the same observer may differ from observation to observation. Indeed, several studies focused on this stage of the process have indicated that each of these factors may work against the attainment of reliable observations. Interpretation is a less studied part of the diagnostic process; obviously, the influence of variable definitions of psychopathological constructs contributes to the possibility of variation in observation. Furthermore, the lack of ideal fits between observed, interpreted data and classes of disease suggests the potential for a further type of variability, which in fact occurs. Numerous studies document the lack of reliability (interjudge disagreement, dissimilarity in diagnostic labeling frequencies, and the instability of clinical diagnosis over time). These studies will not be reviewed here; however, the results of these studies indicate the following conclusions:

1. Observer variation is due in large part to training and orientation, (Thorndike, 1920; Newcomb, 1931; Grinker et al., 1961; Kendall, 1968).

2. There is a lack of a common language for psychopathology, both in terms of description of abnormal behavior and the meaning of various diagnostic labels (Cooper et al., 1972).

3. The error due to patient variation is minimal (Ward et al., 1962).

4. Stability and frequency of diagnosis as means for studying reliability are indirect measures and less useful than looking directly at interjudge agreement (Spitzer and Fleiss, 1974).

5. When given similar definitions for psychopathological behaviors, clinicians improve their agreement on observation (Spitzer and Fleiss, 1974).

6. Agreement is even more likely if systematic interviewing schedules are employed that limit the range of observations to direct observations instead of interpretive ones (i.e., unconscious conflicts, repression, etc.) (Saghir, 1971).

7. Diagnostic agreement suffers when the criteria for placing a clinical state in one category as opposed to another category are not made explicit. Criteria for exclusion and inclusion obviate this difficulty (Ward et al., 1962; Spitzer et al., 1975a).

The implications of these conclusions are straightforward. In fact, attempts to implement standardized techniques for assessing psychiatric patients are under way, with evidence strongly suggesting that diagnostic reliability can be markedly improved. These techniques provide for a sequence of topic coverage in interviews and reduce to a minimum the variability among clinicians in the conduct of interviews. For ratings of psychopathology, these structured interview schedules explicitly define behaviors to be rated, instead of relying on the variable meanings technical terms hold for different clinicians (Spitzer and Fleiss, 1974; Spitzer et al., 1975a).

To summarize, the problems of diagnosis derive from the nosology, or system of classification, how it is organized and defined; and the process of diagnosis itself, which reflects attempts to apply the nosology in the clinical setting. Each of these aspects has been explored in an effort to learn ways to improve on present practice. Some critics argue for abandonment of the present classificatory approach and the substitution of a dimensional one. Specific approaches to nosology improvement include the St. Louis "Feighner" criteria and the Research Diagnostic Criteria. For the improvement of diagnostic process, systematic attempts include a variety of structured interviews (i.e., Schedule for Affective Disorders and Schizophrenia (SADS) and the Present State Examination) that capitalize on operational definitions of observable behavior and organize the scope of clinically derived data.

The implications for clinical training are clear. Psychiatry needs to renew its involvement in psychopathology by teaching it, standardizing its definitions, and, by so doing, ensuring greater reliability among its future clinicians. The mandate for learning the correlates of the defined nosological entities (or the investigation of validity) is also evident.

CLARIFICATION AND MODIFICATION OF THE CONCEPT OF DISEASE

In this analysis of historical and contemporary understandings of disease, psychosis, and diagnosis in psychiatry, there are several key conclusions. First, the complexities of the three concepts preclude simple solutions for the problems of differential diagnosis of acute psychosis. Second, for a variety of reasons, psychiatry has paid more attention to the concept of diagnosis than to the concepts of disease and psychosis, perhaps owing to the fact that diagnosis is an observable, and often required clinical process, not merely a heuristic concept. As a result of this attention, much of the confusion that arises from different orientations, training, and other forms of bias may be reduced in the future. Third, disease and psychosis have not received careful examination as concepts, despite their centrality to the issues of psychiatric practice. (See also Chapter 3 in this volume for discussion of the concepts of illness and deviance from a social scientific perspective.)

In this section, I will deal with the classic Kraepelinian concept of disease entity, in the hope of securing both a clarification and a modification of its meaning that will fit more reasonably the needs of contemporary psychiatric practice. In the next section, I will deal with the concept of psychosis and the requirements for clarification in its use.

This chapter began with the concern that psychiatrists continue to commit serious errors in the facile diagnosis of acute psychosis. I believe this unfortunate practice derives partly from implicit theoretical stances about what psychiatric disturbances are. These stances conceptualize psychiatric disturbances from an orientation different from that of disease. As a result, disease classification becomes, at best, an uninteresting administrative need and, at worst, an unuseful clinical burden. The major schools with orientations that deemphasize the disease concept have been discussed. They include the Meyerians, the psychodynamicists, the interpersonalists and sociotherapists, and the existential groups. Not all psychiatrists within these groups share this ideology, but if they do not, it is likely they have moved away from the mainstream teachings of their school's viewpoint. There are several reasons that help us to understand why these implicit theoretical orientations are maintained:

1. The disease concept implies a certain kind of etiology of psychiatric disturbance (and for Kraepelin this was a clearly biological causality), whereas these schools view other causes as fundamental.

2. The disease concept dehumanizes the individual (a patient's freedom is lost in the mechanistic explanations of disease), say the existentialists.

3. The disease concept tends to lead to the extrication of certain behaviors for treatment (and thus does not deal with the whole person) and deemphasizes the role of crucial environmental and psychological influences (Sullivan, 1931).

4. The disease concept can shackle us unnecessarily by requiring that all cases be fitted into categories, when clinicians see the atypical case as the rule in their practice.

Unfortunately, those who hold these important views have not been able to offer anything that would satisfactorily substitute for the disease concept, particularly in relation to diagnosis. Through the years, the weight of evidence, in effective treatment, in predictions, and even in prevention, has avalanched behind the concept of disease as a valid orienting point in clinical psychiatry; so the idea of throwing this concept away to please those with other views is incredibly shortsighted. Furthermore, one might argue that the implicit disavowal of the disease concept partially accounts for the difficulties in differential diagnosis of acute psychosis. Because of its practical value, clarity in clinical thinking is a mainstay of the disease concept approach in medicine and psychiatry. In practice, the adherents of other views have been less interested in clear clinical descriptions and in making explicit the grounds for treatment decisions. No, the disease concept in psychiatry is here to stay for many reasons. The confusion surrounding it, however, deserves clarification.

Disease entity is a convention, an abstraction, that allows us to order clinical phenomena in meaningful ways. It is "an arbitrary focus" as Panzetta (1974) suggested, for developing a nosology. By introducing such a concept into psychiatry, Kraepelin did not give us the final word on the controversy as to whether there are discrete disease entities. But he did provide us with an approach to organize clinical thinking and develop scientific knowledge, and this is clearly a reflection of the methodology of psychiatry's mother discipline, clinical medicine. As Jaspers (1963) has pointed out, the disease concept represents an ideal formulation of psychiatric disturbance, which may never be reached. Its value lies in the productive research it has motivated, its pragmatic orientation toward treatment and prediction, and its ability to order clinical disturbances in a consistent manner. In considering the issue of whether diseases exist, or whether there are merely quantitative deviations (more or less) from normal in our clinical material, we must conclude that the answers to this controversy are not available. Either or both positions may be right. Both merely represent logical approaches to psychiatric disturbance.

More central to our present concern is the fact that although the qualitative (all-or-none) disease entity position is more in keeping with Kraepelinian formulation, we need not accept Kraepelin's preconceptions about cause in order to reap the benefits of the disease concept as an orienting point in clinical research and practice. The basis for this conclusion is the realization that the core difficulty with the disease entity concept is the notion of causality. The vast majority of psychiatric disturbances at this time have unknown causes. However, the rest of the disease concept provides us with a valuable and realistic means for organizing clinical data and developing research strategies. Etiological investigations probably will remain a central focus for psychiatric research; and biological etiology will continue to be the hypothetical basis for our nosology, but this too will only be an ideal.

Regardless of one's beliefs about etiology, the disease concept has given and can continue to give us the means to order clinical psychopathology in meaningful (homogeneous) groupings, an absolutely crucial feature for diagnosis. The homogeneity that we as psychiatrists discern in the array of disturbances we come into contact with provides several important results. First, it sorts out clinical phenomena for comparative purposes so we may investigate natural history, treatment response, complications, family studies, environmental and other correlates. Second, it provides the bases for meaningful examinations of etiological hypotheses, regardless of biological import. Third, it provides the basis for meaningful interventions for both prevention and mitigation of clinical symptomatology. Although it is a virus, for instance, that is responsible for a certain hepatitis, the most effective intervention in terms of altering the process of disease may be to prevent transfusions of blood from hepatitis victims to the uninfected, or to encourage the careful destruction of needles used in caring for hepatitis victims. Before we understood the "etiology" of scurvy, observations had suggested that citrus fruits in the diet might well prevent its occurrence. The salient causes, the ones over which we may have some influence, may not be looked at unless we develop methods to anticipate them (Leighton, 1967). Fourth, all of these possibilities suggest means by which our total understanding of psychiatric disturbance is enhanced and consequently our total understanding of the individual patient.

In short, the difficulty of using the disease concept in psychiatry lies in the confusion that arises in not recognizing that disease entity is an explanatory model, not a thing. Disease is a concept with explanatory power that provides us with the means to organize our understanding of the relationships between various factors. Science proceeds by generating theoretical models, deducing their observable consequences, and then testing them. The confusion has been that all too often we have confused the concept of disease with a rigid notion of what reality is and what constitutes causes (i.e., biological events), such that diseases have become things (Engelhardt, 1974). The danger in reification is that we lose sight of the bountiful possibilities of such an explanatory model. And this is where I find fault with the contrary viewpoints that have dominated psychiatric thinking in America.

Granted that the disease concept organizes our knowledge in certain directions and that it has some potential for explanatory power in dealing with complex relationships that we investigate in research or clinically, why use this particular model, instead of the dimensional model (the more-or-less, or the quantitative model of behavior disturbance)? This is a far-reaching question, and to answer it, I believe we must examine the differences between medicine and other scientific disciplines. Medicine exists in a context of expectation and value, which is somewhat different from the context of other sciences. At the core of this expectation and value is the notion of health and disease. These concepts are not merely descriptive, but, in fact, normative. As Engelhardt (1974) points out:

> There are no simple, pure facts in medicine, but . . . all facts appear in and are influenced by contexts of expectation and value. . . .
> To engage in medicine is to accept a particular mission to change man, to make him healthy . . . though standards of health are not eternal, culture-free facts. Medicine has a therapeutic imperative.
> A disease concept presupposes judgments concerning natural teleology, what man ought to be, and this influences action.

Thus, we may answer the question in the following manner. First, medicine has a therapeutic imperative; this therapeutic imperative derives from concepts of health and disease, and medicine's relationship to such concepts. With this therapeutic imperative in mind, the goal of psychiatry is to develop knowledge of normality, and understandings of abnormality (disease) that lend themselves to interventions. To meet these goals requires concepts that create the possibility for therapeutic knowledge, not merely knowledge for the sake of knowledge. Thus, the pragmatic emphasis of medicine's concepts is a paramount concern. Pragmatics here relates to the possibility of treatment (to return the patient to the state or status of health), the possibility of prevention (to keep the patient in a state of health), and the possibility of palliation (to reduce suffering by keeping the patient as near a state of health as possible); in psychiatry, as in other branches of medicine, there is a practical value to transmitting a sense of understanding to the patient as well (to reduce suffering through reducing uncertainty about the state of disease). This practice has been the mainstay of much of psychiatric therapy. The genius of the disease concept is that it allows for these pragmatic interventions at each level of its development in dealing with disturbance:

1. We observe the collection of signs and symptoms and discover their relation in patterns. If the observer notices that certain maneuvers act beneficially to change these phenomena, he comes into possession of an empirical therapy. Note that he is ignorant of both the cause of the pattern and the mode of action of the therapy. Further, these observations can be named and identified in the future for the purpose of prediction.

2. We isolate a cause for the pattern; Engelhardt (1974) refers to this as the "provision of an etiological matrix." Predictions about the syndrome can now be made with reference to the laws governing the particular mode of etiology. Clinical disease entities become pathological disease entities.

3. We perform a pattern-relation analysis, in which the pattern of variables is organized into a model of explanation according to the laws of pathology.

The major reason that the disease concept should be preferred over others is its pragmatic consequences. This, of course, assumes that as psychiatrists we act in accordance with the same therapeutic imperative available in the rest of medicine. The dimensional view at present does not fulfill our pragmatic objectives.

But there are peculiar problems for psychiatry and the disease concept. Jaspers (1963), in pointing out the difficulty of extending the Kraepelinian model of disease entity to all psychiatric disorder, thus indicates the limitation of treating psychiatry as merely a branch of medicine. Kraepelin attempted to provide a basis for distinguishing clinical groupings in psychiatry. His etiological bias is reflected in its first characteristic (similar causes), his biological orientation is seen in the last characteristic (similar cerebral pathology). Unmodified, the disease entity model was and would remain an ideal concept for the majority of psychiatric disorders. Unmodified, it has failed to lead to the discovery of new disease entities in psychiatry, save perhaps pellagrous psychosis and general paresis. One might also criticize it for its assumption that similar outcome reflects a similar entity. A number of diseases can cause the syndrome of dementia. Thus, the unmodified concept has limitations. In addition, we should not push it beyond its present applications, so that each case is rigidly subsumed by one of its categories. Thus, this concept has certain dangers: it may obscure atypicality, new diseases, and important observations, if held too rigidly. Nevertheless, it provides a reasonable point for orientation in empirical investigation. In psychiatry, where anchor points in objective knowledge should be highly valued, the significance of this concept should not be underestimated. But the concept requires modification.

Several improvements are possible that might make this concept more relevant to the therapeutic imperative of medicine, more plausible in dealing with the full range of psychiatric disturbance, and more likely to generate practical research hypotheses. Each of the following modifications might be thought of as an attempt to bring greater validity to the notion of disease entity in terms of present-day theory.

First, in view of the difficulties that beset the notion of cause, this concept might best be modified to "significant etiological variables." Let us willingly surrender the concept of unitary causality, be that biological, developmental, or whatever. Causality in disease has become an increasingly sophisticated concept. Moreover, as medicine has progressed, the notion of unitary cause has come to be more and more simplistic. In fact, to talk of cause is, in many instances, the reification of an ontological concept. Causes are concepts, not things. Causality is a relationship, not a thing. (David Hume might bless our field after all.) As a relationship concept, the notion of cause may lead to fruitful understandings of the development, perpetuation, and progression of disease in psychiatry. If a change in A leads to a change in B, then by knowing this we increase our ability to alter situations therapeutically. The notion of cause *qua* cause is not helpful. In fact, in chronic disease epidemiology, where causality is a most complex notion, it is gingerly translated into concepts of risk, or risk factors. Similar investigations in psychiatry, such as family studies, whether they hypothesize social or hereditary transmission of various traits, herald the beginnings of risk factor determinations.

Second, the term "outcome" is too vague. In chronic disorders, for instance, outcome may reflect a very complex interaction of disease process and external factors; the potential for defining outcome may suffer from the heterogeneity of experiences that develop in the course of illness. If we could reduce the time frame or cover it more effectively, this potential for error might be mitigated. For instance, the study of development, pathogenesis, complications, and course of illness may be nearer the mark on this matter than the study of outcome. By reducing the variability of experience by keeping it within certain defined time frames as a first step, we increase homogeneity of clinical samples (Jones, 1973). Response to treatment may be a feature of the disease process that will further delineate homogeneity of clinical groupings, while supplying another criterion for independent validation of our definitions.

Third, the criterion of similar cerebral pathology may eventually be met as technological advances continue in the delineation of the major psychoses. For the present, however, there is no such known pathology, though there is a strong argument to presume biological pathology in "functional" psychoses because of the mimicry of these psychoses by temporal lobe epilepsy, alcohol hallucinosis, and amphetamine intoxication. For the sake of practical orientation, the criterion may be met by any strong biological correlate. The range of correlates might include a biological marker, a very specific response to treatment, a genetic factor, or a reliable cognitive marker.

The modification of Kraepelin's disease entity concept may prove useful in examining psychiatric disorders, because it clarifies the meaning of disease in psychiatry and because it modifies the rigidity of the old concept to fit new times (see below). This modified concept can be a standard for developing the validity of psychiatric syndromes, because it provides meaningful correlates for their definition. This view will be discussed in the next section. As a practical advance, the modified concept emphasizes the range of practical observations in the development of treatment interventions, thus incorporating the insights of those not wedded to the disease approach. As will be pointed out below, the modified disease concept may serve as a basis for developing a strategy of diagnosis and differential diagnosis in acute psychosis.

Modified Disease Concept

1. similar significant etiological variables
2. similar psychological form (cross-sectional clinical features)
3. similar development, course, and complications (carefully defined natural history)
4. similar pathogenesis
5. similar biological correlates (biological or cognitive markers, genetic characteristics, pathology, treatment response)

So modified, the disease concept becomes a tool for psychiatry, rather than a burden. If the tendency to reify it can be avoided, then many psychiatrists can appreciate its usefulness, regardless of the etiological bias of their school or their roles as clinicians or researchers. It offers a logical clinical starting point, in that any psychiatrist must surely determine if specific diseases account for a clinical presentation. Diseases, once having fulfilled all the features of the model definition, lend us potentially the greatest breadth of interventional (therapeutic) information and understanding. When no known disease accounts for a presentation, clinicians must proceed more carefully, recognizing that the validity of diagnosis (and, consequently, the grounds for their treatment intervention) is less secure. In other words, the modified disease concept anchors clinicians' work in the known and serves as a reference point against which to judge their decisions.

The modified disease concept offers a logical starting point for the researcher as well. At present, there is no other consistent model for approaching the task of distinguishing a biological versus a nonbiological cause than the disease model. In sophisticated disease theory, biology has become a less significant aspect of etiology, although obviously it plays a prominent role in diseases such as arthritis, tuberculosis, and diabetes. By modifying the aspect of biological cause, the model becomes a tool for approaching psychiatric disturbances where biological cause is more nebulous or appears remote (e.g., in personality and neurotic disturbances) with a variety of etiological hypotheses. If research discloses that a particular psychiatric disturbance is not biological in origin, this is, nonetheless, acceptable and appropriate. The standard for arriving at that judgment is incorporated in the modified disease concept. That is, the entity is defined initially by criteria other than etiology that constitute the disease concept; and in working out etiological research, there is no logical reason why variables other than biological ones cannot account significantly for the entity. In other words, the modified disease concept anchors the researcher's work through definitional criteria without preconceiving the cause of any disturbance.

This modification should have several useful consequences. By extending the concept of cause in psychiatric disturbance beyond biology, the Kraepelinian idea is not lost, but becomes an idea less contaminated by rigid preconception. While the implications of present knowledge help motivate this change, other concerns lend energy to it as well. Perhaps this qualification of cause can attract some of those psychiatrists of opposing schools to a common enterprise, the development of meaningful research and knowledge in psychiatry, because this concept of disease does not preclude multiple etiological possibilities. Also, the standards for diagnosis may benefit from the provision of an organizing principle—the next section of this chapter will consider this idea more fully. Further, by reducing the significance of unitary or linear causality through the clarification of important and possibly nonbiological sources of disturbance, the modification can effect an increase in therapeutically important knowledge.

A POSSIBLE SOLUTION TO THE GENERAL PROBLEMS IN THE DIAGNOSIS OF ACUTE PSYCHOSIS

I have emphasized that the current state of confusion in the diagnosis of acute psychosis reflects several problems. These were considered in some detail. I then argued that an understanding of the origin of these problems and the shape of potential solutions rested on three central and related concepts in clinical psychiatry: disease, psychosis, and diagnosis. The discussion of these concepts and the clarification and modification of the concept of disease entity are preliminary to the solution I now propose.

One possible solution to the problems is a set of proposals: hypotheses that establish a formal scheme of diagnosis and differential diagnosis of acute psychosis. Implicit in them are the modified concept of disease discussed above; the requirement for standardization of clinical terminology, observations, and interpretation of psychopathology; and the fundamental necessity for clarity in description and coherent thinking undergirded by precision and rigor. As a group, the proposals provide a basis for two functions, namely, the clinical evaluation of patients and the research strategy for deriving increasing homogeneity in sample populations. The key here is the union of clinical and research interests within the same pragmatically based scheme. By specifying the limits of our knowledge through these proposals, we may begin to develop modes of discovery to extend those limits. By pretending to know when we do not, we foster obscurantism and perpetuate confusion.

The proposals to be presented form an argument, if you will, that incorporates several ideas from the earlier discussion. There are several reasons for this approach. First, I wish to make explicit the nature of the problems and the strategy of the solution. Second, I hope to develop a scheme for diagnosis of acute psychosis that provides standards for verification, and a means for distinguishing among different diagnoses. Third, this approach should help us appreciate the limits of our clinical knowledge, and the possibilities for further discovery.

Proposals

1. In order to approach the problems of diagnosis and differential diagnosis of acute psychosis, certain assumptions that guide our work as psychiatrists must be made explicit. By remaining implicit and often obscure, they serve to perpetuate confusion in clinical practice. These assumptions are:
   a. Psychiatry is a medical specialty.
   b. Medicine exists in a context of value; medicine has a therapeutic imperative. Hence, psychiatry also has this imperative.
   c. Therapeutic refers to (1) prevention, (2) palliation or amelioration, (3) cure. It also means "not to harm" by errors of omission or commission.
   d. Therapeutic knowledge derives from the pragmatic appreciation of relations among variables. To be therapeutic requires that we ascertain knowledge of relations among clinically significant variables and that we be able to recognize when they may be put to use.

2. The process of diagnosis in psychiatry has several implicit features:
   a. The precise characterization of the difficulties encountered by the patient.
   b. A concern for avoiding premature closure with facile diagnostic conclusions; this implies an openness to and responsibility for considering all pertinent possibilities for the clinical presentation.
   c. A recognition that diagnosis is the logical beginning of clinical practice and not the terminal point in describing a patient (Maher, 1970; Jaspers, 1963).
3. Two key problems in the diagnosis of acute psychosis are:
   a. The definition of acute psychosis.
   b. The breadth of the concept of schizophrenia.

Much of the problem of diagnosis in acute psychosis lies in the breadth of the concept of schizophrenia (Fish, 1966). Because clinicians generally equate acute psychosis and schizophrenia, this breadth both obscures what schizophrenia is and prematurely closes the process of clinical differentiation of acute psychosis. We must clarify this situation. *In general, the diagnosis of acute psychosis is the differential diagnosis of a state.*

4. We must distinguish clearly between state and disease in psychiatry. There are many states in psychiatry, but as yet few established diseases. A psychopathological state is defined here as a condition of mind in which behavior is abnormally modified. *Modified* here alerts us to the idea that a psychopathological state is not a normal state. (I choose, because of space considerations, to steer clear of a discussion of how abnormality is determined and defined in a general sense, because I feel there is no obvious and clear way to define abnormality. Much of abnormality is established through the imposition of social and cultural norms on behavior. Suffering or pain in the patient or in those with whom the patient interacts also strikes me as a fundamental, if not an entirely satisfying or comprehensive, feature of such behavior. In a real sense, the definition of such abnormality is arbitrary. We must live with the limitation that we do not possess a clear definition of abnormality and must attempt to develop one. See the discussion of diagnosis in this chapter and also Chapter 3.) A psychopathological state may or may not reflect a disease process. Hence, a psychopathological state may have multiple determinants, including social, biological, and psychological determinants; and it may be defined from these three perspectives as well, namely in terms of deviance, pathology, or maladaptation. It is diagnosed on the basis of clinical observation and description. It is, therefore, defined entirely on the basis of cross-sectional evaluation, that is, at a

point in time. A disease, as we have modified its definition, might at any point in time (cross-section) present as a psychopathological state, but it would not necessarily have to, there being the possibility that some diseases are episodic. The distinction between state and disease has to do with the increasing power of specification and explanation in the diseases; to achieve disease status, there must be such an array of relationships in the clinical phenomena that some form of causality is indicated. Disease thus represents a conceptual and practical advance over state by (1) the development of pattern recognition through longitudinal observation (i.e., over extended periods of time, (2) the multiplication of observed, potentially etiological, relationships, and (3) the development of more specific intervention opportunities. A syndrome, in this scheme, is a collection of signs and symptoms that are seen "running together" in a consistent manner—see (1) above. In terms of usefulness, the syndrome would give us more information toward therapeutic intervention than the delineation of a state, and less information than the delineation of a disease. State, syndrome, and disease, then, are three levels of abstraction in the development of a disease model.

5. Acute psychosis, the psychopathological state, should be operationally defined. That is, we need some observable, objective features by which to define psychosis at this level of the disease model. A corollary idea, given the present confusion that marks the use of the terms "schizophrenia" and "acute psychosis," is to define operationally the concept of schizophrenia. Clearly, schizophrenia is more than a psychopathological state, though (cross-sectionally) it may appear indistinguishable from many acute psychoses. As we do not know of an exclusive causal relationship in it, schizophrenia probably best reflects a nonspecific syndrome. Thus, although schizophrenia may present as an acute psychosis, its diagnosis would require longitudinal correlates. We may attempt a definition of acute psychosis:

Acute psychosis refers to a psychopathological state, and has the following characteristics:

a. By definition, it has a cross-sectional determination.

b. The qualifier, "acute," does not necessarily refer to any specific characteristic, such as rapidity of onset or severity; rather, it applies to any psychosis about which the clinician has no longitudinal information. (This feature, by conceptualizing the clinical state generally, yet as precisely as possible, forces the clinician to investigate the multiple possibilities that might account for the disturbance.)

c. It involves a disturbance (disturbances) in thinking or perception that is (are) inexplicable merely in terms of previous experience, and that is (are) severe enough to distort the patient's appreciation of reality.

d. More precisely, it reflects a disturbance (disturbances) in cognitive functioning revealed by either symptom(s) or sign(s) in attention, perception, thinking as expressed in language, memory, orientation, judgment, and the like.

6. At present, the concept schizophrenia should be reserved to refer to the nuclear or process grouping that has gained the greatest validity through thorough study. The criteria, borrowing from Feighner et al. (1972), are that for the diagnosis of schizophrenia, a through c are required:

a. Both of the following are necessary: (1) a chronic illness with at least six months of symptoms prior to the index evaluation without return to the premorbid level of psychosocial adjustment, (2) absence of a period of depressive or manic symptoms sufficient to qualify for affective disorder or probable affective disorder.

b. The patient must have at least one of the following: (1) delusions or hallucinations without significant perplexity or disorientation associated with them, (2) verbal production that makes communication difficult because of the lack of logical or understandable organization. (In the presence of muteness, the diagnostic decision must be deferred.)

c. At least three of the following manifestations must be present for a diagnosis of definite schizophrenia, and two for a diagnosis of probable schizophrenia: (1) single, (2) poor premorbid social adjustment or work history, (3) family history of schizophrenia, (4) absence of alcoholism or drug abuse within one year of onset of psychosis, (5) onset of illness prior to age 40 (Feighner et al., 1972).

This represents a workable and unconfusing definition of schizophrenia. It is a syndrome, and is defined on the basis of longitudinal criteria (a and c), and on cross-sectional criteria (b). These features of the definition provide a basis for moving from the identification of a state to the identification of a syndrome.

Another, perhaps more workable and unconfusing definition of schizophrenia is the following, taken from the *Research Diagnostic Criteria* (Spitzer et al., 1975b). A through c are required for the episode of illness being considered.

a. At least two of the following are required for a diagnosis of definite schizophrenia and one for a diagnosis of probable schizophrenia:

    (1) Thought broadcasting, insertion or withdrawal.
    (2) Delusions of control, other bizarre delusions, or multiple delusions.
    (3) Delusions other than persecutory or jealousy, lasting at least one week.
    (4) Delusions of any type if accompanied by hallucinations of any type lasting at least one week.
    (5) Auditory hallucinations in which either a voice keeps up a running commentary on the subject's behaviors or thoughts as they occur or two or more voices converse with each other.
    (6) Nonaffective verbal hallucinations spoken to the subject.
    (7) Hallucinations of any type throughout the day for several days or intermittently for at least one month.
    (8) Definite instances of formal thought disorder.
    (9) Obvious catatonic motor behavior.
  b. A period of illness lasting at least two weeks.
  c. At no time during the active period of illness being considered did the subject meet the criteria for either probable or definite manic or depressive syndrome (criteria a and b under Major Depressive or Manic Disorders in this manual) to such a degree that it was a prominent part of the illness (Spitzer et al., 1975b).

This definition has the additional advantage of a shorter (though controversial) time frame (i.e., two weeks). Thus, diagnosis may be concluded earlier. It also obviates the difficulties that features in part c of the Feighner criteria provide as possible confounding characteristics of the syndrome, namely, such features as "single" and "poor premorbid social adjustment or work history," which may be the result of social and cultural influences independent both logically and psychiatrically from schizophrenia.

7. The terms "schizophreniform," "schizoaffective," "oneirophrenic," etc., refer to acute psychoses that have cross-sectional characteristics similar to schizophrenia, but that are presumed to have different courses. As nothing but confusion is added by these terms (i.e., they are usually defined with reference to schizophrenia, which has had multiple and often contradictory definitions), I feel they should be abandoned, particularly when developing diagnoses of acute psychotic states. If schizophrenia cannot be diagnosed in these situations without meeting the requirement for longitudinal correlates, these terms certainly cannot be used to diagnose such states at this time either (Bannister, 1968).
8. Among all the psychoses, those in which organic factors form the most significant etiological variable represent the best approximation to the full concept of disease entity as we have modified it.

That is to say that when the clinician can diagnose a biological basis for a psychosis, we have encountered a validating criterion not possible in many psychoses. Biological assessment provides an independent validation of the clinical condition. And, apart from intelligence testing, no other valid criterion exists by which to assess independently a clinical diagnosis.

9. The process of differential diagnosis in acute psychosis is:
   a. To rule out known (validated) disease entities before concluding the diagnostic process. And
   b. Once the former are ruled out (and this means medical disease, intoxications, neurological problems, etc.), and continuing under the guidance of explicit standards—to arrive at a nondisease entity diagnosis. The standards for this further diagnostic endeavor are: (1) the neatness of fit between a genuine case and a defined grouping: (2) definitions of these groups based on the nonetiological features of the disease concept (e.g., natural history, clinical presentation, biological correlates)—definitions based on exclusive and inclusive criteria, which will help us develop therapeutics before we understand etiology; (3) skepticism (should always be a feature of the enthusiasm for any of those diagnoses); (4) when two or more of these groupings may "explain" the particular acute psychosis, and all discriminating features cannot help one distinguish the appropriate one, then the judgment should be to try all treatments for the better prognosis grouping and to assume that this is the acute psychosis until proved otherwise (Ollerenshaw, 1973).

10. The fact that organic psychoses can appear in acute states to be indistinguishable from the cross-sectional characteristics of what has been called "acute schizophrenia" and even from what later turns out to fulfill research criteria for schizophrenia suggests two things. First, schizophrenia may be an organically based syndrome. Second, schizophrenia, although the most common diagnosis (incorrectly) given in acute psychosis, may be a far less specific diagnosis than is possible, particularly if possible multiple organic etiologies are not ruled out. Though certainly many organic conditions are ruled out by the fulfillment of the Feighner definition of schizophrenia, not all are. We must keep this in mind (Bell, 1965; Davison and Bagley, 1969; Slater and Beard, 1963; Stone, 1973; Williams et al., 1974).

11. Acute psychosis should be viewed as a possible organic disease manifestation, particularly in its initial appraisal. Once identified, acute psychosis should be investigated fully to discover the known or treatable causes of such a state. The parallel considerations clinicians have with respect to demented states come to

mind, where the therapeutic imperative strongly motivates exhaustive differential diagnosis and even trial treatment in unclear situations.

12. As a corollary of the above, schizophrenia should be a diagnosis of exclusion. That is, one should rule out known or treatable diseases before applying to a clinical syndrome the label of schizophrenia.

13. Once we have ruled out clearly identified organic disease as the cause of acute psychosis, we then consider clinical entities whose status as diseases is not determined. When we cannot diagnose a disease, our diagnosis must be more tentative, reflecting the fact that we have lowered considerably our capacity to separate out homogeneous groupings. In other words, when diseases, which represent the most validated entities, are ruled out, we step into an area of reduced validity and must consider syndromal or state diagnoses. This further reinforces the importance, in fact the mandate, to rule out known diseases, which can mimic non-specific states or syndromes, before finalizing our diagnostic decision. Further diagnosis proceeds with considerable caution, skepticism, and concern for the error of premature closure. How then should we diagnose these nondisease entities—by what standards of validity? Having made it explicit that we have moved down a hierarchical ladder of validity from disease, we must distinguish among syndromes and states. As etiology is no longer a consideration, we must rely upon other standards for placement of a clinical entity into a particular grouping. The standards are already available (Klerman, 1973); they include the remaining features of the concept of disease entity apart from etiology. But of these criteria, those that are most valid for undergirding and advancing our disease model concept (because they may be independently validated) are the criteria of biological correlation, in terms of biological markers or perhaps treatment response. Genetic transmission might also serve as a criterion, but because of the complexity and lack of conclusive findings in most of these entities, it is currently less useful. Genetic transmission studies rarely can distinguish between socioenvironmental and hereditary transmission. While it is logically possible for a defined clinical entity sample to have a common biological marker and still not be a homogeneous sample, this seems unlikely; yet the existence of even one exception would lower this diagnosis into a less valid category. Until etiology is understood (i.e., all the criteria for disease entity are met), we obscure these issues if we make unqualified assumptions about the validity of syndrome or state diagnoses.

14. Beyond the validation provided by biological correlations of any type, alternatives are less secure. They could include the other

criteria of the concept of disease entity, that is, natural history, development, or pathogenesis, etc. These criteria would constitute the basis for predictive validity (Cronbach and Meehl, 1955). Let us examine one of these possible standards more closely to understand its assumptions and limits as we propose it to be a further standard for delineation of an entity.

Natural history is a possible criterion on the basis of the following assumptions: it is related to biological correlates and even to etiological correlates because of the observation that diseases generally have similar courses, complications, and prognoses. If this criterion is used to diagnose a syndrome, the claim is that clinically observed "entities" with similar natural histories are more homogeneous than those without similar natural histories and that common natural history tends to imply a common substrate, as yet undisclosed. Or, going further, similar natural history presumes a similar etiology, even if the etiology is not known. Of course, there are limitations to this criterion (Strauss and Carpenter, 1972, 1974). First, there is the logical possibility that homogeneity in natural history does not preclude the possibility of heterogeneous entities and etiologies. Hypertensive syndromes may have similar courses, but be due to a variety of known and unknown etiological factors. Second, there is the distinct possibility that natural history may differ with the same disease, as can be the case in so many diseases, such as multiple sclerosis, arthritis, and cardiovascular disease (atherosclerosis). The point is that it may be difficult to fit an individual case to a particular clinical definition. Third, in the clinical situation, learning about the course of a disturbance prior to presentation may be helpful if the information is reliable. With no independent means of confirming the diagnosis and the limitation of the need to observe the patient for long periods of time in order to confirm a diagnosis with longitudinal course criteria, the psychiatrist is forced to make a humble diagnostic decision.

The massing of evidence about natural history in the individual case and for the criteria of diagnosis reduces these problems considerably; the more defined the natural history is in terms of the variables listed, the greater the likelihood of empirical homogeneity. Thus, the refinement of criteria that reflect natural history features enhances the likelihood of developing increasingly validated syndromes. But, clearly, the impetus must be to develop other more exacting and immediately accessible (e.g., laboratory) means of confirming diagnoses.

15. Of the so-called functional psychoses (psychoses without determined etiology), manic depressive psychosis should be ruled out. Typically, the difficult differential diagnosis would be between schizophrenia and manic depression, manic phase. As Ollerenshaw

(1973) points out, the cross-sectional symptomatic picture of mania can be replete with symptoms usually ascribed to acute schizophrenia. This indeed is where great difficulty lies, namely, in the differential diagnosis of acute psychosis with traditionally labeled schizophrenic symptomatology.

Ollerenshaw also notes that this symptomatology is very nonspecific. Ample evidence from the literature (Davison and Bagley, 1970; Reid, 1973; Stone, 1973; Victor and Hope, 1958) underlines this point. We may conclude that schizophrenic symptomatology not only can, but frequently does, occur in known central nervous system disturbances. This being the case, it is useful to draw several other tentative conclusions: (1) the real homogeneity of the clinical sample of symptomatic schizophrenics is questionable; (2) even the poor prognosis group may reflect diverse CNS disturbances; thus, even the carefully defined Feighner criteria may mask a more heterogeneous grouping of entities; (3) manic depressive disturbance, manic phase, represents one common clinical condition with other definable characteristics in which the symptomatoloty strongly mimics schizophrenia. Because manic depressive disturbance can be further differentiated, longitudinally in terms of course and treatment response, and because it prognosis is potentially better than the prognosis for schizophrenia, it must be ruled out before the diagnosis schizophrenia is applied (see 9.b(4) above).

.16. In the situation in which one has excluded known organic disturbances and manic depressive disorder as the basis for an acute psychosis, the next step in clinical differential diagnosis is more difficult. Here validity is least well developed; consequently, reliability in clinical diagnosis may be poor. We are left with the nonspecific syndrome of schizophrenia, and a few other entities that have names but little more in terms of definition along the lines proposed. These include: psychosis felt to arise from psychological stress, the so-called reactive or psychogenic psychosis; hysterical psychosis; atypical psychosis, such as schizoaffective disorder; periodic catatonia; cycloid psychosis; and paraphrenia (Bennett, 1973; Cerrolaza and Cleghorn, 1971; Clayton et al., 1968; Fish, 1964; Gjessing, 1974; Hirsch and Hollender, 1969; Langness, 1967; Leonhard, 1960; Mitsuda, 1965; Perris, 1974; Retterstol, 1966).

Until these entities are better defined in terms of syndrome and later in terms of disease, they must be considered with skepticism. Can we extend the standards of validity suggested above into this confusing area? Yes, but the need for research is clear (Faergeman, 1963; Welner et al., 1974; Croughan et al., 1974). We thus come to understand the limits of our knowledge (by no means an unimportant or negative kind of knowledge in modern psychiatry), and how we can integrate new findings into our diagnostic considerations. Validity is built up from clear definitional criteria, which, when refined, separate populations into groupings as homogeneous as possible. Once this is being done, attempts can be made to develop independent means of assessment and, finally, etiological understandings.

17. The purpose of the disease concept and the scheme outlined here is to develop cogent, reasonable standards for approaching a clinical problem. Because we cannot label an acute psychosis with a particular disease or syndrome diagnosis does not mean that it is neither, merely that we do not know. We must live with this ambiguity, and be aware of it, before we process patients according to our "best experience" in treatment choices. The labels we then choose to apply are the most tentative, least authoritative, and, in the scientific sense of the term, the most tolerant. Even in the case, for instance, where we eventually determine that certain acute psychoses are in fact due to psychological stresses and no necessary biological etiology need be considered, we still will fulfill our role as physicians by ruling out known organic, treatable entities before we stop our search. Our first obligation as physicians is to distinguish and treat known organic disturbances. With full awareness of the ambiguous situation we are in, we carry out our next obligation—to diagnose nondisease entities. Depending on the development of our knowledge with respect to these entities, we may apply therapeutic interventions with varying degrees of success. In fact, our imperative will always be to translate therapeutic knowledge into effective clinical care whether or not we are confronting a disease entity. In order to do this, however, we must understand what is and what is not a disease entity. When we do not know, and are aware of those limits of our knowledge, we will be less likely to proceed with false confidence to premature closure in diagnosis or treatment choice. Within these limits, and they have seldom been made explicit, we may use our limited knowledge in a limited way. The humility of the diagnostic enterprise in acute psychosis is a fundamental lesson. By pretending to know when we do not, we foster obscurantism and perpetuate confusion.

CONCLUDING COMMENTS

This chapter is an attempt to approach a complex clinical problem—diagnosis in acute psychosis—with the intent of settling several confusing matters. We have explored the disturbing problems that vex clinical psychiatrists who deal with acute psychosis. We have seen how these problems reflect fundamental shortcomings in the theory and practice of psychiatry. We then looked at attempts to clarify and solve these difficulties. In subsequent sections, a modification of the disease concept in psychiatry was proposed, and a scheme for evaluating acute psychosis was established. I hope that in the process, certain limits of psychiatry have become apparent. Standardization of clinical terminology, the fundamental necessity for clarity and precision in description and thinking, the importance of research relevant to the context of pragmatic value that motivates our enterprise, the usefulness of strategies that refine our knowledge of clinical disturbances, the explication of the standards that obtain in our work, skepticism, and humility—all these have merited emphasis. The best potential for correcting present abuses and meaningfully extending the frontiers of knowledge in the psychiatry of acute psychosis rests in their realization.

REFERENCES

Abrams, R., M. A. Taylor, and P. Gaztanaga. 1974. Manic-depressive illness and paranoid schizophrenia. Archives of General Psychiatry 31:640-642.

American Psychiatric Association (APA) Committee on Nomenclature and Statistics. 1952. Diagnostic and Statistical Manual of Mental Disorders I (DSM-I). Washington, D.C.: American Psychiatric Association.

American Psychiatric Association (APA) Committee on Nomenclature and Statistics. 1968. Diagnostic and Statistical Manual of Mental Disorders II (DSM-II). Washington, D.C.: American Psychiatric Association.

Baldessarini, R. J. 1970. Frequency of diagnoses of schizophrenia versus affective disorders from 1944 to 1968. American Journal of Psychiatry 127:759-763.

Baldessarini, R. J. 1975. Metabolic hypotheses in schizophrenia. New England Journal of Medicine 292:527-528.

Bannister, D. 1968. The logical requirements of research into schizophrenia. British Journal of Psychiatry 114:181-188.

Bannister, D., P. Salmon, and D. M. Leiberman. 1964. Diagnosis-treatment relationships in psychiatry: a statistical analysis. British Journal of Psychiatry 110:726-732.

Bell, D. S. 1965. Comparison of amphetamine psychosis and schizophrenia. British Journal of Psychiatry 111:701-707.

Bennet, G. 1973. Medical and psychological problems in the 1972 single-handed transatlantic yacht race. Lancet II:747-754.

Bleuler, E. 1950. Dementia Praecox or the Group of Schizophrenias (1911). New York: International Universities Press.

Bowman, K. M., and M. Rose. 1951. A criticism of the terms "psychosis," "psychoneurosis," and "neurosis." American Journal of Psychiatry 108:161-166.

Cerrolaza, M., and R. A. Cleghorn. 1971. Atypical psychosis: a search for certainty in this ambiguous borderland. Canadian Psychiatric Association Journal 16:507-514.

Claridge, G. 1972. The schizophrenias as nervous types. British Journal of Psychiatry 121:1-17.

Clayton, P. J., L. Rodin, and G. Winokur. 1968. Family history studies: III. Schizoaffective disorder, clinical and genetic factors including a one to two year follow-up. Comprehensive Psychiatry 9:31-49.

Cooper, J. E., R. E. Kendell, B. J. Gurland, L. Sharpe, J. R. Copeland, and R. Simon. 1972. Psychiatric Diagnosis in New York and London. London: Oxford University Press.

Copeland, J. R. M., and A. J. Gourlay. 1973. Influence of psychiatric training in the use of descriptive terms among psychiatrists in the British Isles. Psychological Medicine 5:101-107.

Cronbach, L., and P. Meehl. 1955. Construct validity in psychological tests. Psychological Bulletin 52:281-302.

Croughan, J. L., A. Welner, and E. Robins. 1974. The group of schizoaffective and related psychoses: critique, record, follow-up, and family studies. II. Record studies. Archives of General Psychiatry 31:632-637.

Davison, K., and C. R. Bagley. 1969. Schizophrenia-like psychoses associated with organic disorders of the central nervous system: a review of the literature. In Current Problems in Neuropsychiatry. R. Herrington, Ed. British Journal of Psychiatry Special Publication No. 4.

Engelhardt, H. T. 1974. Explanatory models in medicine: facts, theories, and values. Texas Reports on Biology and Medicine 32:225-239.

Everitt, B. S., A. J. Gourlay, and R. E. Kendell. 1971. An attempt at validation of traditional psychiatric syndromes by cluster analysis. British Journal of Psychiatry 119:399-412.

Eysenck, H. 1970. A dimensional system of psychodiagnostics. In New Approaches to Personality Classification, A. Mahrer, ed. New York: Columbia University Press.

Eysenck, S. B. G. 1956. Neurosis and psychosis: an experimental analysis. Journal of Mental Science 102:517-529.

Faergeman, P. 1963. Psychogenic Psychosis. London: Butterworths.

Feighner, J. P., E. Robins, S. Guze, R. Woodruff, G. Winokur, and R. Munoz. 1972. Diagnostic criteria for use in psychiatric research. Archives of General Psychiatry 26:57-63.

Fish, F. 1964. The cycloid psychoses. Comprehensive Psychiatry 5:155-169.

_____. 1966. The concept of schizophrenia. British Journal of Medical Psychology 39:269-273.

_____. 1967. Clinical Psychopathology. Bristol, England: John Wright.

Freud, S. 1949. Outline of Psychoanalysis. New York: Norton.

Gjessing, L. R. 1974. A review of periodic catatonia. Biological Psychiatry 8:23-45.

Grinker, R., J. Miller, M. Sabshin, R. Nunn, and J. Nunnally. 1961. The Phenomena of Depressions. New York: Harper and Row.

Hirsch, S. J., and M. H. Hollender. 1969. Hysterical psychosis: clarification of the concept. American Journal of Psychiatry 125:81-87.

Jaspers, K. 1963. General Psychopathology. Chicago: University of Chicago Press.

Jones, F. 1973. Current methodologies for studying the development of schizophrenia: a critical review. Journal of Nervous and Mental Disease 157:154-178.

Kahlbaum, K. L. 1973. Catatonia (1874). Baltimore: Johns Hopkins University Press.

Kendell, R. 1968. An important source of bias affecting ratings made by psychiatrists. Journal of Psychiatric Research 6:135-141.

Klerman, G. L. 1973. Unipolar and bipolar depressions. In Classification and Prediction of Outcome of Depression, J. Angst, chairman. Stuttgart, New York: F. K. Schattauer Verlag.

Kreitman, N. 1961. The reliability of psychiatric diagnosis. Journal of Mental Science 107:876-886.

Langness, L. 1967. Hysterical psychosis: the cross-cultural evidence. American Journal of Psychiatry 124:143-152.

Leighton, A. 1967. Is social environment a cause of psychiatric disorder? American Psychiatric Association, Psychiatric Research Report 22:337-345.

Leonhard, K. 1961. Cycloid psychoses: endogenous psychoses which are neither schizophrenic nor manic-depressive. Journal of Mental Science 107:633-648.

Maher, B. 1970. Introduction to Research in Psychopathology. New York: McGraw-Hill.

Maxwell, A. 1972. Difficulties in a dimensional description of symptomatology. British Journal of Psychiatry 121:19-26.

Menninger, K., M. Mayman, and P. Pruyser. 1963. The Vital Balance: The Life Process in Mental Health and Illness. New York: Viking Press.

Meyer, A. 1910. The dynamic interpretation of dementia praecox. American Journal of Psychology 21:385-403.

Mitsuda, H. 1965. The concept of "atypical psychoses" from the aspect of clinical genetics. Acta Psychiatrica Scandinavica 41:372-377.

Moriyama, I. 1960. The classification of disease . . . a fundamental problem. Journal of Chronic Diseases 11:462-470.

Newcomb, T. 1931. An experiment designed to test the validity of a rating technique. Journal of Educational Psychology 22:279-289.

Ollerenshaw, D. 1973. The classification of the functional psychoses. British Journal of Psychiatry 122:517-530.

Panzetta, A. 1974. Toward a scientific psychiatric nosology. Archives of General Psychiatry 30:154-161.

Pasamanick, B., S. Dinitz, and M. Lefton. 1959. Psychiatric orientation and its relation to diagnosis and treatment in a mental hospital. American Journal of Psychiatry 116:127-132.

Perris, C. 1974. A study of cycloid psychoses. Acta Psychiatrica Scandinavica Supplement 253:1-76.

Polyani, M., and H. Prosch. 1975. Meaning, Chapter II: Personal Knowledge. Chicago: University of Chicago Press.

Professional Staff of the United States-United Kingdom Cross-National Project. 1974. The diagnosis and psychopathology of schizophrenia in New York and London. Schizophrenia Bulletin 11:80-102.

Reid, A. A. 1973. Schizophrenia: disease or syndrome? Archives of General Psychiatry 28:863-869.

Retterstol, N. 1966. Paranoid and Paranoiac Psychoses. Springfield, Ill.: Charles C Thomas, Chapter III.

Rosenhan, D. L. 1973a. On being sane in insane places. Science 180:250-258.

———. 1973 b. Letter. Science 180:365-369.

Roth, M. 1963. Neurosis, psychosis, and the concept of disease in psychiatry. Acta Psychiatrica Scandinavica 39:128-145.

Saghir, M. T. 1971. A comparison of some aspects of structured and unstructured psychiatric interviews. American Journal of Psychiatry 128: 180-184.

Sandifer, M., A. Hordern, G. Timbury, and L. Green. 1969. Similarities and differences in patient evaluation by U.S. and U.K. psychiatrists. American Journal of Psychiatry 126:206-212.

Shapiro, A. K. 1959. The placebo effect in the history of medical treatment: implications for psychiatry. American Journal of Psychiatry 116:298-304.

Slater, E., and A. W. Bears. 1963. The schizophrenia-like psychoses of epilepsy. British Journal of Psychiatry 109:95-150.

Spitzer, R., J. Endicott, and E. Robins. 1975a. Clinical criteria for psychiatric diagnosis and DSM III. American Journal of Psychiatry 132:1187-1192.

_____. 1975b. Research Diagnostic Criteria. 2nd ed. New York: Biometrics Section, New York State Psychiatric Institute.

Spitzer, R., and J. Fleiss. 1974. A re-analysis of the reliability of psychiatric diagnosis. British Journal of Psychiatry 125:341-347.

Stone, M. H. 1973. Drug-related schizophrenic syndromes. International Journal of Psychiatry 11:391-437.

Strauss, J. S. 1973. Diagnostic models and the nature of psychiatric disorder. Archives of General Psychiatry 29:445-449.

Strauss, J. S., and W. T. Carpenter. 1972. The prediction of outcome in schizophrenia. Archives of General Psychiatry 27:739-746.

_____. 1974. Characteristic symptoms and outcome in schizophrenia. Archives of General Psychiatry 30:429-434.

Strömgren, E. 1969. Uses and abuses of concepts in psychiatry. American Journal of Psychiatry 126:777-778.

Sullivan, H. 1931. Environmental factors in etiology and course under treatment of schizophrenia. Medical Journal and Record 133:19-22.

Thorndike, E. 1920. A constant error in psychological ratings. Journal of Applied Psychology 4:25-29.

Victor, M., and J. M. Hope. 1958. The phenomenon of auditory hallucinations in chronic alcoholism. Journal of Nervous and Mental Diseases 126:451-481.

Ward, C., A. Beck, M. Mendelson, J. Mock, and J. Erbaugh. 1962. The Psychiatric Nomenclature. Archives of General Psychiatry 7:198-205.

Welner, A., J. L. Croughan, and E. Robins. 1974. The group of schizoaffective and related psychoses: critique, record, follow-up and family studies. I. A persistent enigma. Archives of General Psychiatry 31:628-631.

Williams, S. E., D. S. Bell, and R. S. Gye. 1974. Neurosurgical disease encountered in a psychiatric service. Journal of Neurology, Neurosurgery, and Psychiatry 37:112-116.

Woodruff, R. A., D. W. Goodwin, and S. G. Guze. 1974. Psychiatric Diagnosis. New York: Oxford University Press.

World Health Organization (WHO). 1967. Manual of the International Statistical Classification of Diseases, Injuries, and Causes of Death, Revision 8 (ICD-8). Geneva: World Health Organization.

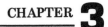

CHAPTER 3

RETHINKING THE SOCIAL AND CULTURAL CONTEXT OF PSYCHOPATHOLOGY AND PSYCHIATRIC CARE

Arthur M. Kleinman, M.D.

INTRODUCTION

In spite of all the evidence attesting to the crucial influence social and cultural factors frequently exert upon psychiatric problems and interventions (evidence that now is indisputable), most psychiatrists remain uncertain about how best to understand and respond to these factors. Though many psychiatrists will now agree that psychiatry rests on social science as well as on biological and behavioral science supports, few are able to define exactly what the first of these consists of, or seem to understand its implications for teaching and practice. The organizational structure of academic psychiatry, of course, has boxes for social and cross-cultural psychiatry, but few individuals, including scholars who affiliate with these labels, can actually delineate the specific scientific foundations of these new disciplines. What is even worse, the very names "social" and "cross-cultural" psychiatry suggest conceptual and methodological links with the social sciences that cannot in fact be demonstrated to exist, except perhaps in only the most superficial and fragile ways.

At present, it is certainly not rash to admit that social and cross-cultural psychiatry, as scientific fields of research and teaching, are fictions. This statement is not at all meant to disparage some

This chapter is based on research supported by grants from the Foundations' Fund for Research in Psychiatry, the Livingston and DuPont-Warren Funds, Harvard Medical School, and the Social Science Research Council.

excellent individual contributions that have been made under those headings. Rather, it signifies the lack of any systematic organization of what knowledge we do possess about the social and cultural aspects of psychiatric questions, and the wide gaps that separate this material from the much larger body of data and theories that comprise modern social science. The absence of systematically organized knowledge is most obvious in the clinical setting, where no frameworks are to be found within which clinicians can conceptualize and communicate their appreciation of social and cultural issues, and where the obvious lack of strategies for applying relevant knowledge is both embarrassing and frustrating. This problem is equally disturbing in the teaching of medical students and psychiatric residents, who rightly demand systematic presentations of principles and methods. Who can honestly say that he or she has met such demands?

If ever an aspect of psychiatry needed to be rethought, that aspect is psychiatry's social and cultural "poor relations." Yet much militates against a rational reappraisal. To begin with, psychiatrists appear to view the social scientific aspects of their profession as marginal concerns, even when they regard social and cultural questions as central to psychiatry. Social science is seen as the venue of social scientists, not psychiatrists. On the other hand, social and cultural questions of practical clinical significance are thought to be the appropriate field for psychiatry, and perhaps also its affiliate psychiatric social work, but not for anthropology, sociology, and social psychology. This view is supported by the unfortunate clinical predilection to think about social and cultural issues in "common-sense" terms, and to ignore the findings and theories advanced by specialists. Such findings and theories are frequently devalued as overly technical, jargonistic, trivial, and clinically irrelevant. This tendency contrasts markedly with typical psychiatric views of biological and psychological science, which are considered to be essential to the practice and teaching of psychiatry. What we usually find, then, are otherwise very competent clinicians ill equipped to talk about, let alone treat, some of the bread-and-butter sociocultural difficulties that require their professional skills. Their simplistic and *ad hoc* concern with the relevant sociocultural reality, no matter how well intentioned, contrasts pathetically with the sophisticated knowledge and methods for testing that knowledge possessed by many contemporary social scientists. The tragic irony behind this disturbing situation is that unless social science is applied by clinicians, the problems that social science is defining with ever more precision and intellectual rigor will never be treated, at least not within appropriate psychiatric settings. Psychiatry, to date, has failed to successfully translate the abstract language of the social sciences into the everyday idiom of clinical practice.

Several other problems contribute to this regrettable situation. Social scientists themselves also have been slow and ineffective to translate their work into forms that can be easily assimilated by their psychiatric colleagues. Furthermore, medical education, until very recently, has kept physicians ignorant of the social science literature, and even more so of its principles and methods. Lacking any significant experience with this field in medical school, many psychiatric clinicians and educators have thereafter avoided confronting a new scientific language and body of readings. The distorted image of social science as basically hostile to the psychiatric profession has made this science more frightening than alluring to psychiatrists, and in the minds of some has justified avoiding even its most relevant contributions.

Nor has this situation been improved by those self-appointed apostles of social truth who implicate "social causes" for just about every problem psychiatrists face, without either specifying precise mechanisms of action by which these factors actually produce their effects or presenting strategies for prediction and control.

Unfortunately, some work in social and cross-cultural psychiatry cannot fail to strike critically minded psychiatrists as trivial, overblown, and pseudoscientific, because it is precisely that. Those psychiatrists who have jumped from casual observations of shamans to the dangerously absurd conclusion that just because all practitioners in the health care field, including shamans and psychiatrists, share some universal psychotherapeutic functions, they are therefore doing exactly the same thing, have done a profound disservice to both psychiatry and anthropology. Similarly, some of the work of social labeling theorists has been an unabashed polemic using psychiatry as a handy scapegoat, and yet, though those abuses hardly qualify as scientific, the social labeling perspective in general has significantly advanced our understanding of psychiatric problems and practices. Even psychiatric epidemiology, which has been virtually the sole outpost of medical science in this area, has been unable to resolve basic questions such as whether the higher prevalence of schizophrenia in lower social classes represents cause or effect. This has not inspired students to pay attention to the epidemiological perspective (important as it is), nor has it demonstrated to clinicians any practical significance of this approach.

The unfulfilled promises and naive misadventures of the community mental health movement, along with its clear failure to build a scientific framework either for systematically studying the problems it attempted to confront or for evaluating the techniques it used to solve those problems, have gone far to undermine the pretenses psychiatry holds about rationally understanding and treating social problems. But the excesses and inadequacies of the community mental health movement should underline the need for bringing social science into psychiatry, not for throwing the little there is out.

Undoubtedly, some social and cultural issues (including poverty, the breakdown of traditional family functions, ethnic prejudice and persecution) go far beyond the scope of psychiatric intervention. The fact that they do is frequently used to support a cynical view of the social and cultural aspects of psychiatry, or to justify dispensing with reason in favor of revolution. These attitudes are clearly unwarranted. There are many important sociocultural concerns that fall squarely within the limits of psychiatric science and practice. Even those broader concerns that relate to realities well beyond the range of appropriate psychiatric interventions per se are important for the better understanding of psychiatric problems and for elaborating appropriate strategies for responding to them.

Finally, the social and cross-cultural streams of psychiatry have suffered from an antitheoretical tradition that has characterized modern medicine in general in recent decades. This positivistic tendency to generate data in the absence of theory has neither encouraged psychiatrists interested in these fields to develop hypotheses that could be tested in field research nor supported the early attempts at conceptualizing these domains within new theoretical systems. And this has occurred at the same time as social science has gone through its period of greatest growth, so that the findings and theories social science has generated, which often are directly related to the interests of medicine and psychiatry, have not been used yet to any significant degree to develop psychiatric concepts. Since psychiatry lacks such concepts, is it surprising that this knowledge has not been assimilated, taught, or used effectively in clinical practice? I would argue that the development of social and cross-cultural fields in psychiatric science requires new conceptual models and translational paradigms in order to make use of social scientific thought and research.

This chapter outlines a framework for understanding and using certain kinds of social scientific knowledge pertinent to basic questions in psychopathology and psychiatric care. By no means is it presented as a complete program for developing psychiatry's social science base. Thus, it does not pretend to fulfill all of the desiderata mentioned above. It is an example of one limited and particular kind of approach that has been found helpful in teaching psychiatry residents and medical students. It has been used as a clinical model primarily in consultative psychiatry, and it also has been used as the theoretical background in a comparative cross-cultural research project. The framework, as we shall see, is narrowed to the cognitive and communicative aspects of illness and health care.

I present this framework here for several reasons. First, it is the product of a deliberate attempt to reconceptualize the social and cultural domains of psychiatry. Second, it deals with certain basic issues that are at the core of social and cross-cultural psychiatry: the relation of psychopathology to deviance and the sick role; the cultural patterning of symptoms—especially the question of somatization; problems in primary psychiatric care and consultation arising from discrepancies in beliefs and difficulties in communication between practitioners and patients; and the question of efficacy of psychiatric care and how that is to be evaluated. Third, these issues have been the subject of actual research that I have been engaged in, and they will be discussed in terms of that research. And, last, it is my hope that this presentation will provide specific examples of "rethinking" certain aspects of social and cross-cultural psychiatry and that it will stimulate larger, more inclusive efforts at defining and advancing that subject.

The reader is cautioned that the framework I present below is not an integrative one. It does not attempt to link the psychosocial and sociocultural spheres with the biological structure of individuals. Instead, it argues for the development of *mid-range*, rather than abstract, high-level, theories in psychiatry, theories that relate to quite specific research problems and that organize relatively small amounts of information in the different subsectors of psychiatric science, but that eschew acting as universal explanations of human behavior. It is my view that we have witnessed far too much of the latter and far too little of the former. Before we can develop macrotheories that integrate the different fields of psychiatry, we must first work out a more developed understanding of these separate domains. This means purposefully refraining from the impulse to build larger and larger integrations, and instead to be concerned with the limits of our knowledge. That implies also concentrating on the theoretical dimensions of each subdiscipline and the fields outside of psychiatry to which they are directly related (e.g., cross-cultural psychiatry and medical and psychological anthropology).

In our case, this means, paradoxically, looking away from psychiatry before we look toward it. The reason for this: the best work in social and cross-cultural psychiatry has not been done by psychiatrists. Anthropologists have provided us with our most important data in cross-cultural psychiatry (see, for example, Levy, 1973; Reynolds, 1976), sociologists with our most productive theories and findings in social psychiatry (see references in Gove, 1975; Jessor et al., 1968; Plog and Edgerton, 1969). In this chapter, I will argue that concepts like social deviance, the sick role, and illness behavior should belong as much to the vocabulary of the psychiatric clinician and teacher as they do to that of social scientists. Similarly, ethnography and cross-cultural psychological research are producing data that are for future psychiatrists to use as much as for future anthropologists and psychologists. Furthermore, ethnographic and comparative cross-cultural methods are appropriate for psychiatrists to use. Social or cross-cultural psychiatrists, then, must be social scientists as well as psychiatrists, and psychiatrists must be just as conversant with social science concepts as they are with psychological and biological ones. I would even go beyond this and suggest that in the next decades we shall witness mainstream psychiatry and medicine becoming increasingly social sciences.

EXPLANATORY MODEL FRAMEWORK FOR MAKING SOCIAL SCIENCE RELEVANT TO PSYCHIATRY

Explanatory models (EMs) are the conceptions about illness and treatment held by patients and practitioners (Engelhardt 1974; Kleinman, 1975a). Although they vary in degree of sophistication, coherence and clarity, and explanatory power, they can be elicited from individual patients, families, and practitioners in all societies and systems of health care (Kleinman, 1975b). A subset of these beliefs, which may be more or less distinct, are those concerning mental illness and its treatment. These beliefs reflect basic social and cultural determinants, including ethnicity, social class, education, religious affiliation, occupation, family and community beliefs, and past experiences with illness and health care. In turn, they influence how illness is defined (i.e., what is labeled illness), what personal and family meaning it has, what decisions are made regarding treatment, the patterns of resort to different health care facilities, and how treatment is evaluated. The behavior of those who are sick and that of those who treat sickness are often a direct outgrowth of these beliefs.

Explanatory models can thus be used as a critical focus for relating theories and findings from a number of social science fields to psychiatric questions. The explanatory model framework can make use of relevant work from cognitive anthropology (Cancain, 1971; Tylor, 1969), ethnoscience (Berlin et al., 1973; Frake, 1961), ethnomethodology (Garfinkel, 1967), social psychology (Jones, 1971; McGuire, 1968; and Zajonc, 1968), and cross-cultural psychology (Berry and Dasen, 1974; Jahoda, 1969). Used in the manner described below, the EM framework becomes a vehicle for importing into psychiatry research and theory from medical anthropology, psychological anthropology, the social labeling and deviance research streams of sociology, and from other social science subdisciplines as well.

Recent publications in cross-cultural medicine and psychiatry have shown how patients' and practitioners' beliefs are a critical focus for studying medical and psychiatric care in different societies, and have made extensive use of anthropological studies (see Fabrega, 1974; Kleinman, 1973a; Leslie, 1976; Yap, 1967). Patient beliefs have been shown to have important effects on illness behavior and health care, and also have allowed a number of anthropologists and sociologists to demonstrate how social science research can provide direct benefit to physicians and psychiatrists concerned with such issues as the psychosocial experience of illness and the communicative context of health care, as we shall discuss in detail below (see Elder, 1973; Freidson, 1970; Harwood, 1971; Mechanic, 1972; Snow, 1974). Fabrega (1974) and Kleinman (1975b) have outlined ways in which behavioral and social science approaches can be used to reformulate our general understanding of the cognitive and communicative aspects of illness and care. Lack of space prevents me from reviewing many other contributions to this subject, but it should be clear that it is a major avenue for social and cross-cultural research in medicine and psychiatry, and one that concerns issues that are fundamental to clinical practice.

One way of analyzing explanatory models is in terms of the components of the local health care systems to which they belong (Kleinman, 1973a). Local health care systems can be conceptualized as composed of three separate but interconnected sectors of care: the modern professional medical scientific sector, the popular sector, and the folk medical sector. Each of these sectors can be described with regard to cognitive structures, social roles, institutions, and the like. The professional medical sector is made up of the social organization of local facilities and practitioners of modern professional medical care. The popular sector includes individuals, families, and communities. The folk sector is composed of various nonprofessional and traditional professional practitioners. Much of health care, and especially psychiatric care, takes place outside of the professional scientific medical institutional structure of mental hospitals and psychiatrists' offices (Freidson, 1970). Psychotherapy, for example, also takes place in families and in the offices of various folk practitioners (secular and religious).

These three sectors of local health care systems can be thought of as interacting dynamically, since individuals move from one sector to the other sectors and back again. Such interactions can be described not simply as the movement of individuals, but also as the interactions between different institutions, social roles, and, as we shall see, explanatory models. Practitioner-patient interactions offer a particularly important focus for using the EM model to study these interactions.

In each of the sectors of local health care systems, beliefs about illness and care help to construct distinct social realities (Freidson, 1970). For mental illness and psychiatric care, for example, these social realities include rules that influence how patients and families come to perceive, define, and experience mental illness; rules for behavior and communication in patient-practitioner interactions; hierarchies of resort to different types of practitioners; and criteria for evaluating treatment practices and their success. Explanatory models label specific patterns of behavior as deviant, define appropriate social roles in response to that behavior (sick roles and healing roles), provide mental illness and its treatment with distinct kinds of personal and social meaning, and set out criteria by which patients and practitioners determine if treatment is effective or not.

Patient and family EMs (here referred to, respectively, as EM_1 and EM_F) are derived from the popular sector of local health care systems. These models not only differ from practitioner models in actual content, but are conveyed in special idioms (Horton, 1967). For example, popular psychiatric beliefs in witchcraft, bad fate, or mental degeneration not only differ from contemporary psychiatric conceptions with regard to these specific attributions but also are expressed in a very different language, that of popular thought as against that of medical scientific thought.

Practitioner EMs (EM_2) are derived from the sector of local health care systems in which a particular practitioner is situated; for example: psychiatric clinic, Christian Science Church, T-group, modern healing cult. We might think of two separate levels of practitioner EMs: theoretical models (EM_{2a}), that is, what is written down in texts, discussed among colleagues, and noted down in patients' records; and practical clinical models (EM_{2b}), that is, what is actually transmitted to patients in the practitioner-patient interaction (be it modern or traditional).

Using ethnoscientific and other ethnographic methods for accurately describing what people think without contamination by the beliefs of the researcher, EMs can be systematically elicited, and described in a fashion that is reproducible and even quantifiable (Fabrega, 1971; Kleinman, 1975a; Metzger and Williams, 1963; Werner and Fenton, 1973). EMs can be elicited for specific categories of illness or for a given case of illness. For example, one can describe the EMs held by individuals, families, and populations for mental illness and psychiatric care. That is, we can describe how people in given cultural contexts name, categorize, and respond to mental illness by eliciting all the names of mental illnesses they know, the types of behavior they associate with these illnesses, and the beliefs they hold about appropriate treatment for each illness defined. Thus, we obtain a description of a particular culture's or social group's popular psychiatric EMs (Kleinman, 1975c).

EMs also can be collected for specific mental illnesses in particular practitioner-patient interactions as single-phrase statements (from practitioners and patients independently) about five parameters: etiology, onset of symptoms, pathophysiology, course of illness (divided into statements about severity and type of sick role), and treatment regimen. These can be elicited both before and after practitioner-patient interactions, and used either to study the impact of these interactions on cognitive, communicative, and behavioral factors, or to compare the EMs of patients and practitioners. We shall discuss below these different ways of studying EMs when we focus first on illness behavior and later on practitioner-patient relationships. In each case, we shall try to demonstrate not only the relevance of EMs for basic problems in psychiatry, but also how they enable us to relate psychiatry's social scientific supports to clinical, research, and teaching concerns. In so doing, I think we can clarify how this framework allows us to reformulate certain social and cultural aspects of psychopathology and psychiatric care. It puts social and cross-cultural psychiatry in a new light: moving them closer to the core of contemporary psychiatric questions and suggesting a different blueprint for the development of these subdisciplines.

EXPLANATORY MODELS AND ILLNESS BEHAVIOR

Social and cross-cultural contributions to psychiatry have generated some extremely difficult problems for psychiatric theory. In fact, they have called into question that theory itself (Plog and Edgerton, 1969; Siegler and Osmond, 1966). Social deviance has been used increasingly as an alternative conceptual approach to psychopathological formulations (Bennett and Sanchez, 1973). Cultural definitions of the same type of behavior—defined as pathological in one setting and as normal in another (now extensively documented in the anthropological, sociological, and cross-cultural psychiatric literatures)—have sensitized people to the important influence of the process of labeling illness, the cultural context, and the beliefs of practitioners and patients about psychopathology (Waxler, 1974). Some problems given a psychiatric diagnosis seem to dissolve entirely when the social and cultural determinants of faulty communication and cognitive discrepancies are understood and responded to (Kleinman, 1975b; and see below). The concept of the sick role suggests that much of what is presently considered disease by psychiatrists may be nothing other than inappropriate uses to which this social role is put. The sick role concept makes clear the widespread phenomenon by which psychosocial problems, and even psychiatric diseases, are socially legitimated by using a medical sick role. Cross-cultural research has stirred major controversy by describing substantial differences in the symptom profiles of the same diseases in distinctly different cultures, and by identifying psychiatric disorders that are reputed to be unique to certain societies (Yap, 1975). These and similar developments have resulted in two separate types of reactions within the psychiatric profession. Most frequently, the reaction is confusion, fear that the central tenets of the discipline are under attack, which could lead to theoretical chaos, and a tendency to either disregard or disparage these issues, so that they have little or no influence on psychiatric ideas and practices. Much less frequently, some psychiatrists have been provoked to rethink fundamental components of psychiatric science and, in so doing, have proposed alternative models for their profession (see, for example, Fabrega, 1974; Lazare, 1974; Yap, 1975). What follows is my attempt to follow the second alternative by using the explanatory model framework to help assimilate into psychiatry some of the social and cultural contributions mentioned earlier as well as others still to be discussed.

From the explanatory model perspective, the question of social deviance versus psychopathology seems easier to understand. All ideas about mental illness are EMs operating within particular sociocultural settings, which we have already described as the different sectors of local health care systems (Kleinman, 1973a). The concepts of social deviance and psychopathology operate in distinct arenas, the former in the popular sector, and outside the health system among social science professionals, the latter in the professional medical care sector. Difficulty arises from conflicts between these EMs when they are both used in the same sector of health care (or another sociocultural context) or when the sectors of health care supporting these EMs interact. The latter occurs when psychiatrists and patients (and their families) interact, the former when psychiatrists and social scientists interact, or when psychiatrists make use of the social deviance EM (and sociologists and anthropologists make use of the psychopathology EM).

The conflict will end either when one of these EMs wins out over the other (e.g., if for scientific or other reasons one is accepted as a better model; see Kuhn, 1974), or when they are superseded by a new EM. But the EM framework also suggests that there is considerable room for their integration. The social deviance model, as initially stated, theorizes that there are two forms of deviance: primary and secondary. The first is that which originates within the individual making his behavior deviate from the existing social and cultural rules governing behavior. This is what most psychiatrists would call individual psychopathology. The second is social deviance brought about by societal reaction to primary behavioral deviance. Examples of this would include the socially deviant roles created by societal reaction to homosexuality, alcoholism, drug abuse, mental illness, etc. This would include the sick role (both medical and psychiatric), which is socially prescribed behavior for sick persons. Most psychiatrists have included some notion like this in their clinical EMs under "course of illness." That these EMs can and in fact need to be integrated is clear. The model of individual psychopathology has much explanatory power and evidence to add to the under-developed concept of primary deviance, while the EM of secondary deviance is a much needed addition to the vague and unsystematic social dimensions of the psychopathological concept of course of illness.

The choice of the words "deviant" and "ill" is largely a matter of external social, cultural, and political factors; that is, it is based on the subsector of the health care system and cultural context in which it is used. For example, "neurasthenia" is a widely used term in Taiwan, but not in the People's Republic of China (P.R.C.). On Taiwan, "neurasthenia" often provides a culturally legitimated medical sick role for psychiatric disease and social problems, while in the P.R.C., it is anathematized as a problem caused by capitalism and therefore impossible in a communist state. People who would be called "ill" on Taiwan are labeled class enemies or malingerers in the P.R.C. On Taiwan, treatment for this problem occurs within a medical setting; in the P.R.C., treatment occurs within a political setting as indoctrination and socially useful work (Kleinman, 1975c).

The question of which is correct, the medical model or the social model of behavioral disorders, is spurious. As we shall show below, the medical model must include social and cultural elements (and probably always has included them when employed by clinicians). More important, these models function in different social and cultural arenas, and the ascendancy of one over the other depends not only on which arena they are used in, but also on the "external" factors already discussed. The history and anthropology of venereal disease, alcoholism, drug abuse, and homosexuality are excellent examples of this. Part and parcel of societal development throughout the world is what Zola (1973) has called the progressive medicalization of society. That is, for political and socioeconomic reasons, more and more psychosocial and biological problems have been legitimated by modern societies as medical (or psychiatric). An obvious abuse of this is the use of the medical term "schizophrenia" to label dissidents' behavior in the Soviet Union. To a certain extent, the question of which EM is in ascendance reflects professional dominance, within or without the health care system, as for example in the cases of the EMs of allopathic medicine and osteopathic medicine in the United States, and Western medicine and Chinese medicine in the P.R.C. prior to the Cultural Revolution.

Several new EMs are emerging both within and at the social

scientific margins of medicine and psychiatry that use the concept of illness behavior as a means for bringing certain social and cultural theories into these fields in clinically relevant ways. Social psychological research on sick persons suggests that a distinction should be made between the terms "disease" and "illness" (Fabrega, 1974; Mechanic, 1962). Disease is defined as a disordered or maladaptive process (physiological, psychological, or psychophysiological) afflicting sick persons. Illness is made to refer then to the psychosocial experience of disease. Illness behavior is essentially interchangeable with illness as defined here. Illness behavior is meant to include the social and cultural patterning of sick persons' perception of illness, the meaning the illness has for them, and their responses to their illness, particularly in terms of their coping behavior, use of a particular sick (or patient) role, and choices of available health care resources from which to seek help.

These new perspectives have tended to focus on different aspects of illness behavior. Thus, Mechanic (1972) has studied the influence of social psychological factors on the presentation of symptoms. Lipowski (1969) has concentrated both on the meaning of the illness in personal and social terms, and on the coping responses the illness calls forth. Both these approaches have been presented in frameworks that could be used by clinicians. More removed from clinical reality are the frameworks worked out by Freidson (1970) and McKinley (1973) to study how people respond to illness from the standpoint of popular (family, social network, and community) help-seeking behaviors. Twaddle (1974) has reexamined the ideas of sick role and health status. Recently, greater emphasis has been placed on the family (Taylor, 1975) and cultural (Snow, 1974) contexts of illness behavior.

Much research has documented the crucial role played by cultural beliefs in structuring and sanctioning particular kinds of illness behavior (see, for example, Harwood, 1971; Rubel, 1964; Snow, 1974; Zola, 1966). The EM framework presented here is perhaps most useful in relating beliefs to actual illness behavior. In order to demonstrate how EMs link social and cultural rules with illness behavior (Colby, 1975; Kleinman, 1975b), and how understanding this linkage within the EM framework enables the clinician to treat health care problems involving faulty communication and cognitive discrepancies, I shall present several case illustrations and a preliminary description of an ongoing research project. These examples will, I hope, make clear how social and cross-cultural insights can be used within clinical psychiatry and medicine. They should indicate how the EM framework allows us to both bring social science into psychiatry and relate social and cross-cultural psychiatry to core issues in health care.

CASE 1 Mr. W. is a 33-year-old Chinese male (Cantonese-speaking) who presented at the medical clinic at the Massachusetts General Hospital with tiredness, dizziness, general weakness, pains in the upper back described as rheumatism, a sensation of heaviness in the feet, twenty-pound weight loss, and insomnia of six months' duration. Patient denied any emotional complaints. Past medical history was noncontributory. Medical work-up was unrevealing, except that the patient seemed anxious and looked depressed. Mr. W. refused to acknowledge either, however. He initially refused psychotherapy, stating that talk therapy would not help him. He finally accepted psychiatric care only after it was agreed that he would be given some kind of medication. During the course of his care. Mr. W. never accepted the idea that he was suffering from a mental illness. He attributed his problem, as did his family, to "wind" (*fung*) and "not enough blood" (*m̄-krá-huèt*).

Pertinent past history included the following: Mr. W. was born into a family of educated farmers and teachers in a village in Kwantung Province, China. He and his family moved to Canton when he was a young child. His father died during the war with Japan, and Mr. W. remembered recurrent feelings of grief and loneliness throughout his childhood and adolescence. At age 10, he accompanied his family to Hong Kong; ten years later they moved to the United States. Mr. W. denied any family history of mental illness. He reported that his health problem began two years before when he returned to Hong Kong to find a wife. He acquired the "wind" disease, he believes in retrospect, after having overindulged in sexual relations with prostitutes, which resulted in loss of *huèt-hèi* (blood and vital breath) causing him to suffer from "cold" (*leūng*) and "not enough blood." His symptoms worsened over the past six months, following his wife's second miscarriage (they have no children) and shortly after he had lost most of his savings in the stock market and in a failing restaurant business. However, he denied feeling depressed at that time, though he admitted being anxious, fearful, irritable, and worried about his financial situation. These feelings he also attributed to "not enough blood."

Mr. W. first began treating himself for his symptoms with traditional Chinese herbs and diet therapy. This involved both the use of tonics to "increase blood" (*po-huèt*) and treatment with symbolically "hot" (*ít*) food to correct his underlying state of humoral imbalance. He did this only after seeking advice from his family and friends in Boston's Chinatown. They concurred that he was suffering from a "wind" and "cold" disorder. They prescribed other herbal medicines when he failed to improve. They suggested that he return to Hong Kong to consult traditional Chinese practitioners there. While the patient was seen at the Massachusetts

General Hospital's medical clinic, he continued to use Chinese drugs and to seek out consultation and advice from friends, neighbors, and recognized "experts" in the local Chinese community. He was frequently told that his problem could not be helped by Western medicine. At the time of receiving psychiatric care, Mr. W. was also planning to visit a well-known traditional Chinese doctor in New York's Chinatown, and he was also considering acupuncture treatment locally. He continued taking Chinese drugs throughout his illness, and never told his family or friends about receiving psychiatric care. He expressed gratitude, however, that the psychiatrist listened to his views about his problem and that he explained to him in detail psychiatric ideas about depression, etc. He remembered feeling bad about his care in the medical clinic where, after the lengthy work-up, almost nothing was explained to him and no treatment was given him. He had decided not to return to the clinic.

Mr. W. responded to a course of antidepressant medication with complete remission of all symptoms. He thanked the psychiatrist for his help, but confided that (1) he remained confident that he was not suffering from a mental illness, (2) talk therapy had not been of help, (3) antidepressants perhaps were effective against "wind" disorders, and (4) since he had concurrently taken a number of traditional Chinese herbs, it was uncertain what had been effective, and perhaps the combination of both traditional Chinese and Western drugs had been responsible for his cure.

I shall now discuss this case solely in terms of illness behavior and culturally sanctioned EMs. In the next section of this chapter, I shall reconsider it from the standpoint of psychiatric care. This case illustrates what I mean by the experience of illness and the cultural patterning of that experience. Mr. W., his family, friends, and local community "experts" defined his problem in terms of local Chinese popular medical EMs, based on the explanatory systems of traditional Chinese folk and classical medicine (see Ahern, 1975; Topley, 1975). Their explanations and actions are based on their belief that he was suffering from a "wind" disorder owing to an underlying "cold" imbalance and "not enough blood." These concepts derive from classical Chinese medical EMs, which state that the healthy body contains a harmonious balance of *yin* and *yang* forces. The former are associated with cold, female qualities; while the latter are associated with hot, male qualities. Imbalance of this harmonious relationship is felt to underlie illnesses and to predispose to causative factors such as "wind" and possession by gods or ghosts. The imbalance itself causes illness as well. Imbalances can be caused by strengthening or weakening either the *yin* or the *yang* in relation to

the other. Treatment involves correcting the imbalance by strengthening and/or weakening the other principle. Mr. W. reinterpreted his
past behavior according to this EM, since it is thought that this
"wind" disorder is brought on by loss of the body's vital essence
(ch'i)—which is almost pure yang—due especially to excessive semen
loss through masturbation or frequent intercourse. Such a loss, it is
held, produces a state of weakness and relative imbalance, with
decreased yang and correspondingly increased yin, such that the body is
"cold," lacks "blood" (which is strong in yang) and is susceptible to
"wind". The characteristic symptoms believed to be associated with
this disorder—general weakness, nonspecific arthritic complaints and
other pains, insomnia, and various emotional complaints, from anxiety
and irritability to anger and loneliness, said to be secondary to the
underlying "physical" disorder—not only accounted for his complaints but, as we shall discuss below, may have helped pattern those
complaints. The belief that this illness is very difficult to cure and
can become chronic again fits with Mr. W.'s actual experience. Because
this problem is not regarded by the Chinese as a mental illness, Mr.
W. sought a medical sick role and treatment for a physical illness
when he turned to modern scientific medicine.

Understanding illness experiences within the context of the popular
EMs that govern them helps us to understand the "internal" meaning
of illness behavior that otherwise seems inexplicable or is wrongly
interpreted by "external" professional medical and psychiatric EMs.
Such an "internal" cultural analysis is called an "emic" analysis by
anthropologists; an "external" cultural analysis is called an "etic"
analysis, based on the linguistic distinction between phonemics and
phonetics. Medicine clearly is an appropriate field for this linguistic-
ally derived approach. From the "etic" perspective, problems labeled
"wind," "cold," or "not enough blood" disorders overlap with a
number of disorders in the modern medical and psychiatric classificatory systems, including depression, anxiety reaction, hysteria,
hypochondriasis, chronic functional complaints, nonspecific arthritis.
In Chinese societies, Western-style medical practitioners often label
these problems "neurasthenia" (shen-ching shuai-jo). By this diagnosis, they mean a psychological or psychophysiological problem, but
their patients generally regard neurasthenia as an organic illness
(Kleinman, 1975c). Nor do these doctors usually correct their
patients' ideas. Neurasthenia in Chinese is a compound term made up
of two characters that denote neurological problems and two that
denote weakness, in the traditional Chinese medical sense. As an
illness, neurasthenia in Chinese societies provides a medical sick role
for problems that are primarily emotional and interpersonal. "Wind,"
"cold," and "not enough blood" disorders and other traditional
Chinese categories of illnesses are associated with psychiatric illnesses

like depression, anxiety reaction, and hysteria, which are commonly manifested by physical symptoms, in addition to psychological complaints. This provides a logical basis for the Chinese categorization of these problems as physical.

In Chinese communities, including Chinatowns in the United States, mental illness carries a marked stigma. Chinese popular EMs state that mental illnesses can be inherited, or contracted through close contact because they are contagious or result from sinful family influences. Thus, it is believed that one should not marry into families that have a member with mental illness. On the other hand, the popular Chinese medical EMs like "wind" and "cold" disorders do not carry such a stigma, nor does the modern medical diagnosis of neurasthenia. The former EM operates in the popular medical subsystem to legitimate mental illness and psychological problems with a medical sick role, while the latter EM shows that professional Western-style medical practitioners in Chinese communities have seen the value of such a special sick role and have created one within the boundaries of the professional medical subsystem. As we shall see in the next section, these EMs have important implications for medical and psychiatric care.

From what is already known about psychocultural aspects of illness among the Chinese, this case clearly illustrates a marked tendency to express emotional problems via somatic complaints (see Kleinman, 1975c; Lin, 1953; Rin et al., 1966; Solomon, 1971; Tseng, 1975b). This phenomenon of somatization is an example of the cultural patterning of the perception of, the affective response to, the cognizing of, and the communication of symptoms, and ultimately of the cultural construction of illness behavior. In my own research with patients with depression and anxiety neurosis in Taiwan, I have found that somatization in these cases relates to a tendency not to define and label dysphoric affects, but to perceive and know them in vague, psychologically naive terms. This is associated with a tendency to attend more to the somatic features of these states, which, in its most marked form results in a label being given only to the somatic component and not to features of the psychological state. Denial, displacement, and dissociation can all be shown to be active. (In Chinese shamanistic treatment, patients are encouraged to enter trance states during which the suppressed or dissociated affect is expressed, but in a culturally sanctioned way.) Similarly, patients with depression and anxiety will not hesitate to define in great detail the external interpersonal, family-based, work, and other social stresses associated with their problem, while denying or suppressing, or just showing much less interest in, and ability to define, their feelings.

Thus, even quite sophisticated Chinese strike Westerners as super-

SOCIAL AND CULTURAL CONTEXT

ficial, nonintrospective, and "enigmatic." Hsu (1971) has presented the most compelling interpretation of this remarkable culturally derived behavior. He attributes it to the fact that Chinese are socialized to place primary investment in family relationships, and also relationships with close friends, and much less investment in their own psychological identity and emotions, or in more distant interpersonal relationships. Thus, they do not acquire sophisticated perceptual, cognitive, and expressive psychological skills to analyze their affective states, but do acquire such skills to analyze their interpersonal situation. Moreover, Chinese are discouraged from expressing affects, including dysphoric affects, since these are considered potentially dangerous to finely balanced interpersonal relations and personal control (Solomon, 1971; Tseng and Hsu, 1969). To express such feelings, even to close friends and relatives, is often considered shameful behavior. And where strong emotions are expressed, they are often expressed only to close family members and friends, and not to doctors or others in distant relationships.

Accordingly, Chinese patients when depressed, for example, often present without feelings of sadness, guilt, and harsh self-criticism, all of which are common in Westerners suffering from depression (Yap, 1965). Most Chinese patients with mental illness go to medical clinics rather than psychiatric clinics. Even very disorderly and frankly bizarre behavior will be tolerated by the family, who prefer the label "eccentric" over the label "sick." Deviant behavior in Chinese culture often is labeled as physical illness in order to give it a legitimate social role. Finally, social stresses such as job failure are pointed to by Chinese as more stressful than many psychological stresses. Stress itself, then, is given a different meaning in Chinese culture. (For extensive coverage of the general issues of cultural patterning of causal factors, symptoms, illness behavior, and sick role, see Dohrenwend and Dohrenwend, 1974; Mechanic, 1972; Yap, 1975; Zola, 1966. Kagan and Levi (1974) have presented a sophisticated model of how cultural factors may play a role in etiology of disease and symptom onset.)

Hsu (1971) has argued that perhaps this Chinese pattern of intrapsychic and interpersonal relations can help correct the distortions produced in behavioral and social science by Western society's excessive valuation of intrapsychic experience and relative devaluation of the interpersonal sphere. He suggests that the Chinese viewpoint might help remove this Western cultural bias, and produce a less ethnocentric and more balanced view of human behavior and its pathologies. This is an example of how cross-cultural studies might help restructure psychological and psychiatric theory.

Further along the spectrum of the cultural patterning of symptoms are those disorders that have been claimed to be unique to

certain cultures. Mr. W.'s case is not an instance of such a
"culture-bound disease," but such disorders have been reported for
Chinese culture (Rin, 1965; Yap, 1975). Although some of these
disorders may be found in only one or a limited number of cultures,
most seem to be examples of marked social patterning of symptoms
of disorders that are universally distributed. In these disorders, it is
often claimed that the content of symptoms may vary (pathoplastic
effect), but the form of the symptoms are unchanging (pathogenetic
effect). Mr. W.'s case, and many others like it that I have studied,
however, raise serious questions as to whether this division can be
maintained. A clearer way of viewing such cases at present is to
distinguish the "emic" and "etic" EMs that are used to classify them,
and the different social and cultural circumstances under which EMs
are applied.

It has been estimated that in 1980 roughly one-fourth of the
world's population will be Chinese and over three-fourths will be
from non-Western cultures, yet the psychological understanding that
we possess in psychiatry, and that is used internationally, is based
largely on Western populations. The case presented above should
argue strongly for the need for cross-cultural psychiatry to advance
substantially our understanding of psychiatric diseases and illness
behavior in non-Western cultures.

There may be a danger, however, in taking an example from a
culture that is represented in our own society in very small numbers,
and that seems so very distinct from most American cultural
traditions. A Chinese example tends to suggest that in our own
culture these issues are esoteric and relatively unimportant, when in
truth they are central to the experience of many and perhaps most
patients. Ethnic beliefs make the EM framework important for
minority groups in the United States (Harwood, 1971; Snow, 1974).
Popular cultural beliefs about illness and treatment, and communicative discrepancies between distinct social groups, make it germane to
the mainstream of American culture. Cross-cultural experiences make
clinicians and researchers much more aware of the impact of these
cultural beliefs and social communication problems in our own
society, where they themselves may share such beliefs and participate
in some of the communicative difficulties. The tremendous specialization of knowledge, so marked in contemporary American and
Western European societies, and characteristic of the health care field,
increases the significance of these factors and lends itself to the EM
conceptual framework, since the social world of modern societies can
be regarded as an almost endless number of isolated EMs. The EM
framework should help to break through our habitual ethnocentrism
and scientific preoccupation with small, fragmented domains of
knowledge. The following cases are included to show how EMs affect

illness behavior in American culture. The cases were encountered in psychiatric consultation in a general medical setting (the medical wards and clinics of the Massachusetts General Hospital). They are extreme examples that led to problems in clinical care. The effect of culture is much wider, of course, producing the various normative integrations of scientific and popular concepts of appropriate sick role behavior which are basic ingredients of all illness experiences in our society (Elder, 1973; Mabry, 1964; Zborowski, 1952).

CASE 2 Mrs. F. is a 60-year-old white Protestant grandmother who is recovering from pulmonary edema secondary to atherosclerotic cardiovascular disease and chronic congestive heart failure on one of the medical wards at the Massachusetts General Hospital. Her behavior in the recovery phase of her illness is described as strange and annoying by the house staff and nurses. While her cardiac status has greatly improved and she has become virtually asymptomatic, she induces vomiting and urinates frequently in her bed. She becomes angry when told to stop these behaviors. As a result, psychiatric consultation has been requested.

Review of the lengthy medical record reveals nothing as to the personal significance of the patient's behavior. When queried about this behavior, and asked to explain why she is engaging in it and what meaning it has for her, the patient's response is most revealing. Describing herself as the wife and daughter of plumbers, the patient notes that she was informed by the medical team responsible for her care that she has "water in the lungs." She further reports that to her mind the physiology of the human body has the chest hooked up to two pipes, the mouth and the urethra. The patient explains that she has been trying to be helpful by helping to remove as much water from her chest as possible through self-induced vomiting and frequent urination. She analogized the latter to the work of the "water pills" she is taking, which she has been told are getting rid of the water in her chest. She concludes: "I can't understand why people are angry at me." After appropriate explanations, along with diagrams, she acknowledges that the "plumbing" of the body is remarkable and quite different from what she had believed. Her unusual behavior ended at that time.

CASE 3 Mr. G. is a 38-year-old university professor with chest pain diagnosed in a cardiology clinic as angina based on coronary artery disease. He has refused to accept this diagnosis, and has demanded that his cardiologist also reject this diagnosis and instead relate the problem to an imagined pulmonary embolus. The psychiatric consultant uncovers not a disease phobia as part of a neurotic disorder, but a popular explanatory model: the belief, shared by his wife and friends, that the development of angina signals the end of an active life style and the onset of invalidism. This patient is trying to prove that his cardiologist has made a mistake and that he has been mislabeled. Unfortunately, his cardiologist was not aware of this hidden explanatory model, and therefore could not attempt to correct or negotiate with it.

Cases such as these, which describe problems resulting from conflicting and undisclosed alternative explanatory models, and which do not represent psychopathology but socially and culturally constructed health belief systems even when they are idiosyncratic, are quite common. They frequently lead to noncompliance, failure to use health facilities, dissatisfaction with medical care, and because of this, poor medical care. Physicians are trained to be blind to the existence of other medical cognitive frameworks. They usually do not examine their patients' understanding of the explanations they give them, much less inquire into their patients' own explanations of illness and treatment. Yet, when these physicians leave the clinic and return to their homes, they too operate with different systems of explanation. When alternative beliefs and unexpected attitudes are uncovered, rarely do modern physicians attempt to discuss seriously and negotiate these alternative views. This seems to represent in the cognitive realm professional medicine's almost total domination of modern health care systems and its disregard for the often very different cognitive orientations of the other sectors of health care systems (see Freidson, 1970; Symposium on the Greater Medical Profession, 1973; Suchman, 1965). In our own society, as in modernizing societies, these sectors, along with their explanatory models, coexist, compete, and cooperate. The interactions that occur between these models, while of little concern thus far to practitioners, are of considerable importance to their patients, and help determine the real quality of health care, as we shall see below.

One corner of psychopathology seems to be much better understood from the standpoint of illness behavior and problems with conflicting (and hidden) explanatory models. That is the spectrum of disorders in which either the factitious production of illness or the inappropriate request to be labeled sick in the absence of demonstrable disease is a central issue. This is an inadequately conceptualized group of problems including hysterical conversion symptoms, hysteria with secondary gain, cases involving compensation, chronic functional complaints, hypochondriasis, Munchausen's syndrome, and malingering. This entire area is a morass of terminological and classificatory confusion. Nor is it clear how such patients are best managed.

The psychiatric clinician consulting with medical and surgical colleagues does not possess an adequate framework for understanding these problems and communicating that understanding to colleagues in primary care or to patients and their families. The psychoanalytic model, while helpful in unraveling some cases of conversion symptoms and their symbolic meaning, is inadequate to deal with this broad range of problems. It also is not very useful in dealing with the social and cultural dimensions of these disorders.

All of these problems concern illness behavior, the sick role, and the EM framework and can be reconceptualized in those terms in a clinically relevant way. Following Lipowski (1969), for example, we note that all illnesses are viewed by patients (and families) as threat, loss, gain, or of no consequence. Gain is best understood as the psychological and social benefits derived from the particular experience of illness and especially the sick role. We can think of gain as motivating illegitimate or inappropriate uses of the sick role. Frequently, the group of illnesses we have mentioned involves misuse or abuse of the sick role. For example, illness is feigned or the sick role claimed in order to gain economic reward, sanction failure, manipulate family members and others, communicate frustration and other psychosocial messages, sanction socially and culturally deviant roles (such as passive-dependent behavior in American society), and the like. Individuals will produce disease in order to experience illness behavior. Thus, several patients whom I have managed with chronic factitious illness experienced no pleasure or relief of anxiety from the actual induction of the illness, but considerable satisfaction from the impact of the self-induced illness on the image others held of them and they held of themselves. The sick role, once achieved, frees one of certain responsibilities and enables one to engage in activities otherwise proscribed (e.g., taking to bed).

However, the sick role usually does not simply come to one for the asking but requires social legitimation from family members, physicians, teachers, employers, etc. (Twaddle, 1974). Problems arise when the individual and others disagree about the social legitimation of behavior via the sick role, and these problems can be conceptualized by the EM framework. That is, when the patient employs an EM involving illness and the sick role while his family or physicians employ an EM that denies that illness is present or that considers the sick role inappropriate, we are in a situation often seen with chronic functional complaints, hypochondriasis, and malingering. On the other hand, when the patient EM does not accept the presence of illness or need for the sick role while the EMs of family or physicians call for the sick role and the labeling of illness, we are in the midst of what is often spoken of as denial, or are witnessing the inappropriate social labeling of illness (e.g., the labeling of social dissidents as schizophrenics in the Soviet Union).

Quite often, patient EMs concerning personal and social gain from the sick role are hidden, and must be systematically searched for by the psychiatric clinician, who then can attempt to explain these EMs to family members and medical personnel, or to change them, or to negotiate a settlement between the conflicting models and the parties holding them.

In this brief space, I cannot develop these notions more fully, but should point out that the EM framework gains further support from work such as that of George Kelly (1963) and his followers (Maher, 1969; Bannister and Fransella, 1974) and Beck 1971 on the impact of personal constructs and cognitive systems, respectively, on psychopathology and psychotherapy.

Systematic research into this subject is only now being carried out. For example, I am presently engaged in a comparative cross-cultural research project describing and comparing concepts of illness behavior, uses of the sick role, specific patterns of labeling behavior as deviant, and responses to particular illnesses in Chinese and American populations (Kleinman, 1975d). I have already mentioned some noteworthy differences between these populations, but the research project has documented large differences in almost all of these areas, differences that are now being analyzed statistically. In addition, similar though less dramatic differences are being documented for patients and families from various ethnic groups in the Boston area. It is hoped that this research will help isolate the cultural rules governing illness behavior in these different groups. Such knowledge would be important for primary care givers and psychiatric consultants working with these groups, for reasons already stated. In the next section, I will detail some of this research as it relates to doctor-patient interactions in medical and psychiatric care. I hope that in the future there will be large-scale ethnographic and comparative epidemiological studies defining and comparing illness behavior and popular EMs in a great variety of social and cultural settings. Such studies should yield data directly applicable to clinical care and teaching in major Western and non-Western societies, and especially in pluralistic societies such as the United States, among distinct ethnic and social groups. Providing such information and translating it into clinical practice would be a major contribution of social and cross-cultural psychiatry, and their social science supports, to both psychiatric care and general health care.

EXPLANATORY MODELS AND PSYCHIATRIC CARE

Earlier, I mentioned that interactions between practitioners and patients can be conceptualized in terms of the EMs they hold and transmit. The doctor-patient relationship (or any other practitioner-patient relationship) can be described as EM_1 (patient explanatory model) $\leftrightarrow$ EM_2 (medical explanatory model). These models can be compared for the five components previously mentioned; that is, beliefs about etiology, onset of symptoms, pathophysiology, course of illness, and treatment regimen. A crude scoring system can then be applied; for example, where two EMs have five components that are congruent and none that are incongruent, the distance between these cognitive models is very small or minimal: 0. Whereas if all five components are incongruent, the distance is very large or maximal: 5. This distance can be determined for EM_1 and EM_2 in any given clinical encounter before doctor and patient actually interact. That initial distance (distance A) is a measure of model discrepancy, or similarity, between practitioner and patient. If the EM transmitted from doctor to patient is then also recorded, and subsequently the patient is asked for his or her EM (that is, the EM following the doctor-patient transaction), a distance can be obtained that measures the discrepancy between these two models. That distance (distance B) is a crude measure of communication between doctor and patient. Successful (or effective) communication in doctor-patient relationships can be very roughly quantified in this fashion and represented by distance B being equal to or less than distance A. When distance A is smaller than distance B, that would roughly measure ineffective clinical communication.

Our research to date has demonstrated that effective communication in a wide range of health care relationships can indeed be measured in this way. We also have the strong impression (now being statistically evaluated) that such effective communication correlates with improved patient compliance and greater patient satisfaction. In addition, studies are being conducted to determine whether effective communication in health care is at all related to improvement in course of illness and treatment outcomes.

A number of factors affect the interaction between EM_1 and EM_2. These include the intensity with which EMs are held, the skill with which they are communicated, whether hidden EMs are uncovered and dealt with, the actual content of EMs, and various key sociocultural factors like ethnic differences and social distance between practitioners and patients. These all act as predictor variables affecting the efficiency of communication and the efficacy of health care.

Most clinicians still look upon the doctor-patient relationship wrongly as the passive transfer of information from expert to client. Modern doctors rarely elicit patient EMs, nor do patients in modern medical care settings usually feel free to relate their own explanatory models. Clinicians may also be unaware that they themselves often shift between distinctly different explanatory models (Lazare, 1973), and that what they actually explain to patients is often quite different from what they think they explain. Where physicians do bother to elicit, analyze, and negotiate with patient EMs, the evidence suggests that problems in clinical communication are reduced and care is facilitated (Lazare, 1974). Interestingly enough, folk practitioners, as is well documented in the anthropological literature, frequently elicit and discuss their patient's EMs, and in such indigenous treatment settings, patients usually feel freer about spontaneously disclosing their own EMs. Indeed, it would seem that from the EM standpoint, such traditional folk medical interactions are generally characterized by better practitioner-patient communication than modern health care relationships, independent of the quality of technical care. The implications of this are considerable, and will be discussed later.

The practitioner-patient relationship is an interaction process, and as such is well conceptualized by a model used to understand the analogous process of translating from one language to another. Nida (Nida and Taber, 1969; Nida, 1974) has described the translational process in five stages: elicitation, analysis, transfer, restructuring, and feedback. Following his terminology, we have seen that elicitation and analysis are infrequently performed by physicians. Similarly transfer, restructuring, and feedback are operations performed by and large only by patients and their families. Contemporary health care has so slighted communication, however, that patients may be forced to actively elicit explanations from clinicians who pay insufficient attention to communication. Patients and families may also find that they are frequently forced to analyze difficult, highly technical, jargonistic communications that may present very real problems for popular (lay) analysis. Having transferred EM_2 to their own indigenous medical belief system or language, patients and families restructure EM_2 in terms of EM_1.

We empirically found four different types of restructured patient EMs following practitioner-patient interactions. These we have called explanatory interaction outcomes (EMIOs). They include: (1) systematic distortion of EM_2 in favor of EM_1 ($EM_1 > EM_2$) such that some or most of the five EM components are congruent with EM_1 and discrepant with EM_2. In this case, the patients hold only one EM which they are unable to divide into indigenously derived and medically derived parts. Preliminary evidence suggests that such distortions make up almost half of all EMIOs, and that they increase over time; (2) the patients hold two distinct and readily separable EMs ($EM_1 + EM_2$), such that they can say which are the indigenously derived and which are the medically derived components; (3) virtually complete loss of one of the EMs, most usually EM_2, such that the patients report only one EM, usually EM_1; (4) the appearance of a new EM (EM_3), which represents something more than just a combination of EM_1 and EM_2. It is the incorporation of new medical knowledge. New knowledge may come from family members, friends, other practitioners, books, etc.

Rarely are physicians aware that restructuring is taking place. They almost never discover EMIOs unless these lead to gross and obvious problems in clinical care. Feedback occurs when patients move from practitioner-patient interactions back to the context of family or community, or on to other practitioner-patient transactions (professional or folk). Such feedback can produce significant changes in patient EMs, such as EM_3, mentioned above. Discrepancies between patient and family EMs often result in major problems for medical and psychiatric care.

The impact of patient EMs on those of clinicians is poorly understood and remains virtually unstudied. However, sensitive and skillful clinicians probably make use of this impact to adjust their interactions with particular patients in the service of good care. We also have a very incomplete appreciation of how clinicians transform their theoretical EMs (EM_{2a}) into the clinical explanations actually given to patients (EM_{2b}). This is a subject perhaps best described as practical clinical rationality. Though of considerable importance to medical and psychiatric care, it is a subject that is not being systematically studied by, nor taught to, practitioners of primary care.

Quite obviously, those who give, and teach, psychiatric care are usually much more centrally concerned with communication and especially explanatory interactions than are others in the health care field. In fact, the EM model would seem quite suited for studying psychotherapy. Psychotherapy might be considered, in part, a process in which EMs can be systematically elicited and studied by both patient and practitioner, and in which more adaptive and personally and socially appropriate EMs can be learned. The work of Bannister and Fransella (1974) supports the view that where patient and practitioner EMs are in apparent harmony, therapy progresses more effectively and quickly than where they are discrepant. It also supports attempts to determine differences between practitioner and patient EMs when psychotherapy is unsuccessful, since efforts of this sort (using the Repertory Grid test) seem to have been effective in promoting therapeutic progress.

But if what we have been saying seems to support the usefulness of the EM framework for understanding and facilitating psychotherapy, we should also note that a great deal of psychotherapy involves views essentially opposed to this framework, since patient and popular EMs are often given little regard by psychiatrists which frequently leads to the same problems as those occurring in general medical care.

I should like to summarize some of the hypotheses that the EM framework generates for health care in general as well as for psychiatric care, and in so doing point out what evidence there is in favor of, or against, these hypotheses. Even though, as we shall see, research findings are still quite limited, this framework receives provisional support as useful for doing clinical research on basic aspects of medical and psychiatric care, aspects of care that heretofore have been largely ignored or inadequately studied.

The EM framework predicts that where distance A is large in practitioner-patient relationships, as in cases where there are significant differences in the cultural beliefs and social status between patients and practitioners, and where distance B remains large, health care outcomes will be poor. The large literature on compliance supports this prediction, as does our current cross-cultural research project, but the evidence for patient satisfaction and especially for impact on course of illness and treatment outcome is still inadequate (see Becker et al., 1974; Davis, 1968; Francis et al., 1969; Haefner and Kirscht, 1970). Conversely, where patients and practitioners share virtually the same social status and cultural background, and where this is reflected in a smaller distance A and an even smaller distance B, health care outcomes should be improved. Again, the studies just cited as well as the work I am involved in support this hypothesis, at least for patient compliance. This hypothesis also suggests that efforts to reduce distances A and B, for example, through patient education, use of indigenous health practitioners and other kinds of health care auxiliaries from the same social and cultural background as patients, and by training practitioners to systematically elicit and respond to patient EMs, should lead to improved health care outcomes. Work by Cartwright (1964), Francis et al., (1969), Harwood (1971), Kane et al. (1974), Lazare (1974), Ley and Spelman (1967), and Stimson (1974) supports this hypothesis. An interesting proviso that has yet to be adequately tested is that those interventions that reduce both distances A and B, or distance B only, should have better results than those that reduce distance A alone; and, therefore, among the interventions mentioned, patient education should be less effective than those interventions involving active elicitation and negotiations with patients regarding EMs. This point, should it prove correct, is an important one, since much of the present thrust in improving the communicative aspect of health care is in the direction of simply increasing patient information via one-way education from health experts to health consumers. Our model suggests that this paradigm may be inadequate and may, in fact, create new problems for medical and psychiatric care.

The clinical cases presented above add support to another hypothesis generated by the EM framework: communicative problems in clinical care result from large distances A and B, and these problems (1) can be predicted by measures of those critical distances and (2) should respond to interventions that narrow those distances. My own clinical experience in consultative psychiatry leads me to believe that many problems in clinical care for which psychiatric consultation is requested relate to these cognitive and communicative discrepancies. The EM framework can be used as a clinical guide for locating and responding to such problems.

A hypothesis currently being evaluated is that psychotherapy, and the psychotherapeutic aspects of medical care (traditional and modern), may be effective largely because the difference between EM_1 (or EMIO) and EM_2 decreases significantly. Research by Bannister and Fransella (1974), Frank (1974), and Tseng (1975a) suggests that something of this kind in fact happens. This framework then appears useful to evaluate and compare different kinds of psychotherapy, especially in the context of general health care. We are studying this subject with regard to the treatment of patients with somatization and various underlying psychological problems in Taiwan by Western-style (general medical and psychiatric), Chinese-style, and folk practitioners.

A closely related hypothesis still to be tested is that the effectiveness of health professionals in handling the communicative tasks of clinical management should be testable by obtaining evidence that distance B is smaller than distance A. Conversely, the lack of effectiveness in these communicative tasks should also be demonstrable. (Later we shall suggest that this would seem applicable to teaching communicative skills and strategies to practitioners of primary medical and psychiatric care.)

Finally, this research approach allows for systematic analysis of the cognitive and communicative interactions taking place between different subsystems of health care systems, and for systematic cross-cultural comparisons between different health care systems, traditional and modern. And the approach can be a practical framework for studying the impact of social development and cultural change on these microscopic aspects of clinical care, in contrast to most other studies of this sort, which tend to illuminate only the macroscopic issues that are far removed from clinical practice.

At this point, clinical examples might help make these issues clearer.

Case 1, described above, illustrates the wide boundaries and multiple components of the pluralistic health care system of which Mr. W. is a part. This patient's initial health care resource was self-treatment, and it remained a very important aspect of his care throughout the course of his illness. When this failed to work effectively, Mr. W. turned pragmatically to .another part of the popular cultural health domain, the family and community-based beliefs and practices available to Chinese-Americans, reflecting in large part traditional Chinese medicine but including as well elements of the mainstream American popular culture's health domain. This also was an important ongoing aspect of his care. Again when he failed to receive full symptomatic relief from this component of his health care system, Mr. W. resorted to professional medical care. Had there been local practitioners of classical Chinese medicine or of Chinese folk medical forms immediately available to him, Mr. W. would have been able to choose (as Chinese patients in Taiwan, Hong Kong, Singapore, and the P.R.C. can) between alternative professional and folk medical institutions. He did not include within his range of alternative health care institutions, however, American folk healing forms, which were available locally but which were not viewed by him as potential resources for care. Mr. W. maintained his empirical orientation while a patient in the modern scientific medical care institutional setting. He saw professional medical care as only one, and not necessarily the most important, component of his health care system. He was prepared to resort to still other treatment forms if he did not receive symptomatic relief there. (Indeed, he continued other treatments while receiving a modern psychotropic agent.) But he was also guided by culturally sanctioned rules concerning the kind of problem he had, the appropriate treatment alternatives, the hierarchy of resort to these alternatives, and the manner in which these agencies were to be evaluated, which provided a logical direction to his movement between the various components of the health care system.

Mr. W. was unhappy with the care he received in the medical clinic because he failed to receive treatment and also because he was not given a meaningful explanation of his problem. This difficulty, which could have led Mr. W. to drop out of this treatment system altogether or to fail to comply with his medical regimen before he received adequate care, occurred in part because he and his physician held very different expectations of the communicative process in the doctor-patient relationship. Fortunately, Mr. W. was acculturated to a sufficient degree to enable him to shift his expectations somewhat and to use technologically based medical care appropriately. I could have reported other examples in which this unfortunately did not occur.

One could very well apply an ecological model to look at the "external" and "internal" factors that influenced Mr. W.'s health care choices and decisions. I have concerned msyelf almost entirely with cultural factors, but one could also look at political, geographic, social class, and "internal" health care system factors that made the course of

Mr. W.'s care very different in Boston from that of other Bostonians and from what his care would have been like in Taipei or Peking.

The Chinese cultural EM that guided the approach to health care of Mr. W. and his family states that "wind" and "cold" disorders are not very effectively treated by modern scientific medicine, but are best treated by traditional Chinese medicines. It is not the talking or supportive aspect of the latter, but the medicines themselves that are felt to be effective. Thus, such patients are often discouraged by their indigenous EMs from seeking help from modern medical care institutions and from Caucasian practitioners. Since Chinese patients often have little understanding of modern psychiatric care, believe that talk therapy by itself is valueless for any problem and does not justify payment, fear being labeled mentally ill, and have a thorough-going psychosomatic and somatopsychic conceptual framework in which great stress is put on bodily problems producing psychological problems that should disappear when the underlying physical problem is successfully treated, it is not surprising that Chinese patients infrequently turn to psychiatrists. In psychotherapy, they expect to be treated also with medicinal agents, and perhaps to have their pulse and blood pressure checked, and they operate under strong cultural sanctions against delving deeply into intrapsychic matters, which makes insight-oriented therapy difficult (cf. Tseng, 1975a; Gaw, 1975). Chinese communities in Asia essentially do without modern psycho-therapy; what they do possess are culturally legitimated forms of indigenous psychotherapy, such as that provided by shamans, fortune-tellers, and religious healing rituals. These treatment forms were, of course, unavailable to Mr. W. in the United States. Finally, Chinese cultural EMs hold that it is proper to make use of several different treatment agents at the same time. Indeed, Mr. W. continued his herbal medicines while taking a Western antidepressant medicine, because he relied upon a traditional Chinese EM that holds that Chinese herbs can refine the effects of Western medicine and can reduce its propensity to produce dangerous side effects. These and other culturally-based beliefs significantly altered Mr. W.'s health care. Thus, his EM led him to evaluate the quality and efficacy of his care from a viewpoint quite different from that of his physicians. This could easily have become the basis for very real problems with the management of his illness, as indeed it does for numerous patients whose EMs concerning the determinants of therapeutic efficacy differ from those of their doctors (Kleinman, 1973b).

Cases 2 and 3, presented above, illustrate both that large distances A and B cause problems for clinical care, and that reducing distance B resolves these problems. Several additional brief case descriptions should illustrate the patterns of interactions between explanatory models and their results (EMIOs), as well as the practical significance of these results in the management of chronic illness. Although the cases are taken from research involving patients with heart disease, I think most psychiatrists will quickly recognize similar situations among patients being treated for psychiatric disorders.

CASE 4 (EM_1 + EM_2) A 39-year-old white married truck driver with three children, suffering from his second documented myocardial infarction, who has a strong family history of this disorder and abnormal serum lipids, reports two models of the etiology of his heart disorder: it has a hereditary component (medical model given to him, EM_2); and it is unrelated to the other cases of heart disease in his family but instead results from past amphetamine abuse (his own model, EM_1). The patient holds both models, can explain each accurately, and admits uncertainty as to which he has more faith in. The medical model has clearly disturbed him because of its implication for his own children, while his own model does not carry the threatening implication. The patient's compliance with his medical regimen varies in relation to these models: he feels less motivated to comply the more he believes in EM_2, since it suggests to him that no matter what he does, he is unable to control the onset and course of his illness. EM_1, on the other hand, stresses his own responsibility for his illness and suggests an active treatment role for the patient.

CASE 5 (EM_1 > EM_2) A 58-year-old single white male machinist of Protestant New England family background is recovering from an uncomplicated myocardial infarction. The patient was raised by his maternal aunt, who was a practicing osteopath. His paternal uncle was a clinical professor of medicine, famous for his diagnostic skills. Most of the patient's work life has been as an inspector of machine parts, an activity he analogizes to medical diagnosis. At the time of hospitalization, and before receiving any medical explanations, the patient held the following model of heart disease: it involves tear or rupture of the heart muscle due to stress, strain, and hypertension (EM_1). Recovery involves healing of the rupture and mechanical restoration of the heart muscle so that the heart can function as a pump. The patient is critical of the initial care he received in the emergency room, since he was sent home with a diagnosis of angina pectoris during a bout of chest pain that preceded his infarction, and because a complete diagnostic work-up was not performed. He compared this to shoddy work done by some machine inspectors. His cardiologist gave him a rather full explanation of his disease and its treatment (EM_2), emphasizing a stress model of its cause and the importance of rest and a slow return to less strenuous work as part of the treatment program. Twenty-four hours later, the patient can recall the entire explanation accurately. Several weeks later, at the time of discharge, the patient reports the following model, which represents a systematic distortion of EM_2 in favor of his original model. (On home visit one month after that, the distortion was even greater.) Heart disease, including his own, is caused by stress, especially hard work. In his own case, heavy labor, which he performed along with his machinist work, apparently was too much for his heart, causing the muscle to pull apart. Now it must heal with formation of a scar. He reports that he cannot go back to heavy labor, or to work that is too much of an emotional strain, since he has hypertension, too much tension, which increases the strain on the heart ($EM_1 > EM_2$). The various explanations used by the patient show the strong influence of family beliefs, which in his case included a mechanical osteopathic model of illness, stressing the impact of strain and tension, high valuation of diagnosis, and devaluation of physical labor as an occupation for family members. The patient's definition of his sick role followed from these beliefs.

CASE 6 (EM_1 or EM_2 alone) A 56-year-old Italian-American former railroad conductor, who is recovering from an acute myocardial infarction in the Coronary Care Unit of the Massachusetts General Hospital, had been evaluated in the same facility two years before for chest pain. At that time, his cardiologist gave him a full explanation of the etiology, pathophysiology, and course of atherosclerotic cardiovascular disease (EM_2). The patient now reports a rather different model of his problem, one that he has never told his cardiologist about, even though it is his chief belief about his illness and was so at the time of his last admission. In his view and that of his family (EM_1), there are two major heart diseases: angina pectoris and coronary thrombosis. The former is mild and self-limited. Since he believes that the former and the latter are *mutually exclusive*, so that to suffer from the milder one is to have the good fortune not to have to worry about experiencing the more severe and dangerous one, he justifies his almost complete failure to comply with his medical regimen on logical grounds understood and supported by his family, who have shared his denial of serious illness.

In order to demonstrate the relevance of the EM framework for psychiatric care, and also its potential as a method for obtaining a much more sophisticated appreciation of the crucial social factors that frequently operate in the treatment of psychiatric patients, I shall briefly discuss a research project involving psychiatric inpatients.

This study was conducted on the inpatient psychiatric unit at the Massachusetts General Hospital from September 1972 through January 1973. The study, which is presently being prepared for publication, began with an ethnographic description of the explanations used by staff members (psychiatrists, psychiatric nurses, nursing aids, and social workers) and patient members of the therapeutic milieu, which the ward functioned as at that time, to justify discharge of patients from the ward. This description was obtained by systematically recording over a one-month period the explanations used to rationalize whether particular patients were to be discharged or were to remain on the ward. These explanations were given by both staff members and patients in the daily ward meetings during which individual cases were discussed by the entire community. From these explanations, I was able to construct a list of ten rules that were most frequently used to assess whether patients were to be discharged or not. These rules, or criteria for discharge, form an articulated set of values by which patient behavior was evaluated: discharge was seen as a "good" that had to be achieved. The therapeutic milieu made explicit use of this value system as a set of polar terms (positively and negatively valued) that were used by staff and patients to judge the behavior of patients. When a patient's behavior was viewed as meeting these requirements, he or she was labeled by the milieu as ready for discharge, which in turn was taken to be equivalent to successfully treated or "cured."

These behavioral rules stated that a given patient should demonstrate: (1) that he/she was able to express his/her feelings; (2) that he was actively working on resolving the problems that had brought him to the hospital; (3) that he was responsible for his personal behavior and was exercising that responsibility; (4) that he was an active participant in the therapeutic milieu; (5) that he showed concern for, and was able to share with, other members of the community; (6) that he was able to confront others about their problems and be confronted by others about his own problems, especially in the large group meetings; (7) that he was making active plans regarding his life after discharge, especially plans for employment; (8) that he recognized his family as both part of his problems and necessary for their resolution; (9) that he could identify some specific change in values and/or behavior that had occurred during his hospitalization; and (10) that in general he viewed the future (i.e., his life after discharge) in more positive terms, and in particular viewed his own life circumstance more positively, than when he had been admitted. These rules were reflected in a large number of polar terms used by both patients and staff to approve or disapprove of individual behavior, including: manipulating/sharing; out of control/in control; responsible/irresponsible; trusting/distrusting; honest/dishonest; open/

closed to others; expressing feelings to others/hiding feelings.

All admissions to this inpatient unit over a six-week period who were not acutely psychotic (after seventy-two hours following admission), demented, or retarded (N = 20) were interviewed during their first, fourth, and final weeks of hospitalization. Average length of stay for this group of patients was six weeks, and this was also the average length of stay of all patients on the ward during the period of this study. During these interviews, patients were asked to explain the criteria for discharge from the unit. The same interview format and questions were used in all interviews.

Findings revealed the following: (1) The ward possessed an organized, coherent set of explanations justifying or rationalizing discharge, which were very frequently articulated and repeatedly demonstrated not as an abstract set of guidelines but as terms used to evaluate specific cases. (2) Patients entered the ward milieu with little or no understanding of these explanations. During the first week of hospitalization, the patients in our sample were able to report an average of less than three of the rules listed above; and they also frequently reported rules that in fact did not apply in this milieu. (3) After approximately four weeks of hospitalization, almost all patients could report most of the chief explanations of discharge. That is nineteen out of twenty patients were able to give at least seven of the ten chief rules; fifteen were able to give eight out of ten; and twelve reported all ten. (4) By the time of their discharge, most patients studied (fifteen out of twenty) could articulate nearly all of these explanations (nine out of ten). (5) At that time most patients (seventeen out of twenty) were able to justify why their own behavior did or did not fit the criteria for discharge: fourteen patients used these explanations to justify discharge, and three patients used them to justify remaining in the hospital. (6) Staff explanations were congruent with patient explanations regarding the discharge of members of this group in all but two cases. In those two cases, patient behavior was felt not to reflect the values these patients espoused. (7) Follow-up via home visits of a small subset of these patients (N = 5) revealed that by six weeks after discharge, three patients were able to report an average of less than five explanations per patient, and all five patients included other explanations that did not belong to the list.

These findings suggest that the therapeutic process in this psychiatric inpatient setting can be described by an alternative model of social learning of a system of rules concerning discharge instead of by the traditional explanatory model of psychiatric healing (or therapeutic efficacy). Being discharged from this ward was almost always automatically equated with therapeutic success by staff and patients. Discharge clearly involved the acquisition and competent use of the therapeutic milieu's ideology. Expressed in the terms used in this chapter, therapeutic efficacy meant the learning of a particular explanatory model—one that was constructed differently from the medical models we have talked about, but that nonetheless followed the same general rules of providing meaning for the illness experience and a means for evaluating treatment. Admittedly, this is an exaggeration of what usually takes place in psychiatric care, but I would argue that such an exaggerated instance gives us insight into the important but unrecognized functions of EMs in both psychiatric and general health care. Such EMs help structure the experience of illness and the criteria for evaluating care, such that the EMs of a given health care system (1) bring the socially constructed experiences of illness and treatment into close approximation, (2) involve an active interchange between popular, professional, and folk systems, and (3) frequently include a process of social learning. But this example also implies that power to make one EM predominant in a particular health care context is what determines both the significance attributed to illness behavior and how healing is evaluated. We do not usually think of power and the struggle for explanatory model dominance in health care systems. Yet this conflict for power assumes many different forms in health care: professional dominance (as in the case of the EMs of psychoanalysts over those of the medical model advocates in an earlier period in psychiatry, or of those of biologically-oriented psychiatrists over those of social workers with social rehabilitation orientation); political ideological dominance (as in examples given above from the Soviet Union and the P.R.C.); and social structural dominance (as in situations where one of the three sectors of the health care system—professional, folk, popular—imposes its EMs on the system as a whole).

Any analysis of health care and psychiatric care, whether conducted at the level of an entire system of care or at the level of individual practitioner-patient relationships, that does not take these factors into account is inadequate. Most studies of health care have not sufficiently examined these issues. These social issues, which are illuminated by the EM framework, show that social science has much to contribute to a better understanding of psychiatric care and general health care.

CONCLUSION: IMPLICATIONS FOR THE TRAINING OF PSYCHIATRISTS AND PRIMARY HEALTH CARE PRACTITIONERS

The preceding sections of this chapter should suggest the value of the explanatory models approach for clinical psychiatric practice and for psychiatric research. This is but one example of a social science framework applied to psychiatric concerns. Other frameworks need to be developed and applied. But the main thrust of my argument has not been simply to present a particular framework, but instead to use that framework as an example of the need to elaborate psychiatry's social science base into conceptual frameworks that can be applied directly to clinical practice, research, and, perhaps most important, teaching.

I have used the explanatory models approach to teach social and cross-cultural psychiatry to medical students, psychiatry residents, and also students of anthropology. It has proved to be a simple and easily used framework that lends itself to clinical case discussions as well as to didactic teaching. I have found that it helps students to understand basic social science concepts that are directly relevant to psychiatry, and it provides clinicians with a means of ordering, communicating, and responding to key social and cultural issues in clinical care.

The EM framework provides a clinical language for talking about psychosocial and cultural issues in general health care; and as such it is a valuable addition to the skills of the psychiatric consultant in the general medical setting and to the psychiatric teacher involved in teaching medical students about psychosocial aspects of medical and surgical care.

Here is an example of how psychiatry might begin to elaborate a behavioral and social science language for translating relevant aspects of those sciences into frameworks that can be used by clinicians, students, and researchers. Obviously, more refined and inclusive frameworks need to be developed. What I have presented is only a tentative first step. That more steps in the same direction are called for seems clear. Whether such steps will be forthcoming, at least from psychiatry, remains uncertain. This challenge, however, seems to me to be a chief one facing contemporary psychiatry. It is an indication of the type of theoretical and research work that critical rationality demands of psychiatric science. The same critical rational direction in psychiatry requires rethinking of all the different subdisciplines of contemporary psychiatry; and that rethinking must take place within the limits of each of those disciplines and must occur prior to attempts at integrating those distinct forms of knowledge into universal theories of human behavior. No area within psychiatry requires a more basic reconceptualization than social and cross-cultural psychiatry. No general, integrating theory in psychiatry can be constructed that is not based on the structure of applied knowledge that results from that reconceptualization. This chapter is intended to be a prologue to that large task.

In closing, I should like to suggest some direct implications of this approach for the training of primary care practitioners and psychiatric residents. First, the education of medical students must include more than a general introductory course on social and behavioral sciences, important as such an introductory course is. Social and behavioral sciences approaches to clinical problems should be taught to medical students as vital components of such learning experiences as the introductory course to clinical medicine, the general teaching of clinical care in the clinics and on the wards, and in the different specialty areas. As such, it should *not* be presented as a separate field or approach, but should be intimately integrated with general clinical teaching around *specific* clinical problems. The same demands need to be made on clinical teachers of behavioral and social sciences as those made on clinical pharmacologists and other specialists. They should be part of the clinical teaching team, along with clinical teachers of medicine and psychiatry. This is the proper stimulus to force teachers of social and behavioral sciences to make their knowledge clinically relevant and practically useful. In order to accomplish this, I believe that such people must themselves be clinicians. That is, they must be physicians or psychiatrists (with special training) who are actively engaged in clinical care. Such clinicians can teach medical students, interns, and residents who train in the context of primary care in a way that social and behavioral scientists cannot, at least at present. But it is also possible that through special clinical training, behavioral and social scientists in the future might perform this task just as well as their clinical colleagues.

Therefore, another important implication is that we must train a generation of clinical teachers of social and behavioral sciences. There are many ways to achieve this end. For example, fellowship programs might be developed for internists and psychiatrists during which they could spend one year in academic work in social and behavioral sciences under the guidance of experts in medically applied anthropology, sociology, and other relevant fields. Then they might spend a second year applying what they have learned in clinical research, practice, and teaching, again under the guidance of experts in the behavioral and social sciences who themselves have had clinical involvement. Alternatively, such clinicians might enter academic degree programs (M.A. and Ph.D.) in medical anthropology and medical sociology. But, unlike the present system, such programs must be restructured toward a central concern with clinical issues. At present, a number of universities in the United States are experimenting with such degree programs, and with building clinical experience into their teaching, but the support for these programs is inadequate, and no general training approach has yet been agreed upon. What I am arguing for is the development of a clinical social science.

Finally, social and behavioral sciences clinical instruction must be brought to the level of residency training. This is especially true in the training of primary care physicians and psychiatrists. I believe that an appropriate training approach for both groups should involve both academic and clinical instructions. The model I have sketched for medical students can also be used for residents in primary care programs, but seminar work would also be desirable so that the depth of knowledge would be greater in the appropriate behavioral and social science literature. Moreoever, it is very desirable that primary care residents have some experience with research that chiefly involves behavioral and social sciences concepts and techniques.

Of all clinicians, I think that psychiatrists require the largest amount of instruction in these fields. Psychiatric residency programs need to have this instruction built in at several levels. There should be a general course in the behavioral and social sciences foundations of psychiatry required of all psychiatrists in the first year of their training. This should involve primarily seminar work organized around some of the concepts covered in this chapter, as well as many others that relate directly to psychiatric issues, and should include involvement with behavioral and social sciences literature. Psychiatric residents should then receive clinical supervision in these fields from teams of clinicians and social scientists or, where available, from psychiatrists specially trained in the social sciences. These supervisory experiences should relate to outpatient and inpatient care, and to psychiatric evaluation, psychotherapy, and community involvements. These teaching interventions should bring social and cross-cultural psychiatry into the mainstream of psychiatric residency teaching, and should be integrated with general residency training in all aspects of clinical work. For those residents with special interests in the social and behavioral aspects of psychiatry, advanced training in these fields as well as in research and teaching opportunities should be made available. Social and cross-cultural psychiatry should not be taught as a separate subject but should be fully integrated into the general training experiences of residents, as suggested above.

More narrowly, the explanatory model approach, discussed above with respect to its clinical and research aspects, might be looked upon as an example of how behavioral and social sciences concepts can be translated into clinical teaching. It can be used to teach medical students and primary care residents how best to communicate with patients and to analyze health care problems that result from faulty clinical communication. Indeed, measuring distances A and B, and relating these distances to simple measures of health care outcomes, can be used as a means of objectifying and grading effective clinical communication. This approach can also be used to isolate specific problems of students and residents, and to evaluate the success of teaching on these same concrete issues.

In the training of psychiatric residents, the EM framework can most readily be taught as an approach for consulting psychiatrists. Obviously, it also lends itself to conceptualizing and applying much of social and cross-cultural psychiatry to contemporary problems in psychiatric care and in general health care, which afterall were among the chief purposes for developing this framework. It can be used as a method for teaching about communication in psychotherapy and in other kinds of practitioner-patient relationships in psychiatric care generally. Moreover, at the risk of claiming too much, I would suggest the EM framework is a model for the kinds of critical behavioral and social sciences approaches that can be elaborated to teach other areas of psychiatry as well, such as comparing systems of psychotherapy and models of psychiatric illness. That is, at a time when psychiatric science, and especially its clinical aspects, are not and seemingly cannot be integrated into a single unifying system, but rather are a field filled with heterogeneous concepts and methods, the EM framework is a quite useful and rather simple means of organizing this disparate material for teaching purposes. Such an organization does not attempt to unify what is presently the ununifiable, fragmented domain of psychiatric theory. Instead the EM framework allows that material to be presented as the bundle of heterogeneous bits of information that it is, while taking away some of the dread of confronting this kind of complex and chaotic knowledge because it provides a practical framework for comparing and making clinical use of much of this material. Although the explanatory model approach described in this chapter is still somewhat crude and not nearly inclusive enough, I believe further attempts in the same direction, but probably of rather different kinds, will prove significant as vehicles for teaching residents in psychiatry as it now exists and probably will exist for some time. Nor should this be surprising, since the explanatory model approach, and behavioral and social sciences approaches generally, must take as an appropriate subject the explanatory concepts and language of psychiatry itself.

REFERENCES

Ahern, E. 1975. Sacred and secular medicine in a Taiwan village: a study of cosmological disorder. *In* Medicine in Chinese Cultures: Comparative Studies of Health Care in Chinese and Other Societies, A. Kleinman et al., eds. Bethesda, Md.: Fogarty International Center, N.I.H; 91–114.

Bannister, D., and F. Fransella. 1974. Inquiring Man: The Theory of Personal Constructs. Baltimore: Penguin Books.

Beck, A. 1971. Cognition, affect and psychopathology. Archives of General Psychiatry 24:495–500.

Becker, M., 1974. A new approach to explaining sick-role behavior in low-income populations. American Journal of Public Health 64:205–216.

Bennett, R., and E. Sanchez. 1973. Psychopathology or deviance: treatment or intervention? *In* Psychopathology, M. Hammer et al., eds. New York: Wiley.

Berlin, B. 1973. General principles of classification and nomenclature in folk biology. American Anthropologist 75:214-242.

Berry, J., and F. Dasen. 1974. Culture and Cognition: Readings in Cross-Cultural Psychology. London: Methuen.

Cancain, F. 1971. New methods for describing what people think. Sociological Inquiry 41:85.

Cartwright, A. 1964. Human Relations and Hospital Care. London: Routledge and Kegan Paul.

Colby, B. 1975. Culture grammars. Science 187(4180):913-919.

Davis, M. 1968. Variations in patients' compliance with doctors' advice. American Journal of Public Health 58:274-288.

Dohrenwend, B., and B. Dohrenwend. 1974. Social and cultural influences on psychopathology. Annual Review of Psychology 25:417-451.

Elder, R. 1973. Social class and lay explanations of the etiology of arthritis. Journal of Health and Social Behavior 14:28.

Engelhardt, H. T. 1974. Explanatory models in medicine. Texas Reports on Biology and Medicine 32:225-239.

Fabrega, H. 1971. Some features of Zinecantecan medical knowledge. Ethnology 9:25-43.

_____. 1974. Disease in Relation to Social Behavior. Cambridge, Mass.: MIT Press.

Frake, C. 1961. The diagnosis of disease among the Subanum of Mindanao. American Anthropologist 63:113-132.

Francis, V. et al. 1969. Gaps in doctor and patient communication: patients' response to medical advice. New England Journal of Medicine 280:535-540.

Frank, J. 1974. Persuasion and Healing. 2nd ed. Baltimore: Johns Hopkins University Press.

Freidson, E. 1970. Profession of Medicine: A Study of the Sociology of Applied Knowledge. New York: Dodd, Mead.

Garfinkel, H. 1967. Studies in Ethnomethodology. Englewood Cliffs, N.J.: Prentice-Hall.

Gaw, A. 1975. An integrated approach in the delivery of health care to a Chinese community in America. *In* Medicine in Chinese Cultures: Comparative Studies of Health Care in Chinese and Other Societies, A. Kleinman et al., eds. Bethesda, Md.: Fogarty International Center, NIH., pp. 327-349.

Gove, W. 1975. The labelling of deviance. New York: Wiley.

Haefner, D., and J. Kirscht. 1970. Motivational and behavioral effects of modifying health beliefs. Public Health Reports. 85:478-485.

Harwood, A. 1971. The hot-cold theory of disease: implications for treatment of Puerto Rican patients. Journal of the American Medical Association 216:1153-1158.

Horton, R. 1967. African traditional thought and Western science. Africa 27:50-71.

Hsu, F. L. K. 1971. Psychosocial homeostasis and *Jen*: conceptual tools for advancing psychological anthropology. American Anthropologist 73:23-44.

Jahoda, G. 1969. The Psychology of Superstition. Baltimore: Penguin Books.

Jessor, R., 1968. Society, Personality and Deviant Behavior. New York: Holt, Rinehart and Winston.

Jones, E., ed. 1971. Attribution. Morristown, N.J.: General Learning Press.

Kagan, A., and L. Levi. 1974. Health and environment—psychosocial stimuli: a review. Social Science and Medicine 8:225-241.

Kane, R. 1974. Manipulating the patient: a comparison of the effectiveness of physicians and chiropractic care. Lancet 1:1333.

Kelly, G. 1963. A Theory of Personality. New York: Norton.

Kleinman, A. 1973a. Toward a comparative study of medical systems. Science, Medicine and Man 1:55-65.

_____. 1973b. Some issues for a comparative study of medical healing. International Journal of Social Psychiatry 19:159-165.

_____. 1975a. An explanatory models approach to the study of the communicative aspects of health care: an appendix. In Medicine in Chinese Cultures: Comparative Studies of Health Care in Chinese and Other Societies, A. Kleinman et al., eds. Bethesda, Md.: Fogarty International Center, N.I.H., pp. 645-658.

_____. 1975b. Explanatory models in health care relationships. In Proceedings of the International Health Conference on the Health of the Family, C. Taylor, ed. Reston, Va. November 1974. Washington, D.C.: National Council for International Health; pp. 159-172.

_____. 1975c. Social, cultural and historical themes in the study of medicine in Chinese societies. In Medicine in Chinese Cultures: Comparative Studies of Health Care in Chinese and Other Societies, A. Kleinman et al., eds. Bethesda, Md.: Fogarty International Center, N.I.H., pp. 589-644.

_____. 1975d. Cross-cultural studies of illness behavior and health care: a preliminary report. Bulletin of the Chinese Society of Neurology and Psychiatry 1(2):1-5.

Kuhn, T. 1974. The Structure of Scientific Revolutions. Chicago: University of Chicago Press.

Lazare, A. 1973. Hidden conceptual models in clinical psychiatry. New England Journal of Medicine 288:345-351.

_____. 1975. The customer approach to patienthood: basic concepts. Archives of General Psychiatry 32:553-558.

Leslie, C. ed. 1976. Asian Medical Systems. Berkeley, Calif.: University of California Press.

Levy, R. 1973. Tahitians: Mind and Experience in the Society Islands. Chicago: University of Chicago Press.

Ley, P., and M. Spelman. 1967. Communicating with the Patient. London: Staples Press.

Lin, T. Y. 1953. Anthropological study of the incidence of mental disorder in Chinese and other cultures. Psychiatry 16:313-336.

Lipowski, Z. 1969. Psychosocial aspects of disease. Annals of Internal Medicine 71:1197-1206.

Mabry, J. 1964. Lay concepts of etiology. Journal of Chronic Disease 17:371.

Maher, B., ed. 1969. Clinical Psychology and Personality: Selected Papers of George Kelly. New York: Wiley.

McGuire, W. 1968. The nature of attitudes and attitude change. In Handbook of Social Psychology, G. Lindzey and E. Aronson, eds. Vol 3. 2nd. ed. Reading, Mass.: Addison-Wesley.

McKinley, J. 1973. Social networks, lay consultation and help-seeking behavior. Social Forces 51:275.

Mechanic, D. 1962. The concept of illness behavior. Journal of Chronic Diseases 15:189-194.

———. 1972. Social psychological factors affecting the presentation of bodily complaints. New England Journal of Medicine 286:1132-1139.

Metzger, D., and G. Williams. 1963. Tenejapa medicine: the curer. Southwestern Journal of Anthropology 19:216-234.

Nida, E. 1974. Toward a science of translating. Leiden: Brill Press.

Nida, E., and C. Taber. 1969. The Theory and Practice of Translating. Leiden: Brill Press.

Plog, S., and R. Edgerton, eds. 1969. Changing Perspectives in Mental Illness. New York: Holt, Rinehart and Winston.

Reynolds, D. 1976. Morita psychotherapy. Berkeley, Calif.: University of California Press.

Rin, H. 1965. A study of the etiology of Koro in respect to the Chinese concept of illness. International Journal of Social Psychiatry 11:7-13.

Rin, H., 1966. Psychophysiological reactions of a rural and suburban population in Taiwan. Acta Psychiatrica Scandinavica 42:410-486.

Rubel, A. 1964. Epidemiology of a folk illness: Susto. Ethnology 3:268-283.

Siegler, M., and H. Osmond. 1966. Models of madness. British Journal of Psychiatry 112:1193-1203.

Snow, L. 1974. Folk medical beliefs and their implications for care of patients. Annals of Internal Medicine 81:82-96.

Solomon, R. 1971. Mao's Revolution and the Chinese Political Culture. Berkeley, Calif.: University of California Press.

Stimson, G. 1974. Obeying doctor's orders. Social Science and Medicine 8:97-104.

Suchman, E. 1965. Social patterns of illness and medical care. Journal of Health and Human Behavior 6:2-16.

Symposium on the Greater Medical Profession. 1973. New York: Josiah Macy, Jr., Foundation.

Taylor, C., ed. 1975. Proceedings of the Internal Health Conference on Health and the Family. Reston, Va. November 1974. Washington, D.C.: National Council for International Health.

Topley, M. 1975. Chinese and Western medicine in Hong Kong. In Medicine in Chinese Cultures: Comparative Studies of Health Care in Chinese and Other Societies, A. Kleinman et al., eds. Bethesda, Md.: Fogarty International Center, N.I.H.; pp. 241-271.

Tseng, W. S. 1975a. Traditional and modern psychiatric care in Taiwan. In Medicine in Chinese Cultures: Comparative Studies of Health Care in Chinese and Other Societies, A. Kleinman et al., eds. Bethesda, Md.: Fogarty International Center, N.I.H.; pp. 177-193.

———. 1975b. The nature of somatic complaints among psychiatric patients: the Chinese case. Comprehensive Psychiatry 16:237-245.

Tseng, W. S., and J. Hsu. 1969. Chinese culture, personality formation and mental illness. International Journal of Social Psychiatry 16:5-14.

Twaddle, A. 1974. The concept of health status. Social Science and Medicine 8:29-38.

Tylor, S., ed. 1969. Cognitive anthropology. New York: Holt, Rinehart and Winston.

Waxler, N. 1974. Culture and mental illness: a social labeling perspective. Journal of Nervous and Mental Diseases 159:379-395.

Werner, O., and J. Fenton. 1973. Method and theory in ethnoscience and ethnoepistemology. *In* Handbook of Method in Cultural Anthropology, R. Naroll and R. Cohen, eds. New York: Columbia University Press, pp. 537-580.

Yap, P. M. 1965. Phenomenology of affective disorders in Chinese and other cultures. *In* Transcultural Psychiatry, A. de Reuck, ed. Boston: Little, Brown.

_____. 1967. Ideas of mental disorder in Hong Kong and their practical influence. *In* Some Traditional Chinese Ideas in Hong Kong, M. Topley, ed. Hong Kong Branch of the Royal Asiatic Society.

_____. 1975. Comparative Psychiatry. Toronto: University of Toronto Press.

Zajonc, R. 1968. Cognitive theories in social psychology. *In* Handbook of Social Psychology, G. Lindzey and E. Aronson, eds. Vol. 3. 2nd ed. Reading, Mass.: Addison-Wesley.

Zborowski, M. 1952. Cultural components in response to pain. Journal of Social Issues 8:16.

Zola, I. 1966. Culture and symptoms. American Sociological Review 31: 615-630.

_____. 1972. Medicine as an institution of social control. Sociological Review 20:487-504.

_____. 1973. Pathways to the doctor—from person to patient. Social Science and Medicine 7:677-684.

A CONCEPTUAL MODEL OF DRUG DEPENDENCE

Peter Mansky, M.D.
Jack Altman, Ph.D.

INTRODUCTION

Drug dependence as discussed in this chapter will refer to "compulsive" drug self-administration, that is, repeated drug use often at high cost to the individual. We shall present the terms "addiction" and "habituation" in historical context as antecedent to the use of the term "drug dependence" and the associated terms "physical" and "psychological dependence." We shall attempt to apply behavioral principles to the phenomena of drug dependence, using primarily the concepts of operant conditioning, but also relying on other conceptual explanations when appropriate.

Much of the discussion will be illustrated by describing the specific action of opiates, opiate agonist-antagonists, and opiate antagonists as they relate to drug dependence. We have chosen this spectrum of drugs for major illustration because they are among the most thoroughly studied drugs in humans. Repeated self-administration of these compounds has been related to their subjective, behavioral, and physiological effects. In addition, investigation of these drugs has demonstrated a unique dissociation between physical dependence and drug dependence. We shall also discuss other classes of drugs when their properties appear pertinent to our conceptual model.

This chapter will present a model of drug dependence and attempt to predict and suggest applications of the model to treatment and prevention. We are hopeful that the hypotheses generated by this model will be testable in specific treatment situations.

HISTORICAL BACKGROUND

The word "addiction" is used frequently to describe the phenomenon in which a drug interacts with a living organism to promote its continued self-administration. Used in this manner the word "addiction" is synonymous with the term "drug dependence" as defined in 1969 by the World Health Organization Expert Committee on Addiction-Producing Drugs (WHO-ECAD). However, the word "addiction" has been used to connote several different patterns of drug use. An understanding of the terms used to describe drug dependence can be facilitated by examining historically the definition of terms promulgated by WHO-ECAD and by observing the changes in the pattern and description of drug use that occurred during the same time.

In the early 1950s, WHO-ECAD defined drug "addiction," but it soon became evident that the definition was too restrictive to include the many diverse patterns of frequently repeated drug self-administration that had formerly been discussed as "addiction." Thus, in its Seventh Report (WHO-ECAD, 1957), the committee used the additional term "habituation" to describe various patterns of nonmedical continuing drug self-administration that could not be described as addiction. The terms "addiction" and "habituation" were defined by the committee as follows:

> *Drug addiction* is a state of periodic or chronic intoxication produced by the repeated consumption of a drug (natural or synthetic). Its characteristics include: (1) an overpowering desire or need (compulsion) to continue taking the drug and to obtain it by any means; (2) a tendency to increase the dose; (3) a psychic (psychological) and generally a physical dependence on the effects of the drug; (4) detrimental effect on the individual and on society.

> *Drug habituation (habit)* is a condition resulting from the repeated consumption of a drug. Its characteristics include: (1) a desire (but not a compulsion) to continue taking the drug for the sense of improved well-being which it engenders; (2) little or no tendency to increase the dose; (3) some degree of psychic dependence on the effect of the drug, but absence of physical dependence and hence an abstinence syndrome; (4) detrimental effects, if any, primarily on the individual.

As can be seen from the definitions, addiction and habituation could be construed to describe two different poles of drug use, one being pernicious and difficult to alter, the other being less harmful to the individual and society and easily treated or changed. Addiction, although not requiring physical dependence, was frequently considered to imply physical dependence. Many investigators considered this to be the most important component of drug dependence.

During the late 1950s and early 1960s, several drug-use patterns emerged that did not conform to the above definitions. Amphetamine and methamphetamine use produced marked dependence in selected individuals but was not considered to produce physical dependence. In addition, a class of drugs known as narcotic antagonists or agonist-antagonists (nalorphine and cyclazocine) were found to produce physical dependence but no drug-seeking behavior upon withdrawal (Martin and Gorodetzky, 1965; Martin et al., 1965).

Although the patterns of drug self-administration of stimulants such as amphetamine and cocaine and of LSD and marihuana appear frequently in both technical and lay literature, observations related to the opiate antagonists are less widely disseminated and appreciated.

The opiate antagonists nalorphine and cyclazocine differ from pure antagonists such as naloxone and naltrexone in that they have some agonist activity in addition to their antagonism of opiates such as heroin or morphine. Thus, nalorphine and cyclazocine have been termed agonist-antagonists by some investigators. Others have differentiated the two groups by lumping them all under the category of opiate antagonists, calling naloxone and naltrexone "pure" antagonists. With this distinction in mind, we will refer to nalorphine and cyclazocine simply as opiate antagonists.

Nalorphine when administered to non-opiate-dependent subjects produces a unique constellation of subjective effects. Low doses (1 to 5 mg) have little effect, or at the most produce a mild degree of euphoria and analgesia, but higher doses (3 to 10 mg) produce a combination of sedative-hypnotic and psychotomimetic effects that are considered by most subjects to be dysphoric. The state produced is rather like that of being "overtired," that is, feeling sleepy and tired but unable to sleep because of the excitant effects of the drugs. Subjects appeared drunk or ataxic and sleepy but were not able to sleep for any length of time sufficient to feel rested.

This constellation of subjective effects was seen to decrease if the same dose of antagonist was given repeatedly. If the dose was then slowly increased, the antagonists could be administered in very large doses with apparent complete tolerance to their subjective and physiological effects. If the antagonist were then withdrawn, a clearly observable physiological abstinence syndrome was observed.

Both cyclazocine and nalorphine have been studied intensively to carefully observe and describe this abstinence syndrome. Interestingly enough, the abstinence syndrome from nalorphine and cyclazocine resembles physiologically the morphine abstinence syndrome. Physical examination reveals lacrimation, rhinorrhea, and gooseflesh, along with increased pupil size, and pulse rate and body temperature above prewithdrawal levels. Notably, subjects being withdrawn from nalorphine or cyclazocine feel uncomfortable but do not ask for any medication to relieve their symptoms; that is, they do not exhibit drug-seeking behavior, nor do they report drug craving.

The withdrawal syndromes of nalorphine and cyclazocine do differ from morphine withdrawal in time course, intensity of symptoms as measured on the standardized Himmelsbach Scale (Andrews and Himmelsbach, 1944; Himmelsbach, 1941), and prominence of specific signs and symptoms. The onset and duration of nalorphine and cyclazocine abstinence syndromes are more prolonged than those seen after morphine withdrawal. In addition, the intensity of the withdrawal of comparable maintenance doses of the antagonist is much less than that seen after morphine withdrawal. The specific signs of hyperpnea and increased blood pressure are not prominent after withdrawal of the antagonist but are prominent after morphine withdrawal; hyperthermia, mydriasis, and tachycardia are more prominent after withdrawal from the antagonists. Furthermore, "shocks," myoclonic jerks, and scratching are seen frequently after withdrawal of the antagonists (Martin and Gorodetzky, 1965; Martin et al., 1965; Martin, 1967).

Although the withdrawal syndrome from opiate antagonists is quite unpleasant, it does not lead to drug-seeking behavior. The difference in intensity discussed above cannot account for this lack of drug-seeking behavior, since it has been noted that withdrawal from maintenance doses of morphine as low as 30 to 40 mg daily (period of maintenance three weeks) leads to low-intensity physiological withdrawal but prominent drug-seeking behavior[1] (Andrews and Himmelsbach, 1944; Himmelsbach, 1941; Jasinski, 1975). The qualitative differences alluded to above are significant, but the withdrawal syndrome from the opiate antagonist has been noted to be at least as unpleasant as the withdrawal from opiates. If this physical unpleasantness can be associated with a negative reinforcer (i.e., an event whose removal or delay supports behavior) inherent in the withdrawal syndrome, then we should expect the withdrawal syndrome from both morphine and the opiate antagonists to be a negative reinforcer leading to drug-seeking behavior. Strikingly, this is not the case.

The historical and theoretical importance of this observation was to demonstrate that physical dependence alone would not act as a negative reinforcer and lead to drug-seeking behavior and drug

---

[1] The studies cited by Himmelsbach show conclusively drug-seeking behavior and measurable physiological withdrawal in a subject taking 40 mg of morphine daily. Jasinski's communication (1975) needs further confirmation. Nonetheless, in well-documented isolated cases, subjects taking 30 and 40 mg of morphine daily were withdrawn with the observation of low-intensity physiological withdrawal but *prominent drug-seeking behavior*. Consistent physiological withdrawal has been described in several subjects maintained on 60 mg of morphine daily and is discussed by Jasinski and Mansky (1972).

craving. Thus, it seemed evident that at this time, some drugs such as amphetamines and LSD promoted "compulsive" drug use (repeated use often at a cost to the individual) in certain individuals without producing physical dependence, whereas other drugs such as nalorphine could produce physical dependence without "compulsive" drug use.

This evidence allows us to reflect on the definitions of drug dependence presented earlier in this chapter. We see clearly that physical dependence is neither a necessary nor sufficient negative reinforcer to account for compulsive drug use in opiate-like drugs, whereas it has been postulated that psychological dependence is both necessary and sufficient. There are no drugs among the opiates that do not produce physical dependence but do lead to "compulsive" drug use, so that other classes of drugs must be examined to postulate psychological dependence as a sufficient condition to lead to drug dependence. The nonopiates investigated have included marihuana, LSD, cocaine, amphetamine, and amphetamine-like drugs. In summary, then, the evidence indicated that psychological dependence was both a necessary and sufficient condition for drug dependence, whereas physical dependence was neither a necessary nor a sufficient condition for drug dependence.

Considering this evidence, in 1969 WHO-ECAD abandoned the use of the terms "addiction" and "habituation" and used instead the term "drug dependence," the sine qua non of which was psychological dependence. Isbell and Chrusciel (1970) attempted to clarify the new definitions as follows:

Drug dependence: A state, psychic and sometimes also physical, resulting from the interaction between a living organism and a drug, characterized by behavioral and other responses that always include a compulsion to take the drug on a continuous or periodic basis in order to experience its psychic effects, and sometimes to avoid the discomfort of its absence. Tolerance may or may not be present. A person may be dependent on more than one drug.

Psychic dependence: A compulsion that requires periodic or continuous administration of a drug to produce pleasure or avoid discomfort. This compulsion is the most powerful factor in chronic intoxication with psychotropic drugs, and with certain types of drugs may be the only factor involved in the perpetuation of abuse even in the case of most intense craving. Psychic dependence, therefore, is the universal characteristic of drug dependence. Operationally, it is recognized by the fact that the dependent person continues to take the drug in spite of conscious admission that it is causing harm to his health and to his social and familial adjustment, and that he takes great risks to obtain and maintain his supply of the drug.

Physical dependence: A pathological state brought about by repeated administration of a drug and that leads to the appearance of a characteristic and specific group of symptoms, termed an abstinence syndrome, when the administration of the drug is discontinued or—in the case of certain drugs—significantly reduced. In order to prevent the appearance of an abstinence syndrome the continuous taking of the drug is required. Physical dependence is a powerful factor in reinforcing psychic dependence upon continuing drug use or in relapse to drug use after withdrawal.

The use of the term "drug dependence" as defined above with a modifying phrase linking it to a particular type of drug was supported by the WHO Scientific Group on Evaluation of Dependence Producing Drugs (1964; and see Isbell and Chrusciel, 1970) and has also been supported by the Committee on Drug Addiction and Narcotics of the National Academy of Sciences—National Research Council.

Although these definitions appear to be an improvement over the 1957 WHO-ECAD formulations, they have serious weaknesses. Goldberg (1976) has noted that they are of little scientific value in relying upon such vague terms as "pleasure" and "craving," which, due to their long history of popular use, are difficult to define operationally and to quantify. The most severe deficiency, however, is the circular use of terms, such as "compulsion" (Skinner, 1953). The assumption is made that some inner state or compulsion is responsible for continued drug taking. Yet the presence of this inner process is inferred from the repeated drug-taking behavior—that is, the behavior is supposedly caused by some hypothetical construct (compulsion) that is known to exist only from the behavior. There are other problems with these definitions, but they did attempt to separate clearly physical dependence from drug dependence. Physical dependence was important only in that it could exacerbate the phenomenon of repeated drug consumption. The emphasis was now placed upon psychological dependence.

In addition, Isbell and Chrusciel (1970) added a behavioral component to the definition of psychological dependence. According to them, the concept of psychological dependence contains two major variables. The first describes a drug action that would "produce pleasure or avoid discomfort" quite analogous to Kolb's definition (1925) of positive and negative euphoria. The second adds to the definition the observable component of psychological dependence. This component can be thought of as the "price" (or response cost) an individual is willing to pay to continue drug taking. It is this price feature that offers some measure of the degree of psychological dependence. A similar analysis could measure the degree of "psychological dependence" one sees in other behavioral disorders (for example, "compulsive" gambling, obesity) and permit comparisons between drug dependence and dependence on other environmental events.

In the final analysis, defining psychological dependence may prove valuable only insofar as the term refers to observable and measurable events. Whereas previous work has emphasized the physical components of drug dependence, attention should now, in addition, focus on behavioral and environmental variables that influence drug use. This is especially important, since it is clear that drug dependence can occur in the absence of physical dependence.

A BEHAVIORAL APPROACH

It is the contention of reinforcement theory (operant conditioning) that behavior (including drug use) is controlled by consequent events in the environment. Although this statement reiterates a simple concept, it also implies the following: (1) to control behavior (that is, to establish it, increase it, maintain it, or decrease it), one must concentrate on observable environmental events and not on the person's inner self or feelings; (2) behavior does not occur spontaneously, but is controlled by environmental factors that are often obscure, due to an inadequate knowledge of the individual's history; and (3) given our ignorance of a person's prior history, there is no such thing as irrational behavior, since even odd or peculiar behavior must be controlled by environmental events.

This well-known theoretical framework utilizes the now common concepts of reinforcement. Consequent events that tend to establish, maintain, or increase preceding behaviors are then called *reinforcing events* or *reinforcers* and can be divided into two categories. If presentation of the events increases or maintains the preceding behavior, the consequences are *positive reinforcers*. For example, work behavior will increase when money is the consequent event. Behavior will also increase or continue if it results in the delay or removal of certain consequent events called *negative reinforcers*—for example, driving slowly to avoid a speeding ticket. The application of these examples to drug-abuse behavior is readily apparent. Individuals may be ingesting drugs to (1) avoid negative reinforcers—physical discomfort, disapproval from peers, psychological distress—or (2) gain positive reinforcers—the "high" or intoxicating effect of the compound, approval from peers, increased pleasure from other events while intoxicated (for example, eating, listening to music, self-analysis). The advantages of this conceptual approach are that it forces one to define the behavior and environmental events precisely and that it yields measurable data. In other words, one can verify (theoretically, at least) what variables might be responsible for continued drug-seeking behavior. What initiated drug use may then be more important in an epidemiological framework and in prevention, while the factors maintaining drug consumption may be the critical elements in treatment.

The theory becomes infinitely more complex by considering another significant variable affecting the strength of behavior, the schedule by which the behavior is reinforced. Intermittent presentation of reinforcing events produces much greater control over preceding responses than regular reinforcement. Since it is often extremely difficult to discover the schedule of reinforcement that might be responsible for drug use in humans, changing or extinguishing the drug-taking pattern becomes quite difficult. Also, not only is the schedule of drug administration important, but the schedule of delivery of other reinforcers in the individual's life can be crucial as well. For example, Falk (1964) in lower animals and Katchinoff et al. (1973) in humans have demonstrated that individuals responding to reinforcers according to certain schedules of reinforcement will often engage in *adjunctive behaviors* (including consumption of drugs). Individuals who have pressing duties only at certain times each day may visit a nearby bar during the times when they are free. Altering this drug-seeking pattern might be very difficult without shifting the temporal distribution of their job requirements. It may be that for many people who are abusing substances, the important variables are not related to drugs but to the schedules of reinforcement controlling other aspects of their lives.

The use of positive and negative reinforcement paradigms may allow us to formulate a unified theory of drug abuse incorporating the negative reinforcing properties of physical dependence with the positive reinforcing drug-induced states (subsumed under psychological dependence). In addition, other physiological factors, coping behaviors, and environmental conditions antedating drug use but promoting the drug self-administration could also be expressed in operant terminology. The degree of drug dependence could then not only be measured as suggested earlier by the behavioral "price" one is willing to pay for drug use but by the difficulty associated with the extinction of drug-seeking behavior or compulsive drug use. In like fashion, the use of a unified terminology would be helpful in assessing the neurophysiological substrate of drug dependence. Since positive and negative reinforcing neural sites have been well established (Olds and Olds, 1965), investigators interested in the role of the brain in drug dependence have turned to these brain areas (median forebrain bundle, periventricular system) for possible involvement.

This approach of relating behavior to specific brain structures is by no means new. Pavlov (1927) argued emphatically for a physiologically based explanation for behavior, in opposition to the psychological and philosophical explanations of feelings and consciousness prominent in the late nineteenth century. The formulation of drug dependence in terms of classical and operant conditioning by Abraham Wikler (1973) has also revealed the impressive utility of conditioning theory in leading to unified theoretical constructs, relating these constructs to physiological and environmental events and formulating theories that can be investigated experimentally in the hopes of developing better treatment of drug dependence.

In contrast to Wikler's formulations, ours will be based primarily on the concepts of operant conditioning, using the phenomenology of opiate action and dependence as a major illustration of the complexities involved. We shall continue to use the terms psychological and physical dependence as defined by WHO-ECAD (1969), but only as long as they permit functional analyses.[2] The use of operant terminology to describe the phenomena of drug dependence will, we hope, lead to the discovery of relationships between "final common pathways" of the brain and observable behavior. The use of the terms psychological dependence and physical dependence will allow us to best segregate the phenomenology of drug dependence, and the use of operant terminology within both constructs of dependence will, we hope, lead to a unified theory.

The utility of the use of separate terms for psychological and physical dependence has been essential in our discussion of the opiate antagonists nalorphine and cyclazocine. The dissociation of physical dependence from psychological dependence in these two opiate antagonists has led us to state that a withdrawal syndrome can act as a powerful negative reinforcer for continued self-administration only if the drug can also function as a positive reinforcer in other situations. In other words, physical dependence is not enough to ensure continued drug use.

Practical clinical considerations have also indicated the usefulness of separating the description of physical dependence from the description of psychological dependence. This has been evident in the consultation work of Peter Mansky at Massachusetts General Hospital and other Boston-area hospitals. Many clinicians are hesitant to give opiates to patients in amounts that will induce physical dependence. Apparently, many primary clinicians equate physical dependence with the concept of "addiction" described in the historical presentation of WHO-ECAD definitions. These physicians feel that once a patient is physically dependent on opiates, he or she

---

[2] Functional analysis refers to a description of behavior with regard to its controlling factors—e.g., consequences, scheduling of consequences, stimulus events, etc.

will be unable to stop using them. This is contrary to existing evidence (which will be discussed later in this chapter) that of the many patients who are apparently physically dependent on opiates in the hospital, few seek the drugs from illegal sources after discharge (O'Donnell, 1969). A related phenomenon may be the large number of American soldiers who were drug dependent in Vietnam yet stopped drug use after they returned to the United States (Robins et al., 1975).

A possible explanation for these results may be derived from an area of operant conditioning not yet discussed—stimulus control. When behavior is reinforced only in the presence of specific stimuli of events (discriminative stimuli), these stimuli come to control the occurrence of the response. That is, the behavior is emitted only when the discriminative stimuli are present and is withheld in their absence. Thus, individuals who become drug dependent in one environment and under one set of circumstances may exhibit little or no drug-seeking behavior when the environment is considerably altered—for example, hospitalized patients returning home or soldiers coming back to the United States. We shall attempt alternative explanations for these phenomena later in the chapter.

FORMATION OF THE MODEL

In the preceding sections, we have attempted to demonstrate that drug dependence is determined by various factors (reinforcing properties of the substance, schedule of drug administration, schedules of other consequences, stimulus control) and that physical dependence is neither a necessary nor a sufficient condition for drug dependence. There has been little objective research, however, examining these variables, due to their complexity and the difficulty of data acquisition. Information concerning the factors influencing drug use would be invaluable, since it could be applied both to treatment and to predicting which individuals or which compounds may result in drug dependence.

The positive reinforcing properties of certain drugs may be related to their subjective effects in humans. The subjective effects of opiates have been investigated after single-dose administration by measuring verbal responses to structured questionnaires. Many of the studies have been conducted using a sample population of former opiate "addicts." This selection of subjects certainly adds a bias to the collected data but appears justified in that it is clear that the positive reinforcing properties of opiates are not universally perceived in a population of subjects selected from nonopiate addicts (Lasagna et al., 1955). Whether this is due to learning, social pressure, or intrinsic neurological factors is unclear, but nonetheless the opiate agonists do act as reinforcers of drug-seeking behavior in former opiate "addicts."

Much of the systematic work investigating the subjective effects of opiates and opiate antagonists has been conducted at the National Institute of Mental Health (NIMH) Addiction Research Center (now a section of the National Institute of Drug Abuse). The subjective and behavioral effects of opiates and opiate antagonists have been extensively investigated and quantified in former opiate addicts, using the 550-item Addiction Research Center Inventory (ARCI) (Hill et al., 1963; Haertzen et al., 1963a, 1963b). This inventory is patterned after the MMPI, using short, single-sentence items and requiring a response of true (+) or false (−). A shortened form of this questionnaire containing forty highly discriminating items has been used to quantify the subjective effects of single-dose administration of various drugs (Jasinski et al., 1971). This shortened form allows multiple presentation after single-dose drug administration (usually at 1/2, 1, 2, 3, 4, and 5 hours) in order to determine the time action curve of subjective effects. Three scales derived from the ARCI are represented by the forty items of the single-dose questionnaire. These scales are the MBG (morphine-benzedrine group) scale, the LSD (lysergic acid diethylamide) scale, and the PCAG (pentobarbital-chlorpromazine-alcohol group) scale. In a technical and restriced sense, responses on these scales refer only to verbal or written behavioral responses to the items. In a broader sense, these scales have been considered to represent three different classes of subjective effects. Thus, the MBG scale represents euphorogenic effects, the LSD scale psychotomimetic effects, and the PCAG scale sedative effects (Jasinski et al., 1971).

In many studies, morphine and other opiate agonists have been shown to have a prominent and dose-related effect on the MBG scale. On the other hand, nalorphine rarely produces any significant response on this scale. In the few studies in which nalorphine elicited a significant response on the MBG scale in a sample population of former "addicts," the response was significantly less than that for morphine in the given population. Furthermore, nalorphine did not elicit a dose-related response on the MBG scale. In fact, as the dose of nalorphine was increased, the response on the MBG scale did not increase but became indistinguishable from placebo (Jasinski et al., 1971; Mansky and Jasinski, 1970). Unfortunately, the MBG scale is undirectional, and the dysphoria so frequently reported with higher doses of nalorphine was not measured quantitatively.

As just illustrated, the MBG scale appears to measure the euphorogenic effects of opiates. Reference to the concept of opiate euphoria recalls Kolb's use of positive and negative euphoria mentioned earlier. Since euphoria may be either positive or negative, the MBG scale may be measuring either the drug's ability to act as a positive reinforcer or its ability to counteract the action of a negative reinforcer (e.g., withdrawal). It must be noted that this scale has been administered to former addicts under special but varying circumstances. The items in the questionnaire refer to a comparison to "normal" feelings ("I feel better than normal") and to feelings associated with being high in previous settings. Some of the tested addicts have been drug free for greater than six months, the longest period physiological abnormalities have been noted post opiate withdrawal (Martin and Jasinski, 1969). Therefore, it appears unlikely that the MBG scale measures the opiate ability to relieve an external negative reinforcer or a physiological abnormality associated with former physiological dependence. It is possible that the opiate use relieves some chronic dysphoric state of the addicts, thus acting as an operant in a negative reinforcement paradigm. Although this cannot be ruled out, no psychological scale has been able to measure a subjective feeling of chronic dysphoria in the subjects participating in the studies. Thus, we conclude that it is justified and useful to assume that the MBG scale measures positive euphoria or, more precisely, the subjective effects induced by opiates in former addicts identified with positive reinforcing properties of opiates.

An astute observer may note that in the data described, not only was nalorphine unable to produce dose-related responses on the MBG scale, but it often produced dysphoric responses not measured by the MBG scale. Relief of these dysphoric responses upon discontinuation of chronic nalorphine or cyclazocine administration could explain the lack of drug-seeking behavior described earlier. Indeed, this may hold for some subjects, but it has been noted that nalorphine, cyclazocine, and related opiate antagonists may be given in such a way as to produce few, if any, unpleasant effects during slow dose build-up and that many subjects fail to exhibit drug-seeking behavior upon withdrawal of the antagonists.

Thus, again, it appears that among the opiate-like drugs and the opiate antagonists, only the drugs that act as positive reinforcers reflected by a dose response score on the MBG scale lead to drug dependence. It may be that the MBG scale measures only the positive reinforcing properties of opiates and amphetamines. However, in the future, the MBG scale may be shown to measure the properties of other drugs that lead to positive reinforcement associated with drug dependence. Experiments employing the MBG scale in measuring the subjective effects of various classes of drugs may eventually establish or refute this point.

We have described one aspect of psychological dependence, the ability of the drug to act as a positive reinforcer. This aspect of drug reinforcement may be learned but more likely is due to an innate reaction of organisms to drug administration. Psychological dependence, however, includes not only the positive reinforcement properties of the drug, but also the ability of drug use to act as an operant in escaping or avoiding negative reinforcers. The negative reinforcement paradigm could represent the relief of an intrinsic dysphoric condition (e.g., pain, psychotic disorder, affective disorder, or situation-induced feelings of dysphoria such as depression or anxiety) or an environment-induced dysphoric state (e.g., living in a slum area, poor family or other interpersonal relationships, assignment to Vietnam). It is then logical to question the different properties of the negative reinforcement paradigms of psychological dependence in leading to compulsive drug-seeking behavior and likewise to examine the difficulty or ease of extinction of drug-seeking behavior by the removal of the negative reinforcer.

Several observations concerning opiate-dependent subjects could be examined in order to hypothesize the effect of the negative reinforcing paradigm of psychological dependence. It is now known that physical dependence on opiates develops after the daily administration of 30 to 40 mg of morphine (or equivalent) for probably a minimum of twenty-one days (no studies to date have established an absolute minimal time period) (Andrews and Himmelsbach, 1944; Himmelsbach, 1941; Jasinski, 1975). Thus, it is evident that many hospitalized patients who experience relief of a negative reinforcer, pain, by opiates may also become physically dependent on the opiates. Yet the number of iatrogenic opiate addicts remains small in comparison to the large number of opiate addicts treated for pain during hospitalization (O'Donnell, 1969). Examination of the large group of subjects dependent on opiates in Vietnam has revealed that only a small percentage have exhibited frequently repeated drug use leading to drug dependence upon returning to the United States. One explanation, already discussed, relates to the massive change in environmental stimuli that may be controlling drug ingestion. Another explanation is that drug-related psychological dependence may involve both a positive and a negative reinforcement paradigm. The positive paradigm would be related to direct drug effects (upon brain structures) as formerly postulated. The negative reinforcement paradigm would depend upon intrinsic or extrinsic reinforcers (usually dysphoric conditions). Removal of these negative reinforcers by means other than opiates would then extinguish the drug-seeking behavior promoted by the negative reinforcement paradigm. Total extinguishing of the drug-seeking behavior would then depend upon the ease of extinguishing the positive reinforcing properties of the drug in the individual.

Moreover, the positive reinforcing properties of peer group approval and acceptance (present in some urban subcultures and in Vietnam) in addition to the negative reinforcement of social disapproval (a veteran returning to a small rural town) may play a role in either initiating use upon return to the United States or in reinforcing drug abstinence, respectively. Although these particular social pressures are strong reinforcers, it is our contention that they play a prominent role in reinforcing *initiation* or *non-initiation* of drug use but play a less prominent role once repeated use has been established.

Opiates, and other drugs such as alcohol, evidently may act as positive reinforcers in some individuals and may be negative reinforcers for other individuals. The positive reinforcement may be graded such that some individuals find drug use very rewarding, others just slightly so. Thus, when the negative reinforcers inherent in psychological dependence are removed (e.g., return from Vietnam, relief of pain), the positive reinforcing properties of the drug may be easily extinguished. This extinguishing may occur by covert conditioning, and may be influenced by self-concept and cognitive labeling (Wisocki, 1973; Haertzen and Hooks, 1971; O'Donnell, 1969). This will be discussed in greater detail later in this chapter.

In completing our discussion of operant conditioning paradigms associated with compulsive drug use, we note that it would be interesting to determine which varieties of negative reinforcement antedate use and which result from it. Those which antedate it include primarily the extrinsically and intrinsically induced dysphoric states discussed earlier, whereas those which result from it involve almost exclusively the drug withdrawal abstinence syndrome or the conditioned abstinence syndromes.

The prominent role of the opiate abstinence syndrome and conditioned abstinence in leading to relapse of drug use has been discussed at length by Wikler (1973). He states that descriptions of drug use and relapse often concentrate on the positive reinforcing properties of the drug. These descriptions of relapse often fail to ascribe relapse to the dramatic abstinence syndrome. The opiate abstinence syndrome and the conditioned abstinence syndrome (negative reinforcers) may play a more prominent role in relapse to opiate use than the "remembered" euphorogenic effects (positive reinforcement).

Wikler also argues this in discussing the treatment of opiate dependence using opiate antagonists or blockers. A frequently used antagonist today is naltrexone. This drug has little agonist activity, but when given over a period of time, it retains antagonist activity to the euphorogenic effects of opiates such as morphine and heroin (Martin et al., 1973). The theory underlying the use of an antagonist contends that continued drug self-administration without the concomitant reinforcement of the euphorogenic effects would lead to the extinction of self-administration and related drug-seeking behavior. Recent evidence, however, indicates that extinction does not occur with antagonist treatment either on an inpatient (Altman, 1975) or an outpatient (Kleber et al., 1974) basis. Individuals receiving the antagonist simply stop opiate use and rarely challenge the blockade. Since behavior must be emitted for the extinction contingency to operate, drug self-administration does not extinguish during the period of antagonist consumption, but is merely absent. Once antagonist treatment is discontinued, the behavior reappears and relapse is rapid. Nevertheless, antagonists may be useful in the treatment of opiate dependence since their continued ingestion represents an important step in treatment—the elimination of opiate use.

In summary, psychological dependence, operationally measured by the "price" one is willing to pay for drug use or by ease of extinction of drug-seeking behavior, appears to be linked to the capacity of the drug to act either as a positive reinforcer of acquisition and administration behavior or as an attenuator of the effects of an intrinsic or extrinsic negative reinforcer such as pain or a dysphoric social situation. These properties of a drug are linked to its pharmacological action and the biological and environmental states of the individual taking the drug.

Physical dependence can then be seen as a condition arising from previous drug use and dependent upon the negative reinforcing properties of the abstinence syndrome. The drug taking acts as an operant in relieving this syndrome. The abstinence syndrome may be related to pharmacological withdrawal of the drug or may be conditioned to environmental or internal conditions contingent upon previous withdrawal experience. The negative reinforcing properties of physical dependence appear unique in that they are inoperative in promoting continued drug use unless the drug has positive reinforcing properties.

The reinforcing properties associated with psychological dependence have been studied most extensively in street addicts who claim to feel a positive euphoria, or a negative euphoria, related to relief of feelings contingent upon social or environmental conditions. These addicts have been shown to respond to single-dose opiate administration with subjective reports of liking the drug along with dose-related responses on the putative euphorogenic scale (MBG). These same addicts have also exhibited drug-seeking behavior after chronic administration and withdrawal of drugs that they liked but not after similar drugs that they disliked. Thus, as stated earlier, addicts have to like drugs in order for their physical dependence producing properties to promote continued drug use.

It appears that the positive reinforcement inherent in psychological dependence (probably related to direct drug effects upon the brain reward system) provides the all-or-none switch that then determines whether the abstinence syndrome will act as a negative reinforcer. In no way does this explain the intensity of the negative reinforcement of withdrawal. This intensity, however, may be related to both the degree of physical dependence as shown by intensity of the withdrawal syndrome and the degree to which the drug acts as a positive reinforcer.

USE OF THE MODEL

"Cognitive labeling" and "self-concept" are terms that can modify the effects of reinforcers in a given individual and deserve some discussion in this section, which relates our model to the treatment of drug use. The degree to which withdrawal acts as a negative reinforcer could be influenced by the cognitive label applied to drug withdrawal. Certainly, the recognition that one is suffering from a dramatic but non-life-threatening and time-limited withdrawal syndrome may be a necessary condition for opiate-dependent subjects to discontinue drug use on their own. They may fear the uncomfortable withdrawal effects but may be willing to endure them with the knowledge that they are time limited. Also, limits to the intensity of the withdrawal syndrome in a detoxification program may lead to a dependent subject's acceptance of slow detoxification.

Far more disturbing and less acceptable may be the milder but unpredictable episodes of conditioned abstinence of opiate users (Wikler, 1973; Wikler, 1965; Wikler and Pescor, 1965; Goldberg and Schuster, 1970; Whitehead, 1974). The intensity of conditioned abstinence may be sufficient to be cognitively labeled as drug withdrawal. It may be puzzling to the opiate addict in that it may occur while he or she is taking an opiate and thus be considered an indication for more opiate. This phenomenon has been observed and reported specifically in methadone maintenance programs (Whitehead, 1974). The conditioned abstinence syndrome may occur, also, months to years after opiate use and withdrawal. As such, it may be interpreted by the former addict as indicative of a continuing "need" for opiates, possibly due to a cognitively labeled "permanent need" for opiates, generated by former use.

The conditioned abstinence syndrome may also present minor signs and symptoms of withdrawal such as restlessness and anxiety. These minor signs and symptoms may be indistinguishable in intensity and quality from restlessness and anxiety experienced in nondrug situations. As such, the former addict may not ascribe these signs and symptoms to opiate use but may scan his or her "feelings" and environment to explain these signs and symptoms. As such, the addict may consider that these signs and symptoms are indicative of his or her inability to cope with internal conflict or external stresses present in daily living. Thus, he or she may feel inadequate to cope and turn to drug use for relief of this dysphoric feeling.

Akin to the phenomena of conditioned abstinence at minimal

intensity seen with opiates may be the minor signs and symptoms (minimal abstinence) of withdrawal seen several days after the termination of the use of relatively low doses of a sedative-hypnotic (Covi et al., 1973). This has been frequently observed and eloquently reported by Goldiamond (1973) after the discontinuation of a benzodiazepine used to treat muscle spasm.

In the case of sedative-hypnotics such as the benzodiazepines or alcohol, anxiety may be experienced several days after discontinuation of drug use. Although this anxiety is a minor symptom of withdrawal, the time separation between the termination of drug use and the emergence of the minor symptom of withdrawal may be so long that no cognitive link is established to relate the minor abstinence signs and symptoms (e.g., anxiety, restlessness) to the *discontinuation* of the drug. In this case, it is possible that the individual may scan his or her external environment or internal feelings and ascribe the symptom to either external or internal conflict. This cognitive process may lead to the decision to use the drug to relieve the conflict and may be stated as: (1) "I am an *anxious person* because I have conflicts. I better resume drug use to relieve this defect in my internal makeup"; or (2) "I live in a situation that provokes feelings of anxiety. These feelings can be relieved by the drug I have been taking." This may be especially pertinent when initial use of the drug was associated with an internal or external negative reinforcer that was perceived affectively as anxiety. Since most anxiety is time limited, it may be that the anxiety experienced after drug withdrawal does not originate from the original transient source but is now solely drug related. In this latter case, the cognitive recognition that within a very short period after drug withdrawal one may experience anxiety that is solely drug related and transient may be useful in stopping drug use.

The cognitive labeling may be a modifying factor of the effect of the abstinence syndrome upon continued drug use. Cognitive labeling in terms of self-concept may also affect continued drug use. This hypothesis has been supported by the work of O'Donnell (1969), concerning the role of self-concept in the relapse of Kentucky addicts discharged from the Public Health Service Hospital at Lexington. His postulate involved only two supposedly opposing self-concepts, that of a medical addict (taking the opiate as medicine, in the sick role) and that of perceiving oneself as healthy and taking the opiate for "kicks" (for discussion of sick role, see chapters 1 and 3). Among the subjects who had no involvement in the drug subculture were those who maintained the sick role. When the sick role was no longer supported by a physician, some of the subjects stopped opiate use and did not become involved in the drug subculture; others did become involved. O'Donnell states that his sample is drawn in such a manner that he was

not able to make a definitive statement concerning the number of
people who may have stopped opiate use after having to give up the
sick role, since this group would tend not to be hospitalized at the
Public Health Service Hospital. Nevertheless, he did find differences in
drug-use patterns among those who received their opiates from one
physician only (assumed to be the sick role "addicts") and other
"addicts."

In the same way the marked decrease in drug use seen among
returning Vietnam veterans may be due to their self-concept as
"nondeviant" citizens and may make continued involvement in the
criminal subculture incompatible with their self-concept. Again, an
easily acceptable alternate explanation is that removal from the
negative reinforcement of Vietnam service, along with minimal
positive reinforcement of direct drug effect, may explain the ease of
extinction of drug-seeking behavior upon returning home. This
explanation may be more likely, since it has been shown that many
veterans had easy access to opiates without becoming intimately
identified with a criminal or "deviant" subculture (Robins et al.,
1975). The example of the Vietnam veterans and O'Donnell's
follow-up studies also indicate that self-concept as applicable to group
identification may be an important factor in promoting, or at least
initiating drug use.

SUMMARY AND CLINICAL UTILITY
OF THE MODEL

The conceptual model of drug dependence discussed in this chapter
provides a framework of organization in considering the various forms
of treatment used in helping individuals to alter patterns of behavior
associated with repeated drug self-administration.

We might first consider the area of prevention. Using the basic
tenets of our theoretical model, one would want to examine the
internal and external events that tend to initiate drug use. There are
many examples of external positive and negative reinforcers that
would include peer group pressure with a sense of group membership,
desire to have new and different experiences, living in a slum area,
poor family and other interpersonal relationships, and so on. Altering
these external factors is an indeed difficult, but important, activity
mostly unrelated to the specific goal of preventing drug use. Clearly,
many of the external reinforcers are inherent in the structure and
functioning of a society and culture. They play a role in influencing
much of the behavior exhibited in a given society and are not
specifically related to drug self-administration; that is, they may lead
to other behaviors, some of which may be to the advantage of the
individual and society and others of which may not. To prevent the

initiation of drug self-administration by changing the external reinforcers of society would be an impossible task and would greatly affect other behaviors.

Another approach in prevention has been to limit the availability of drugs that act as positive reinforcers. This again may have varying results when the external reinforcers referred to above can affect a wide range of observable behavior. Thus, when a drug is not available, other behavior may easily be reinforced. In addition, we have noted that the use of the drug alone, even if it is reinforced initially, does not lead inevitably to lifelong drug dependence.

Identifying the drugs that may lead to dependence may be very useful. The well-known examples of the use of heroin as the cure for opiate dependence and the belief that newer drugs in similar classes did not produce dependence (meperidine and meprobamate being just two of these newer drugs) indicate a need for identifying the drugs that may lead to dependence. Although laws making the possession of certain drugs criminal can be one result of such identification, the identification of new drugs with the potential to lead to drug dependence may be more effective in the long run. The knowledge of the potential of various drugs to produce dependence can lead to less cavalier prescription and distribution of the identified drugs by physicians. Much of the work done by the ARC, alluded to earlier, has been to investigate new drugs in comparison to known standards of drugs of the same class. Indeed, this may supply valuable information to physicians, affecting the distribution of drugs.

The medical model of disease with epidemiology of spread is a model not cited in the text that may suggest ways to prevent initiation of repeated drug self-administration. We mention it in this section only to include it in our discussion of prevention. This model along with very stimulating observations is presented by Hughes et al. (1972).

Internal or intrinsic reinforcers associated with both the initiation and continuation of repeated drug self-administration should also be considered in treatment. The complete psychiatric examination of a patient could identify intrinsically determined negative reinforcers promoting continued drug use. Indeed, considering a well-defined intrinsic condition such as a major affective disorder can be illustrative. For example, many cases of alcohol dependency have been related to a major affective illness (Winokur et al., 1970). Alcohol self-administration has often been decreased or eliminated by effective medical treatment of the affective disorder.

Psychiatric evaluation may lead not only to the use of medication but also to psychotherapy. Individual-oriented psychotherapy has been well known to be an inefficient and frequently ineffective treatment for drug dependence. Perhaps, however, therapies centered on altering self-concept and cognitive labeling as discussed in this chapter may be useful. The identification of the environmental events controlling drug use would be essential. The ideal psychotherapy would, of course, involve training the patients to carry out a functional analysis of their drug use so that they could alter either their responses or the environmental factors themselves controlling their drug-taking behavior. In addition, it has been found valuable to examine the behavioral events that could influence drug use as *adjunctive* behavior.

Certainly, the concepts discussed here have played a prominent role in self-help groups (such as Synanon, Alcoholics Anonymous, Odyssey House), which readily use self-concept and cognitive labeling to alter drug-seeking behavior. Peer group pressure may also be a prominent feature in the self-help organizations to prevent initiation of drug use. Moreover, the full range of time-consuming activities promoted by many of these organizations may prevent drug dependence as adjunctive behavior.

To complete our brief discussion of model application, we should mention the possible use of opiate antagonists and antabuse[3] in treatment. Recent evidence (Altman, 1975; Kleber et al., 1974) indicates that the use of narcotic antagonists can effectively eliminate opiate abuse. Addicts pretreated with cyclazocine, naloxone, or naltrexone will not challenge the antagonist. When they wish to "get off," they will simply stop antagonist consumption. Relapse is usually rapid once antagonist self-administration becomes intermittent, and irregular. Although this appears discouraging, antagonists do offer one striking advantage over other forms of treatment: one can be sure that the individuals are not abusing opiates as long as they take the antagonist. In effect, the patients are presented with a daily decision. If they take the antagonist (e.g., naltrexone), they are "safe" for the day no matter where they go or what they do. If they do not take it, they run the risk of opiate abuse. This represents an especially interesting development to those applying a behavioral model since the drug-abuse problem has shifted. Therapists can now concentrate their skills on establishing one clear behavioral sequence (terminating in the consumption of antagonist) rather than on attempting to train the individuals (an exceedingly difficult task) to avoid the many environmental factors leading to drug use. This treatment procedure can be (1) the major treatment component for those individuals who have few behavioral deficits other than their weakness for drugs, and (2) the essential first step in treatment for those who possess other severe behavioral deficiencies. Although administration of the antagonist will ensure an opiate-free individual, there is still the possibility of abuse of other drug classes, and rehabilitation may remain very

[3] The possible treatment efficacy of antabuse is very similar to that discussed for narcotic antagonists (Wilson, 1975).

difficult. However, antagonist treatment will have accomplished a very important step—cessation of opiate use.

Reexamination of treatment modalities and their effectiveness using our model will be the test of the utility of the model of drug dependence presented here. Ultimately, our model will stand or fall on its ability to organize the information we know about drug dependence and to apply it to hypothesis development, to hypothesis testing, and eventually to treatment.

REFERENCES

Altman, J. L. 1975. Laboratory modification of heroin acquisition: implication for narcotic antagonist treatment. Proceedings of the Conference on Biomedical Research in Narcotic Abuse Problems, 131-149. Sponsored by NMUDD, Ottawa, Ontario, Canada.

Andrews, H. L., and C. K. Himmelsbach. 1944. Relation of the intensity of the morphine abstinence syndrome to dosage. Journal of Pharmacology and Experimental Therapeutics 81:288-293.

Covi, L., R. S. Lipman, D. H. Pattison, L. R. Derogatis, and E. H. Uhlenhuth. 1973. Length of treatment with anxiolytic sedatives and response to their sudden withdrawal. Acta Psychiatrica Scandinavica 49:51-64.

Falk, J. L. 1964. Studies on schedule-induced polydipsia. In Thirst: First International Symposium on Thirst in the Regulation of Body Water, M. J. Wayner, ed. New York: Pergamon Press, pp. 95-116.

Goldberg, S. R. 1976. The behavioral analysis of drug addiction. In Behavioral Pharmacology, S. D. Glick and J. Goldfarb, eds. St. Louis: C. V. Mosby, pp. 283-316.

Goldberg, S. R., and C. R. Schuster. 1970. Conditioned nalorphine-induced abstinence changes: persistence in post morphine-dependent monkey. Journal of the Experimental Analysis of Behavior 14:33-46.

Goldiamond, I. 1973. A diary of self-modification. Psychology Today. November:95-102.

Haertzen, C. A., H. E. Hill, and R. E. Belleville. 1963. Development of the addiction research center inventory (ARCI): selection of the items that are sensitive to the effects of various drugs. Psychopharmacologia 4:155-166.

Haertzen, C. A., and N. T. Hooks. 1971. Contract effects from simulation of subjective experiences: a possible standard for behavioral modification. British Journal of Addiction 66:225-227.

Hill, H. E., C. A. Haertzen, A. B. Wolbach, and E. J. Miner. 1963a. The addiction research center inventory: standardization of scales which evaluate subjective effects of morphine, pentabarbital, alcohol, LSD-25, pyrahexyl and chlorpromazine. Psychopharmacologia 4:167-183.

———. 1963b. The addiction research center inventory: appendix. Psychopharmacologia 4:184-205.

Himmelsbach, C. K. 1941. The morphine abstinence syndrome; its nature and treatment. Annals of Internal Medicine 15:829-839.

Hughes, P. H., E. C. Senay, and R. Parker. 1972. The medical management of a heroin epidemic. Archives of General Psychiatry 27:585-591.

Isbell, H., and T. L. Chrusciel. 1970. Dependence liability of "non-narcotic" drugs. Bulletin of the World Health Organization 43(Supplement):1–111.

Jasinski, D. R. 1975. Personal communication concerning unpublished studies of subjects maintained on morphine 30 mg/day and then withdrawn.

Jasinski, D. R., and P. A. Mansky. 1972. Evaluation of nalbuphine for abuse potential. Clinical Pharmacology and Therapeutics 13:78–90.

Jasinski, D. R., W. R. Martin, and R. Hoeldtke. 1971. Studies of the dependence-producing properties of GPA-1657, profadol and propiram in man. Clinical Pharmacology and Therapeutics 12:613–649.

Katchinoff, R., R. Leveille, L. T. McClelland, and M. G. Wagner. 1973. Schedule-induced behavior in humans. Physiology and Behavior 11:395–398.

Kleber, H., J. K. Kinsella, C. Riordan, S. Greaves, and D. Sweeney. 1974. The use of cyclazocine in treating narcotic addicts in a low-intervention setting. Archives of General Psychiatry 30:37–42.

Kolb, L. 1925. Pleasure and deterioration from narcotic addiction. Mental Hygiene 60:699–724.

Lasagna, L., J. M. Von Felsinger, and H. K. Beecher. 1955. Drug-induced mood changes in man, 1. observations on health subjects, chronically ill patients and "post addicts." Journal of the American Medical Association 157:1006–1020.

Mansky, P. A., and D. R. Jasinski. 1970. Effects of dextromethorphan in man. Pharmacologist 12:231.

Martin, W. R. 1967. Opioid antagonists. Pharmacological Reviews 19:463–521.

Martin, W. R., H. F. Fraser, C. W. Gorodetzky, and D. E. Rosenberg. 1965. Studies of the dependence-producing potential of the narcotic antagonist 2-cyclopropylmethyl-2'-hydroxy-5,9-dimethyl-6,7-benzomorphan (cyclazocine, win-20,740, ARCII-C-3) Journal of Pharmacology and Experimental Therapeutics 150:426–436.

Martin, W. R., and C. W. Gorodetzky. 1965. Demonstration of tolerance and physical dependence on N-allynomorphine (Nalorphine). Journal of Pharmacology and Experimental Therapeutics 150:437–442.

Martin, W. R., and D. R. Jasinski. 1969. Physiological parameters of morphine dependence in man—tolerance, early abstinence and protracted abstinence. Journal of Psychiatric Research 7:9–17.

Martin, W. R., D. R. Jasinski, and P. A. Mansky. 1973. Naltrexone, an antagonist for the treatment of heroin dependence. Archives of General Psychiatry 28:784–791.

O'Donnell, J. A. 1969. Narcotic addicts in Kentucky. Public Health Service Publication Number 1881, 297 pages.

Olds, J. S., and M. E. Olds. 1965. Drives, rewards and the brain. New Directions in Psychology—II. New York: Holt, Rinehart and Winston, pp. 329–410.

Pavlov, I. P. 1927. Conditioned Reflexes—An Investigation of the Physiological Activity of the Cerebral Cortex, G. V. Anrep, ed. and trans. New York: Dover.

Robins, L. N., J. E. Helzer, and D. H. Davis. 1975. Narcotic use in Southeast Asia and afterwards. Archives of General Psychiatry 32:955–961.

Skinner, B. F. 1953. Science and Human Behavior. New York: The Free Press.

Whitehead, C. C. 1974. Methadone pseudowithdrawal syndrome: paradigm for a psychopharmacological model of opiate addiction. Psychosomatic Medicine 36:189-198.

Wikler, A. 1965. Conditioning factors in opiate addiction and relapse. In Narcotics, D. M. Wilner and G. C. Kasselbaum, eds. New York: McGraw-Hill, Chapter 6, pp. 85-100.

_____. 1973. Dynamics of drug dependence: implications of a conditioning theory for research and treatment. Archives of General Psychiatry 28:611-616.

Wikler, A., and F. T. Pescor. 1965. Factors disposing to "relapse" in rats previously addicted to morphine. Pharmacologist 7:176.

Wilson, A. 1975. Disulfiram implantation in alcoholism treatment: a review. Journal of Studies on Alcohol 36:555-565.

Winokur, G., T. Reich, J. Rimmer, and F. N. Pitts. 1970. Alcoholism III. Diagnosis and familial psychiatric illness in 259 alcoholic probands. Archives of General Psychiatry 23:104-111.

Wisocki, P. A. 1973. The successful treatment of a heroin addict by covert conditioning techniques. Journal of Behavioral Therapeutics and Experimental Psychiatry 4:55-61.

World Health Organization Expert Committee on Addiction-Producing Drugs (until 1969 when changed to World Health Organization Expert Committee on Dependence Producing Drugs). 1957. Seventh Report. World Health Organization Technical Report, Series 116.

_____. 1964. Thirteenth Report. World Health Organization Technical Report, Series 273.

_____. 1969. Sixteenth Report. World Health Organization Technical Report, Series 287.

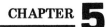
LOOKING AT SICK CHILDREN
A Comprehensive Formulation of Childhood Illness and Review of the Experience of a Psychosomatic Unit in a Children's Hospital

Timothy M. Rivinus, M.D.
Gordon P. Harper, M.D.

INTRODUCTION

The way that clinicians look at their patients is one of the crucial variables in medicine and health care. Such "mental sets" may be implicit or explicit, stated in the vernacular, or formalized as a conceptual model. They influence how clinicians perceive problems and formulate treatment plans. Clinical research has shown that the way doctors view their patients (and themselves and their work) influences treatment and outcome (Korsch et al., 1968; Heagarty and Robertson, 1971). Historically, the categories into which the sick and the deviant have been classified have reflected the aspects of human life that are of most concern to those doing the classifying (such as redemption or perdition, good or bad inheritance, or characterological

We wish to thank Dr. Eugene Piazza for his help in assembling part of the clinical data and for sharing with us his view of the developmental history of the Psycho-Somatic Unit at The Children's Hospital Medical Center, Boston. We alone take responsibility, however, for any errors of fact or interpretation of this material. This work was supported by grants from the Commonwealth Fund.

163

sloth or industry), as well as presumed mechanisms of illness (black or yellow bile, colic or melancholic, "body disease" or "mind disease").

The unprecedented expansion of the biological and psychological bases of medical practice in this century has created new areas of specialized knowledge and determined the current shape of this age-old question: Is the patient to be viewed in terms of a specialty, or comprehensively? Although everyone subscribes in principle to the goal of caring for the whole patient, that goal is made difficult both by the burden implicit in knowing a great deal about a particular system and by the ethical burden implicit in the specialist's ability to *do* a great deal to restore proper functioning.

The current balance between the specialized and comprehensive views can be assessed in two ways: by review of the clinical literature and by surveying the institutional arrangements developed for clinical care. In the area of child health, institutional development during the last two decades has, with notable exceptions (Janeway, 1968, 1974; Richmond, 1968, 1971), seen a trend toward more and more specialization. While primary physicians continue to confront all aspects of illness, the secondary and especially the tertiary facilities where most of the growth in child health services has occurred in this period have promoted patterns of training and of service delivery in which people and institutions become highly competent to assess one aspect, such as pediatric cardiovascular physiology, in a way not possible twenty years ago. But the role of the *integrative* child doctor or, perhaps, the health specialist of the whole child has not flourished to the same extent. Such a trend has been evident both in medical schools and residency training and in institutional arrangements for the provision of service (Duff and Hollingshead, 1968). Pediatricians who have concentrated on assessing common (but complicated) problems like headache or abdominal pains from a comprehensive point of view have reflected that while the generations of future pediatric neurologists, hematologists, and so on, are easily identified, it is harder to see where the future *comprehensive* pediatricians are coming from (MacKeith, 1974).

Child mental health specialists, especially child psychiatrists, have at times identified themselves as the advocates of the "whole child" and have brought to attention many features of children's life not otherwise appreciated. But they are located for the most part, both conceptually and in practice, far from their colleagues in child health. Child psychiatrists, for the most part, work in settings, such as child guidance clinics and private offices, tenuously (or not at all) attached to medical facilities and affording few daily interactions—either personal or intellectual—with clinicians who are attending to the nonpsychological aspects of their patients. It is hardly surprising that little common language and much mutual misunderstanding have arisen in these circumstances.

Such a split in institutional and professional practice is reflected in the literature on child health as well. Despite sporadic voices in the medical wilderness calling for appropriate attention to the needs of the "whole child" (Apley and MacKeith, 1962; Prugh, 1963), most literature is clearly directed toward audiences in one specialty or another. The split, reflecting the separate paths of investigation and therapeutics in each field, occurs particularly along the lines dividing those interested in psyche and those interested in soma. An article describing a new medical or surgical advance is unlikely to discuss its possible *meanings* to the children for whom it is intended, or offer relevant clinical advice for helping such patients and their families with predictable fears and fantasies. (The medical editors' complicity is reflected in the fact that the same articles would not be accepted if they neglected to discuss method and technique in adequate detail.) An article in the child psychiatric literature is just as unlikely to come to grips with the questions of genetic, physiological, or neurological contribution to the psychological dysfunction reported.

In such a climate, it is perhaps not surprising that the word "psychosomatic," at times promoted as the key to a holistic view of patients and illness (Apley and MacKeith, 1962; Lipowski, 1973; Pinkerton, 1972; Prugh, 1963), retains with some tenacity several narrow meanings over which the partisans of the psyche and the soma find it easy to struggle.[1] "Psychosomatic illness" thus has meant either physical symptoms of presumed psychological origin or illness in which current medical techniques do not reveal a specific somatic diagnosis and treatment. For others, "psychosomatic illness" has meant that which lies beyond one's understanding or special field of interest. In some situations where patients' unexplained suffering lies beyond one's special competence to understand and treat, frustration, exasperation, and finally resentment are the result. At those times, the term "psychosomatic" may be invoked to imply that the complaints are not "real," that the patients are in some sense dissimulating or "putting it on," and that they do not deserve the sick role to which they aspire. An interpersonal communication of hostility and rejection can then be conveyed in such ostensibly neutral comments as "There's nothing wrong with you," or "Our tests don't show anything—everything must be all right," or "I guess it's psychosomatic," as well in the more obviously hostile "It's not real," or "It's all in your head." All of these uses of the term

---

[1] In contrast to the emphasis on "psychosomatics," Richmond (1967) has proposed "child development" both as a focal point for those interested in the whole child and as a "basic science for pediatrics."

underline the clinical bankruptcy of an approach that involves both clinical overspecialization and a certain dualism of mind and body. It is as if the classical *"Nihil humani a me alienum puto"* (Nothing human can be foreign to me) had been changed in the century of science to *"Nihil a me alieni humanum puto"* (Nothing foreign to me can happen to people", "No illness I can't understand can be real").

In the last decade, a different, more specific, and yet wider definition of "psychosomatic medicine" has been proposed and with it a new conceptualization according to which all the aspects of any illness must be considered. Most notably, Lipowski (1973) has proposed that "psychosomatics" is the study of the *interactions* of social, psychological, and biological factors affecting illness. He stakes out this ground for the term in particular because of the obsolescence of older uses: "psychosomatic," meaning psychogenic, reflects the intellectual activity of the forties and fifties in which "psychogenicity" seemed the pressing issue; and the notion of a discrete roster of "psychosomatic illnesses" (Alexander et al., 1968) suggests incorrectly that the set of illnesses in which psychological factors are relevant is limited and definable. Lipowski identifies, according to this more comprehensive definition of psychosomatics, three aspects to the field: an analytic area, for researching *relationships and interactions* among social, psychological, and biological factors in illness; a synthetic area, for developing higher-order formulations of environment-mind-body transactions from the analytic data; and an applied, practical area, concerned with translating such knowledge into guidelines for clinical action (preventive, therapeutic, and rehabilitative).

We see such a redefinition of the field as a creative recognition that struggles over etiology, especially primacy of etiology, are both intellectually limiting and of diminishing usefulness to patients.

Lipowski (1973) and others (e.g., Reiser, 1975), however, working with adult medicine and psychiatry, have not applied this new formulation to illness in childhood. In this chapter, we intend to do so. In other words, we define psychosomatics as concerned with *all* illness—not just a discrete group of illnesses—and specifically with the *interaction* or *relationships* of many factors in illness.

The model requires the addition of two notable features of childhood and adolescence that can, as we will show, bear heavily on all aspects of health and disease. The first of these is the *developmental* aspect, the fact that individuals during the years of childhood and adolescence are undergoing the most dramatic (or at least the most noticed) psychobiological changes in the entire life cycle. The second is a consequence of the first: during the years of dependency, children and adolescents are necessarily involved, residentially, economically, and emotionally, in *families* or family surrogates.

DEVELOPMENTAL AND FAMILY ASPECTS OF
ILLNESS IN CHILDREN

Any clinician approaching any child, whether from the point of view of diagnosing illness or assessing health, must to some extent make explicit, and thereby clinically useful to him or her, a set of expectations of what is expected at any given age or stage of development. As with many parts of "common sense" that are translated both from and into explicit, professionally organized bodies of information, such expectations may appear trivial, concealing their importance in distinguishing normality from pathology. A few examples make the point, and the possible complications, clear. The nine-month-old infant is not expected to walk; the eighteen-month-old infant, generally, is. What of the ten-month-old who does walk? What of the fifteen-month-old who does not? Is the one precocious, the other retarded? At which point does either precocity or slowness suggest pathology? What of the fifteen-month-old who has been walking, but "gives it up" when he or she becomes ill? What of the fifteen-month-old who doesn't yet walk, but was born three months premature? When one adds to the variables of chronological age, age since conception, past medical and developmental history, and current stress, such variables as family and cultural expectations, it becomes clear how complicated developmental assessment can be.

The questions "When should a developmental milestone normally occur?" and "What does it mean when it has not?" apply in every area of the child's growth and development. "Which of them are 'absolute' cross-culturally and which are culture bound or influenced?" is a further area of concern. Any weight and height in a child are meaningful only when related to age norms and to the child's personal history. Conditions in every part of the body and the child's behavior that are pathological at one age are normal at another: the patent ductus arteriosus is physiological, "normal" throughout fetal development, and unremarkable through the first weeks of extrauterine life. Spontaneous voiding and stooling is normal until the age when neurodevelopmental maturation (usually around 2 years) permits and social and family expectations facilitate the acquisition of voluntary control; a definition of "enuresis" must include an age coordinate. The same applies to other "milestones," such as developmental motor skills (like clear speaking, tying shoes, and writing), changes in mental life (such as arrival at the Piagetian stage of formal operations), the physiological changes of puberty, and the psychosocial changes of adolescence. The content and context of each of these changes continue to be spelled out by investigators and clinical guidelines developed for understanding deviations from statistical norms.

Such clinical work clearly differs from the situation in adult medicine, where, for the most part, an "ageless" person is considered to be the "host" of a disease process. The progress of the child himself, vis-à-vis someone's idea of what he *should* be doing at his age, is of central concern to the clinician in the area variously called developmental assessment, developmental diagnosis or, in our view, developmental psychosomatics. The corresponding diagnostic issue of distinguishing "normal for age" from "developmental lag," and of deciding when "developmental lag" shades over into "illness" is clearly crucial. And the notion of "illness" involved here is different in one important way from the other kinds of "illness" we consider: in this case, the standard we use in identifying ill health or dysfunction must by necessity include some reference to age and carefully defined developmental expectations.

The relevance of the developmental frame of reference applies to the study of cognitive, emotional, and social growth of the child as well as of physical growth and psychological maturation (Erikson, 1950; Freud, 1965; Kohlberg, 1969: Piaget, 1952).

Two examples of problems in pediatric practice may illustrate the developmental perspective in some detail.

The changing pattern of life-threatening infections in infants and young children relates to the development of their immunological competence. The newborn, with limited experience with exogenous antigens, has initially only those antibodies that cross the placenta from the maternal circulation during gestation. Only antibody molecules of the Gamma G group cross and appear in the newborn circulation. Gamma M molecules, which mediate resistance to gram-negative bacteria, do not make this passage and are absent from the circulation of the infant for the first weeks of life. At this stage, accordingly, infants are susceptible to gram-negative infections at a rate that will not be matched at any other point in the life cycle. The maternally derived Gamma G antibodies, however, provide passive immunity against other bacteria, such as pneumococcus and *Hemophilus influenzae*, and so these infections rarely appear until the infant is at least six months old. By mechanisms less clearly understood, a developmental change in immunity to *H. influenzae* probably accounts for the observed decreased incidence of that infection following age 4 or 5. To explain the changing age incidence of other common infections of childhood, psychosocial milestones may be relevant. For instance, for most children, school entrance at age 5 or 6 means acquaintance not only with new peers, but with the multiple viral agents of common upper respiratory infections and exanthems those peers bring from *their* homes.

School entrance is a milestone from another point of view; problems here illustrate another kind of developmental pathology. School avoidance, initially masquerading as a host of diverse complaints, many involving physical symptoms, occurs especially at times when getting to school involves a developmental separation from home and parents (Eisenberg, 1958; Waldfogel et al., 1957). Looking just at the school years, one sees the peaks of school phobia to coincide with the milestones of separation; at age 5 or 6, when most children first enter school, and at puberty, when physiological maturation and environmental pressures distance the child from the psychosocial protection of family and latency and expose him or her to the increasing independence of adolescence. The many psychological problems of late adolescence, including first psychotic episodes, may be seen as analogies to another crisis of separation.

Developmental psychobiology affects every aspect of illness. We have cited age-specific incidences; other examples include idiopathic nephrotic syndrome of childhood, which rarely occurs before age 1 or after age 7; febrile seizures, which frequently accompany high temperature during infancy, rarely thereafter; and intussusception (passage of one segment of bowel into another, leading to ischemia and sometimes gangrene), which occurs principally around age 2, hardly ever thereafter. The same illness can also present at different ages with different symptoms: otitis media may be evident in the infant only as fussiness and poor feeding, in the older child as localized ear pain, and becomes quite rare after the configuration of the developing Eustachian tube changes. In the view of some, a single disease process, atopy, considered to be a constitutional predisposition to various allergic manifestations, accounts for eczema in infancy, for frequent respiratory infections with or without asthma in young children, for bronchial asthma in older children, and later still (after the asthma may clear in adolescence) for a predisposition to diverse allergic reactions such as to medications, foods, etc. Physicians must also consider *age-specific pathophysiological implications* of illness: the same gram-negative sepsis that is serious but not puzzling in a newborn raises the serious possibility of underlying immunological or hematological disorder when it occurs in a 5-year-old.

Once a diagnosis is established, there may be *age-specific therapeutic implications*. A fracture through a metaphyseal growth plate in the years when active skeletal growth remains must be managed differently from the same fracture at a later age. And mild degrees of congenital dislocation of the hip, recognized at birth before the acetabulum is fully formed, may be treated with special diapering; club foot recognized at the same age, with casts. At later ages, the hip would require prolonged casting; the club foot, surgery.

The physician must also be aware of *age-specific meanings* of illness or, rather, of interactions between illness, especially chronic illness, and psychosocial development. Because of developmental changes in body image, a preadolescent reacts to a transplanted kidney with different feelings and concerns from those of an adolescent. An illness like diabetes mellitus may present little apparent problem to a 10-year-old. A few years later, it can become the major focus of an adolescent's struggle to find a balance between dependence and independence, to reassess his body image and bodily integrity, and to renegotiate relationships with his parents and other authority figures (including doctors).

Other illness, or "illness behavior," may express *specific developmental concerns*. The adolescent's complaints to his or her physician of vague genital or perineal symptoms may serve as an entry ticket to a discussion of larger developmental issues such as genital integrity, anxiety over masturbation, or the implications of sexual intercourse. The challenge for the doctor is to tease out the developmental concerns behind the more easily presented concerns with illness.

The notion of developmental progression necessarily implies the concept of *developmental regression*. All children grow by forward movement, regression, and then resumption of forward movement. Any crisis (whether it be birth of a sibling, a family move, a frightening event, or illness itself) may produce regression. The regression in turn may constitute or contribute to illness: enuresis or sleep disturbance in a younger child who has previously mastered toilet training and night fears, or the exacerbation of a chronic illness like seizure disorder or diabetes in an older child.

THE FAMILY AND ILLNESS

Children will bring developmental concerns, and all health and illness issues, to physicians primarily through the medium of their families (Anthony and Koupernik, 1970). (A broader definition of "family" includes nonfamily caretakers.) The familial component of childhood psychosomatics concerns the interaction of family and child around illness phenomena. In a simple example, a child complains of a (seemingly) random abdominal sensation to his or her mother. If the mother happens to have her own concerns about either the child's health, or abdominal pain in general (related, say, to family experience with abdominal malignancy), or unrelated intercurrent worries (which may in some way be stimulating the child's pains), the child's complaint may make her anxious. Her anxiety, even if she tries to reassure the child, in turn may be communicated to the child and make him or her more anxious about the sensation. Though the child may be the identified patient, the two come to medical attention as a family.

Factors in the family that will influence the family response to children's symptoms include the following: personal experience with illness; culturally determined attitudes to illness (Fabrega, 1974); the parents' own coping strengths; specific relationships to the child in question; the developmental stage at which parents and other children find themselves; any intercurrent crises; and the objective resources for health maintenance and health and other services available to the family, including notably the relationship with, and attitude toward physicians and other health care personnel. That relationship will be influenced in turn by the developmental stage of the physician—how able he is to respond to the demands the child's illness leads the family to place on him (Balint, 1957).

In the child, the following factors may be relevant: any constitutional disposition (genetic or acquired in ways not identified) to illness, the child's own developmental stage, specific strengths and weaknesses with which the child has emerged from earlier developmental stages and previous life stresses.

Minuchin (1974) has described the "family structure" of families of children with complicated illnesses—illnesses where the presence or exacerbation of physical symptoms in a child seem involved in some kind of interpersonal pathology in the family as a whole. He describes such families as characterized by "enmeshment" (overinvolvement in each other's personal lives), "overprotection," "rigidity in conflict resolution," and the use of the child to express parental conflict, especially where the parents' repertory of conflict-resolving techniques is limited. Minuchin and his colleagues (1975) have presented persuasive evidence that this view of the family is both conceptually useful and clinically effective. Although Minuchin has used this kind of model with regard to children with anorexia nervosa, diabetes mellitus, and asthma, it seems likely that such issues are relevant for the understanding of *all* children with chronic illness.

THE MODEL OF PSYCHOSOMATICS IN CHILDREN

We define psychosomatics in children as the study of the interaction of *all factors affecting all illness* in children, specifically including *biological* endowment and current status; *psychological* state, including both cognitive and affective components; *social* situation, including cultural, school, and community influences; and *family* factors, both as to specific family traditions and attitudes and current healthy or pathological relationships and functioning. Finally, all of these must be considered along a *developmental* axis, which places the child, with regard to each of these issues, in the context of normal or disturbed growth and development.

CLINICAL REVIEW

An illustration of the conceptual framework presented here can be drawn from the experience of the Psycho-Somatic Unit of The Children's Hospital Medical Center, Boston, Massachusetts.

Description of the unit In 1965, a ward was designated at The Children's Hospital Medical Center as an extended-care facility for children requiring chronic nursing care for orthopedic and neurological conditions. Pediatricians and psychiatrists began to utilize this unit for long-term hospitalization of patients with asthma, ulcerative colitis, and anorexia nervosa. It was apparent that these patients were easily lost and alienated in hospital wards oriented more toward acute care. Their long hospitalization generated discouragement and frustration among the hospital staff. In addition, comprehensive evaluation and rehabilitative planning were difficult to organize on wards whose model was acute illness, rapid turnover of patients, and conditions in which the emphasis was on fast diagnosis and medical and/or surgical treatment.

In 1970, the unit was renamed the "Psycho-Somatic Unit," and an admission policy was established, and the first concerted effort made to create a therapeutic milieu. Teachers from the Boston public schools offered limited instruction for the patients. Therapeutic groups were established for the patients on the unit and for their parents. In 1971, a job category new to the hospital was created with the introduction of "child care workers." This role, borrowed from clinical experience in the residential care of children, was filled mostly by young men, intended to augment and complement the (mostly) female nursing staff in the care of children with difficult behavior as well as medical problems. In 1972, the Psycho-Somatic Unit was made a joint operation of The Children's Hospital Medical Center and the affiliated Judge Baker Guidance Center, drawing on the clinical resources, interests, and skills of the medical hospital and the child guidance–residential treatment traditions. The school of the Judge Baker Guidance Center provided special instruction for the children on the unit, including those with learning disabilities and emotional disturbance.

Each patient was assigned a psychotherapist drawn from staff or trainess in child psychiatry, clinical psychology, and social work at the two institutions. A case worker (usually a social worker) was assigned to each set of parents. In addition, by 1972, a referral net had been established by which pediatricians and psychiatrists throughout eastern New England referred patients to the unit. Other patients continued to come from other wards and outpatient clinics at The Children's Hospital Medical Center.

In 1974, the unit capacity was doubled and now has twenty-seven beds. A full census and a large waiting list suggest that the unit fulfills an otherwise unmet need for the patients, their families, and their referring doctors.

The ideas behind the unit included: (1) autonomy of the unit in terms of admissions (no "dumping" of inappropriate patients from other wards); (2) the importance of a cohesive milieu staff (no indiscriminate "floating" of staff to and from the unit); (3) the team approach with pediatrician, therapist, case worker, and milieu staff; (4) sustained ties with the rest of the hospital (consultative services, laboratories, research), avoiding the nonmedical residential treatment model; (5) total involvement of the child in a milieu program that included medical and psychiatric treatment, school, and activity programs; (6) involvement of the family in the treatment program; (7) emphasis on the "therapeutic leave of absence," using graduated lengths of return home to test the gains made in the treatment program; and (8) new approaches to the funding of a longer hospitalization for children with complicated and interrelated medical and psychological problems.

The unit evolved as much through necessity as through design. This necessity operated in several areas. First, with regard to admissions, the original plan was to admit a group of patients with a discrete group of "classical" (Alexander et al., 1968) psychosomatic (meaning psychogenic) conditions. This policy was modified through the *needs* of the referring medical and hospital community into the present policy: to take children with illnesses in which a variety of medical and psychological problems were intermingled (avoiding the narrow argument of "psychogenicity"). This policy is reflected in widely ranging diagnoses as shown in Table 1. Second, such a heterogeneous group of patients, with severe medical and psychological problems, created a demand for clinicians who could relate to both. Third, full evaluations revealed the severity of their school and learning problems (see Table 2), and the educational part of the program had to be expanded from brief visits to the ward by public school teachers to a fully developed special educational program for all the children, on a full-school-day basis. Fourth, acquaintance with these children brought to light the difficult family problems involved in the chronicity of their illnesses and led to the expansion of the family treatment component of the program.

Analysis Our analysis of the clinical experience of the Psycho-Somatic Unit is presented in two parts. Table 1 presents, for the entire period September 1970 to December 1975, a breakdown by diagnostic groups of the admissions. Diagnosis here refers to the major problem. A more detailed examination of a smaller group of patients is presented in the review of the admissions between July 1973 and December 31, 1973 (Table 2). Data for these thirty-one

TABLE 1   Admissions to the Psycho-Somatic
Unit, the Children's Hospital Medical
Center, Boston, Mass., September
1970–December 1975 (64 Mos.)[a]

	Total	Female	Male
Anorexia	64	56	8
Asthma	32	10	22
Obesity	28	18	10
Encopresis and enuresis	28	8	20
Ulcerative colitis and regional enteritis	16	6	10
Seizures	25	14	11
Conversion reactions	18	10	8
Miscellaneous (e.g., sickle cell anemia, ileal loop)	17	7	10
Abdominal pain— school phobia	17	9	8
Cyclic vomiting	12	10	2
Diabetes	10	4	6
Collagen diseases	6	2	4
Children at risk, failure to thrive	29	14	15
Eczema	5	3	2
Headaches	6	3	3
Myelodysplasia	6	2	4
Neurological diseases	10	3	7
Lead poisoning	3	0	3
Post-op cardiac surgery	5	2	3
Total	337	181	156

[a]Including 17 readmissions.

cases are presented (two were omitted because records were inadequate or unavailable). They were tabulated for review under the following headings: age, sex, medical diagnoses (primary, secondary, etc.), age at onset of symptoms, psychiatric diagnosis, pathological family relationships, developmental deviations, school problems (behavioral and academic), and disturbances in the social environment of the child. Data were tabulated if felt to contribute significantly to the child's problems and to the outcome. Such impressions are necessarily subjective; they represent an unfolding, as well as a retrospective, picture. Examples may illustrate the degree of disturbance reflected in the table. Under pathological family relationships

TABLE 2 Psycho-Somatic Unit Case Review July–December 1973

Case number	Age on admission (years)	Sex	Medical diagnosis	Age onset of medical symptoms (years)	Psychiatric diagnosis[a]	Disturbance[b]				Outcome (at end of hospitalization and at 12-month follow-up)
						Family	Developmental	School	Social	
1	4	M	Gait disturbance; fecal soiling; ? seizure disorder; failure to thrive	10 months	Psychoneurotic disorder, anxiety type	+	+	−	+	Improved
2	7.5	F	Eczema; alopecia; asthma; strabismus	Infancy	Social developmental deviation	+	+	+	+	Dramatic improvement
3	8	F	Asthma; eczema; short stature	Infancy	Integrative developmental deviation	+	+	+	−	Dramatic improvement
4	8	F	Asthma	1	Affective developmental deviation	+	+	+	−	Improved
5	8	F	Post infectious encephalopathy; ? cerebral vascular accident; with severe regression	7.75	Brain syndrome	+	+	+	−	Improved
6	8.5	M	Primary encopresis; asthma	Toddler years	Psychoneurotic disorder, phobic type	+	+	+	−	Improved
7	10	F	Myelodysplasia; encopresis	Birth	Motor developmental deviation	+	+	+	+	Improved
8	11	F	Secondary encopresis	4	Personality disorder	+	+	+	−	Improved
9	11.5	M	Anorexia nervosa	11	Psychoneurotic disorder, depressed type	+	−	−	−	Improved

175

TABLE 2 (*continued*) Psycho-Somatic Unit Case Review July–December 1973

Case number	Age on admission (years)	Sex	Medical diagnosis	Age onset of medical symptoms (years)	Psychiatric diagnosis^a	Disturbance^b Family	Developmental	School	Social	Outcome (at end of hospitalization and at 12-month follow-up)
10	11.5	F	Obesity	Infancy	Social and psycho-sexual developmental deviation	+	+	–	+	Not improved
11	12	F	Epilepsy and hysterical behavior	9	Hysterical personality disorder	+	+	+	+	Not improved
12	12	M	Obesity; abdominal pains; headaches; ? duodenal ulcer; fainting spells; serous otitis	Varied; mostly of long standing	Social developmental deviation	+	+	+	–	Improved
13	12	F	Anorexia nervosa	12	Personality disorder	+	+	–	–	Dramatic improvement
14	13	F	Anorexia nervosa	11.5	Psychoneurotic disorder, obsessive-compulsive type	+	+	–	–	Improved
15	12	M	Primary encopresis	Toddler years	Psychoneurotic disorder, depressed type	+	+	+	–	Dramatic improvement
16	13	M	Small stature; epilepsy	1	Psychoneurotic disorder, depressed type	+	+	+	+	Improved
17	14	M	Ulcerative colitis	9	Psychoneurotic disorder, depressed type	+	+	–	–	Improved

No.	Age	Sex	Complaint	Age of onset	Psychiatric diagnosis					Outcome
18	15	F	Anorexia nervosa	13	Personality disorder, compulsive type	+	+	+	−	Improved
19	15	M	Asthma	1	Psychoneurotic disorder, phobic type	+	+	+	+	Dramatic improvement
20	15	M	Abdominal pains	14	Psychoneutrotic disorder, depressed type	+	−	+	−	Dramatic improvement
21	15.5	F	Anorexia nervosa	14.5	Psychoneurotic disorder, depressed type	+	+	−	−	Improved
22	15	M	Obesity; abdominal pain; recurrent vomiting	14	Psychosis of late childhood	+	+	+	+	Not improved
23	15.5	M	Diabetes mellitus; seizure disorder	11	Personality disorder	+	+	+	+	Improved
24	16	F	Recurrent vomiting; obesity	14	Personality disorder, mixed	+	+	+	−	Improved
25	16	F	Obesity; abdominal pain	Always obese	Psychoneurotic disorder, depressed type	+	+	+	−	Improved
26	16	F	Leg pains; metromenorrhagia; alleged rape; ran away from orphanage	15	Personality disorder, mixed	+	+	+	+	Improved
27	16	M	Regional enteritis	13	Psychosis of late childhood	−	+	+	−	Improved
28	16	F	Anorexia nervosa	15	Psychosis of late childhood	+	+	+	−	Improved

177

TABLE 2 (*continued*) Psycho-Somatic Unit Case Review July–December 1973

Case number	Age on admission (years)	Sex	Medical diagnosis	Age onset of medical symptoms (years)	Psychiatric diagnosis[a]	Disturbance[b]				Outcome (at end of hospitalization and at 12-month follow-up)
						Family	Developmental	School	Social	
29	17	F	Obesity; chronic active hepatitis with post-necrotic cirrhosis; hematologic problems; steroidism	4	Personality disorder, overly dependent	+	+	+	−	Not improved
30	17	F	Anorexia nervosa	16	Psychoneurotic disorder, depressed type	+	−	+	−	Not improved
31	17	M	Primary encopresis and enuresis	Toddler years	Developmental deviation, mixed	+	+	+	+	Improved

[a]Committee on Child Psychiatry, 1966.
[b]+ = presence of disturbance; − = absence of disturbance.

were listed paternal absence, and maternal abandonment at time of hospitalization; chronic family scapegoating of the patient (for example, the favorite daughter of the deceased father, by the widowed mother and two sisters) and father-daughter incest. Less overt but equally damaging family pathology of the kind described by Minuchin (1974) was common. Developmental deviations included severe temper tantrums at age 8 in a child with asthma; pica at age 4; hydrocarbon ingestion at age 5; uncompleted toilet training in a 12-year-old; severe separation problems in many older children, and infantile manner and way of relating in an 8-year-old. School problems included truancy, school phobias, specific and global learning disabilities that were previously undetected and untreated, and other antisocial behavior at school. Examples of significant social disturbance were: inner-city families with absent or inadequate financial support living in slum dwellings and rural families in debt and legal difficulties.

There were fourteen boys and seventeen girls. The age range was from 4 to 17. Of the thirty-one, twenty-nine had established a medical diagnosis prior to their arrival. Two presented medical diagnostic problems; investigation yielded a diagnosis of post-ictal encephalopathy in one case, and multiple conversion reactions in the other. Fifteen of the cases had a single medical diagnosis upon admission, sixteen had multiple medical diagnoses upon admission. Of the thirty-one, twenty-one had, before referral, psychiatric diagnoses or behavioral symptoms clearly described. Of the remaining ten, although behavioral problems were suspected at the time of referral, these were not well described. During the hospitalization, it became clear that these ten had psychopathology worthy of diagnostic record.

Table 2 lists these patients in order of chronological age with associated medical diagnoses, age of onset of medical symptoms, psychopathological diagnoses, presence or absence of significant findings in the areas mentioned, and outcome.

Previous treatment and referral From an examination of the age of onset of initial medical symptoms all but one (Case 5) of the diagnoses would appear chronic. Hospitalization in other settings for the presenting problem had occurred two or more times in fourteen cases, once in ten cases (this includes transfers from other wards at The Children's Hospital Medical Center); and seven had never been hospitalized for the presenting problems and were direct outpatient referrals to the unit. Two were second admissions to the unit. Thirteen were direct transfers from other hospital wards at The Children's Hospital Medical Center. Three were direct transfers from other hospital inpatient services. Nine were referrals from The Children's Hospital Medical Center Out-Patient Departments. Seven were direct out-patient referrals from other sources.

Although the thirteen cases transferred from other wards at The Children's Hospital Medical Center were made in consultation with a staff psychiatrist, the major impetus for referral came from a pediatric subspecialist. Five cases were referred by a single hospital-based pediatrician who is a specialist in behavioral disorders. Two cases were referred by local pediatricians. Five cases were referred by psychiatrists. Four cases were referred jointly by psychiatrists and pediatricians. Five cases had been in psychiatric care for some time prior to the referral for the presenting problem or related problems.

These data highlight the large amounts of professional attention that these cases required prior to their referral and the high medical cost of their care. They also, we believe, show the high degree to which these patients have frustrated the well-meaning professional attempts at their rehabilitation.

Family, developmental, school, and social problems Thirty of the thirty-one patients had significant family pathology. In none of the referral material on these patients were family factors mentioned as important problems or contributing factors. In twenty-seven of the cases, there were past or present developmental deviations. In twenty-four of the thirty-one patients, there were significant school problems. All twenty-four were associated with impaired academic performance of long standing or with recent academic deterioration. Eleven of the twenty-four children with school disturbances also had problems of school nonattendance. Only rarely (five cases) were school problems mentioned in the referral. In eleven of the thirty-one cases, there were significant environmental or social factors that contributed to the presenting symptom complex. It is noteworthy, however, that although poor socioeconomic background appeared of less significance than family and school problems when the whole group was reviewed, it was emphasized in eight of the eleven cases in the referral material.

Outcome The outcomes of patients in this sample, as can be seen from Table 2, are varied. The patients were rated at the end of hospitalization and at one year after discharge. The category of "dramatic improvement" indicates a complete clearing of the presenting problem and significant improvement in other areas after hospitalization and at one-year follow-up. Of these, there are a gratifying number: six. There were also twenty "improved" cases in which there was significant amelioration of presenting problems, other uncovered difficulties, and no further hospitalizations necessary. The remaining five cases were unimproved or worse. A clinical example of one of each of these categories is given below.

One of the dramatically improved cases, fourteen of the improved cases, and one of the unimproved cases remained in individual therapy or family therapy at one-year follow-up. Of the five unimproved patients after hospitalization, three have improved in outpatient psychotherapy at one year, one is in a state hospital, and one is lost to all but telephone follow-up.

CASE 1 R. C. is a 15-year-old black youth from an inner-city welfare family. His father was said to have had asthma before his violent death when the patient was 3. His mother has chronic asthma. The patient himself had had chronic respiratory difficulties since the age of eighteen months and had been hospitalized nine times for asthma. He had had three hospitalizations in the six months prior to admission. He had had many emergency-room visits. Therapy had been arranged for him and his family by mental health workers in three other institutions, but each time follow-up was lost. He had missed eighty-six days of school in the prior year. Although well into puberty, he was still locked in a dependent struggle with his mother. The family was socially disorganized and his one-year-older sister had recently become pregnant out of wedlock. They lived in a slum dwelling that was often without heat. He was diagnosed to be of borderline intelligence with severe anxiety and phobic neuroses in addition to his asthma. He had advanced restrictive and constrictive lung disease by the time of admission. He had been on steroids for a year prior to admission. In four months of hospitalization, intensive physiotherapy, individual psychotherapy (including relaxation and desensitization therapy for phobias that precipitated attacks), family case work, school help, and special education were offered. Significant improvement occurred: he was weaned from steroids, had no further asthma attacks, and continued to do well following discharge. In the year since discharge, he has had no hospitalizations and no emergency-room visits for asthma. He remains off steroids and has grown four inches in one year. He is employed in a vocational workshop. His family has been aided in a move to better housing. His case can be considered a dramatic improvement.

CASE 2 F. T. is a 17-year-old boy with diabetes mellitus and seizure disorder. In the year prior to admission he had had two hospitalizations for insulin overdoses. He was an angry young man with suicidal thoughts and intentions. There was significant family pathology. His father was an alcoholic and often abused his children. Diabetes, depression, and family problems had made him miss much school and fail academically in recent years. His management of his diabetes mellitus was inconsistent, defiant, and, at times, self-destructive. He had a stormy course on the Psycho-Somatic Unit, but his attitude slowly improved. He became more consistent and positive toward management of his diabetes. He still displayed hostility and anger toward members of his disturbed family. He was transferred to another psychiatric hospital, and he remained there for two months. Upon discharge, he was engaged in an outpatient group therapy program at a state hospital. He continues there and attends school regularly while living at home. There have been no further insulin overdoses, the management of his diabetes mellitus has presented no problem, and his follow-up clinic appointments have been regular. This can be considered to be an improved case.

CASE 3 H. N. is a 12-year-old girl with a seizure disorder dating from the age of 9. She had been treated with anticonvulsants as an outpatient in The Children's Hospital Neurology Clinic. She had also had two hospitalizations for seizure control. Her mother had an immature and disturbed personality, had been married and divorced three times, was sexually intemperate, and had incurred many debts. Her younger brother presented behavior problems at home and at school. H. N. was doing poorly academically and behaviorally in school for at least one year prior to her admission. She had had two hospitalizations within the previous year for seizures that in retrospect are suspected to have been conversion episodes. She was admitted to Children's Hospital for seizure control, then while on the acute medical ward, demonstrated aggressive, sexually provocative, and histrionic behavior as well as hysterical epileptiform attacks. She was then transferred to the Psycho-Somatic Unit, where she remained for four months. There were two runaway incidents. After the second runaway from the unit, it was felt that an open ward could not contain such behavior and she was discharged home. Her mother never cooperated in the inpatient or outpatient treatment program or follow-up as arranged. After four months at home, H. N. overdosed herself with seizure medication and was admitted in an acute condition to a general hospital. She was not readmitted to Children's Hospital but was transferred to a state hospital children's unit. She remains there, still evidencing hysterical and aggressive behavior, an uneven hospital course and an uncertain future. Her case can be considered to be in the category of not improved or worse.

Conclusions The patients described represent complex medical and psychological problems that defied comprehensive treatment in other settings sometimes over many years. They represent cases that generalist and specialist pediatricians and child psychiatrists felt at the time of referral required more than traditional settings could offer. They are patients who demand much financially, physically, and emotionally from themselves, from their families, and from the professionals caring for them. The complexities of their medical and behavioral difficulties necessitated a team approach. Severe and often chronic cases, they required much time to unravel diagnostic knots and to plan for future management. In many cases, disturbed areas of functioning previously unsuspected were uncovered during the diagnostic work-up. These areas included family, school, developmental, and social disturbance. With a holistic approach to the patient, including team cooperation of medical, psychological, family, social, and school disciplines, encouraging results in many of these chronically ill and disturbed children with multiple problems could be achieved.

DISCUSSION

The demanding and difficult group of patients presented here illuminates two points: first, frequently our most intractable patients are those who "fall through the cracks" of our expertise; and, second, our difficult diagnostic and treatment problems as often represent what we have not considered as what we do not know. We contend that clinicians in no field are at present specifically trained to consider clinical phenomena from several shifting points of view. That is, neither in medical or psychiatric training, nor in clinical social work or dynamic psychotherapy, is the ability to shift from one point of view to another and to consider data not just from different systems, but from different *kinds* of systems, deliberately cultivated. One description of this kind of mental exercise is in Erikson's essay (1964) "The Nature of Clinical Evidence." In it, he describes the analytic therapist's scanning attention, moving partly by design and partly by free association to consider historical data, psychological test findings, the patient's present and past situation, feelings in the patient, and feelings in the therapist—and then trying to integrate all of these kinds of information in a way that can help the patient.

The kind of exercise we describe differs from the familiar process of medical differential diagnosis in two ways: first, differential diagnosis attempts to reveal physiological mechanisms of illness, but not necessarily the contributions of different *kinds* of systems (such as the psychology of the individual, and family dynamics); second, the goal of differential diagnosis is a unitary diagnosis, the "right" diagnosis, and a "name" even if it is as nonspecific as "idiopathic." We are suggesting here, on the other hand, that a *plurality of diagnoses* from different areas of the child's life is inevitable in many cases, particularly the difficult ones, and that it is expressly the *interactions* among the problems in these different areas that are clinically relevant.

The lucidity and organizational efficiency of the Problem-Oriented Method of Record Keeping promoted by Weed (1971) has in recent years appealed to many concerned with issues of medical diagnosis and treatment planning. Our proposal differs from the "Weed System" in that we do not take for granted the increasingly specialized clinician's inclination to look into *all* relevant areas of the patient's life and recognize them as areas of potentially unrecognized significance to the patient's medical and psychological dysfunction.

Another critique of traditional medical diagnosis came in Balint's proposal (1965) for "overall diagnosis," in which he hoped to combine an "autogenous" diagnosis (what the patient complains of) and an "iatrogenous" diagnosis (what the doctor feels he or she can recognize and treat). We would push clinicians treating "intractable," "chronic," or "recidivist" patients to go even further, beyond both their own spontaneous survey of the patients' problems, and beyond what the patients themselves might complain of, to a fuller examination of everything going on in the patients' lives that may be of relevance to illness.

Our work may bear comparison with that of Lazare (1973). He identifies four "hidden conceptual models" in psychiatry (behavioral, social, medical, and psychological) and attributes much of the frequent misunderstanding of psychiatrists, by each other and by other physicians, to their failure to make explicit which of these models is being used. His purpose in identifying these models is to encourage clarification of thinking and communication. In a sense, we are offering an extension of his model—to a new age group, with different kinds of illnesses (here, all childhood illness), and invoking two new sets of considerations: family and development. While he suggests that the several models may operate alongside each other, we would raise a more difficult challenge to the clinician: not just to set different ways of thinking next to each other, but to *integrate* the findings from each in order to best organize a treatment plan for the patient.

As medical educators have not promoted training in this integrative clinical work (Janeway, 1974)—with the exception of the current resurgence of family medicine—so medical administrators have not appreciated the challenge of developing institutional expression for integrative medicine. Rather, institutional growth has often seemed a captive of the specialty services (reflecting current "academic" medical trends and fiscal arrangements that make specialized laboratory and diagnostic services especially attractive to hospital administrators). It is as if specialty services were the only setting in which scientific knowledge could be translated into patient care.

The Psycho-Somatic Unit reviewed here has tried to provide an institutional framework within which integrative, or comprehensive, care can take place. Specifically, the goal has been a medical ward that has a psychiatric orientation as well. We would emphasize again the way that this unit arose *by necessity* rather than by design. If there was an original design, it was that children with "pure psychosomatic" (meaning psychogenic) illnesses would be admitted; the name Psycho-Somatic Unit was adopted in that sense, and only the needs of the referring medical community, including a pediatric hospital and the internal logic of having such a unit located in the pediatric hospital, led to the unit's development into a unit offering children comprehensive care.

One way to view the unit's evolution-by-necessity is to review its development as a gradual acknowledgment that it was, indeed, a psychiatric unit, as well as a medical ward, and to make provisions, in several ways, for that fact. This "coming of age" has involved many administrative and clinical arrangements undreamed of on other hospital wards.

On a policy level, the need of each child for a psychotherapist, and of each set of parents for a psychiatric social worker, was accepted. It soon became clear that the kind of therapy and family case work provided had to be sophisticated and intensive. The decision to arrange special education through a liaison with the Judge Baker Guidance Center School was made in the same spirit. Team work and time for communication and supervision were built in at all levels. The details of the particular problems recognized as part of the job, and of the special support systems built accordingly, for milieu staff and for the pediatric house officer, go beyond the scope of this article and are described elsewhere (Harper and Rivinus, 1976). The emotional development of staff and leadership was recognized to be a crucial therapeutic ingredient. Administrative issues for the hospital as a whole ranged from the complex financial arrangements necessary for such hospitalizations to special flexibility in the face of troubling behavioral symptoms (such as fire setting and running away).

This part of the development of the unit can be seen both as an acknowledgment, inside and outside the unit, that the psychiatric problems here were not "something added" to be treated in a secondhand or part-time way, but a coequal part of the clinical work. This acknowledgment was difficult because of the inevitable tendency of ward staff, off-ward physicians, and hospital administration to deny the severity of the children's problems. It has been difficult for everyone in the hospital, as it is for parents and all clinicians, to acknowledge the pain, sorrow, and anxiety of children both physically ill and emotionally disturbed. The understandable wish that one could care for such children only by treating their wheezing, weight loss, or impacted colon makes all clinicians eager to try to "make do" with as little emotional involvement as possible. Gradually, it was seen, however, that progress for the children could only come if it were possible for the staff to *live* with the children, understand how they felt beneath their symptoms, and then accept and work with them and their families.

The therapeutic program was not simply the marriage of a psychiatric and a medical ward. The whole was indeed greater than the sum of its parts, just as the cases could not be described simply as one child with two illnesses—medical and psychiatric. Two examples may illustrate how the program worked. The 8-year-old girl (Case 5) with severe developmental regression following post-infectious and post-ictal encephalopathy received more than just medical rehabilitation services. As she gradually recovered the ability to swallow, to walk, to use the toilet, and to control her impulsiveness in play with other children, there was continual interchange between pediatrician, school, psychotherapist, and milieu staff, so that the demands made in the milieu were carefully paced to her progress and needs. Just as recovery of her developmental losses involved neurological, cognitive, and emotional progress, so the contributions of specialists in each of these areas had to be coordinated. In the meantime, case work with the parents (and gradually increasing home stays) helped them to cope with a situation that had initially left them feeling completely overwhelmed. They were then more ready to help their child at home at the time when she was ready to leave the hospital. The patient's involvement in a real-life setting (and its transfer to the real-life setting of home), as opposed to a traditional ward in which most of the patients would be bedridden, was crucial for her redevelopment of adaptive skills and for the parents' ability to see that she could, indeed, reenter a normal life situation.

In another case, a 12-year-old boy (Case 15) with primary encopresis had been treated for five years by a pediatrician and a psychotherapist as an outpatient. In his case, a concerted use of the Therapeutic Life Space (Redl, 1966) as a therapeutic tool, especially around his soiling, in coordination with psychotherapy and family case work, produced change in a symptom that had determinants in his bowel physiology and his personality development, both of which had been refractory to other treatment over many years.

The usefulness of this unit can be measured, as we have indicated, in the outcome of the presenting illnesses. Another kind of outcome criterion is the frequency of new diagnoses, especially those bearing on personal adjustment and school problems. A third kind of usefulness, which applies both to a conceptual model and to such a unit, is the *heuristic* purpose: whether it helps clinicians, patients, and families to *make sense* of children's illness and suffering. Frequent comments at time of referral to the unit expressed the bafflement engendered by these patients' illnesses of conscientious and skilled physicians as well as parents. As treatment progressed, the uniform outcome was that some understanding of what was going on was indeed possible. The benefit derived by simply adding *understanding* of the child's total situation to therapeutic management cannot be underestimated, especially in dealing with medically ill and disturbed children to whom the personal experience of not being understood is all too well known.

An implication of this argument for medical education is that *all* medical and psychiatric training should explicitly cultivate and encourage the ability to integrate data from many points of view in clinical work. It goes without saying that such a habit is useful in preventive medicine as well as in difficult diagnosis and treatment. Furthermore, the importance of the developmental and family aspects of illness suggests that clinical vision should expand to include these issues, perhaps most conspicuous in childhood, but in fact relevant at all points in the life cycle. Systematic exploration of developmental issues in the years of adulthood has begun (Haan, 1972; Levinson et al., 1974; Valliant and McArthur, 1972).

A final implication lies in the use of a residential unit as a medical ward, and of the medical usefulness of longer lengths of stay (average: around ninety days) than are customary on acute services. The fact that the children were up and out of bed and expected to take part in the daily activities of a healthy child including school was useful in both diagnosis and therapy. For example, many children's chronic scapegoating in school was understood through the repeated observation on the unit of the subtle but unmistakable ways that they provoked such responses from other patients. Recognition of this pattern made possible therapeutic intervention in the Therapeutic Life Space (Redl, 1966) of the unit.

SUMMARY

Recent reformulations of psychosomatic illness in general have departed from the conceptualizations of the 1940s and 1950s in two ways: They have extended the *content* of psychosomatics well beyond a concern for psychogenicity (or its absence) and for hypothesized intrapsychic mechanisms of symptom production (Reiser, 1975). At the same time, the *range* of conditions considered in psychosomatics has been broadened to include all illness in psychiatry and medicine. From this viewpoint, the idea of a discrete roster of "classical" psychosomatic disorders is rejected as obsolete. In its place, psychosomatics is redefined to deal with all illness and specifically with the interaction of biological, social, and psychological factors in illness (Lipowski, 1973). These redefinitions come (significantly) at a time of increased medical subspecialization, which lures clinicians away from a comprehensive view toward patient care.

Such reformulations have not reached, thus far, into childhood and adolescence. Pediatricians and child psychiatrists, in applying this work to their own concerns, will see the need to include two additional factors specific to childhood, namely, the changing situation of the *developing child* and the child's place *within the family*. We present a formulation of psychosomatics in children that takes into account these specific features of childhood.

To illustrate this theoretical formulation from a clinical point of view, thirty-one cases are presented (three in detail), representing a review of patients admitted during a seven-month period to the psychosomatic inpatient unit of The Children's Hospital Medical Center, Boston, Massachusetts. These were cases refractory to medical and (sometimes) psychiatric therapy exclusive of each other in other settings. They also represented considerable medical, emotional, and financial expenditure and frustration. The review demonstrated that a conceptual framework restricted to one set of factors (physical or psychological) was inadequate to understand these children's problems, and that a treatment program focused on multiple facets of the child's life and illness was necessary. The developmental circumstances and *modus operandi* of this treatment setting were reviewed in order to emphasize the needs that the unit met and the methods that contributed to its success.

REFERENCES

Alexander, F., T. M. French, and G. H. Pollock. 1968. Psychosomatic Specificity. Chicago: University of Chicago Press.

Anthony, E. J., and C. Koupernik, eds. 1970. The Child in His Family. New York: Wiley.

Apley, J., and R. MacKeith. 1962. The Child and His Symptoms—A Psychosomatic Approach. Philadelphia: Davis.

Balint, M. 1957. The Doctor, His Patient and the Illness. New York: International Universities Press.

———. 1965. Overall diagnosis: the doctor's therapeutic function. Lancet 1:1177-1180.

Committee on Child Psychiatry. 1966. Psychopathological Disorders in Childhood: Theoretical Considerations and a Proposed Classification. New York: Group for the Advancement of Psychiatry.

Duff, R. S., and A. B. Hollingshead. 1968. Sickness and Society. New York: Harper & Row.

Eisenberg, L. 1958. School phobia: diagnosis, genesis, and clinical management. Pediatric Clinics of North America 5:645-666.

Erikson, E. H. 1950. Growth and crises of the healthy personality. In Symposium on the Healthy Personality, Supplement II: Problems of Infancy and Childhood, J. E. Senn, ed. New York: Josiah Macy, Jr. Foundation.

———. 1964. Insight and Responsibility. New York: Norton.

Fabrega, H. 1974. Disease and Social Behavior: An Interdisciplinary Perspective. Cambridge, Mass.: MIT Press.

Freud, A. 1965. Normality and Pathology in Childhood. New York: International Universities Press.

Haan, N. 1972. Personality development from adolescence to adulthood in the Oakland growth and guidance studies. Seminars in Psychiatry 4:399–414.

Harper, G., and T. M. Rivinus. 1976. The psycho-somatic unit. Paper presented at the American Orthopsychiatric Association meeting, Atlanta, Ga.

Heagarty, M. C., and L. S. Robertson. 1971. Slave doctors and free doctors: study of physician-patient relations. New England Journal of Medicine 284: 636–641.

Janeway, C. A. 1968. Preface to Ambulatory Pediatrics, M. Green and R. J. Haggerty, eds. Philadelphia: Saunders.

———. 1974. Family medicine—fad or for real? New England Journal of Medicine 291:337–342.

Kohlberg, L. 1969. Stage and sequence: the cognitive-developmental approach to socialization. In Handbook of Socialization Theory and Research, D. A. Goslin, ed. New York: Rand McNally.

Korsch, B. M., E. K. Gozzi, and V. Francis. 1968. Gaps in doctor-patient communication. Pediatrics 42:856–871.

Lazare, A. 1973. Hidden conceptual models in clinical psychiatry. New England Journal of Medicine 288:345–351.

Levinson, D. J., C. M. Darrow, E. B. Klein, M. H. Levinson, and B. McKee. 1974. The psychosocial development of men in early adulthood and the mid-life transition. In Life History Research in Psychopathology, D. F. Ricks, A. Thomas, and M. Roff, eds. Vol. 3. Minneapolis, Minn.: University of Minnesota Press.

Lipowski, Z. J. 1973. Psychosomatic medicine in a changing society: some current trends in theory and research. Comprehensive Psychiatry 14:203–215.

MacKeith, R. 1974. Personal communication.

Minuchin, S. 1974. Families and Family Therapy. Cambridge, Mass.: Harvard University Press.

Minuchin, S., L. Baker, B. L. Rosman, R. Liebman, L. Milman, and T. C. Todd. 1975. A conceptual model of psychosomatic illness in children. Family organization and family therapy. Archives of General Psychiatry 32:1031–1038.

Piaget, J. 1952. The Origins of Intelligence in Children. New York: International Universities Press.

Pinkerton, P. 1972. The psychosomatic approach in pediatrics. British Medical Journal 3:462–464.

Prugh, D. G. 1963. Towards an understanding of psychosomatic concepts in relation to illness in children. In Modern Perspectives in Child Development, A. L. Solnit and S. A. Province, eds. New York: International Universities Press.

Redl, F. 1966. When We Deal with Children. New York: The Free Press.

Reiser, M. 1975. Changing theoretical concepts in psychosomatic medicine. In American Handbook of Psychiatry. S. Arieti, ed. Vol. IV. New York: Basic Books.

Richmond, J. B. 1967. Child development: a basic science for pediatrics. In Annual Progress in Child Psychiatry and Child Development, S. Chase and A. Thomas, eds. New York: Brunner-Mazel.

———. 1968. Preface to Ambulatory Pediatrics, M. Green and R. J. Haggerty, eds. Philadelphia: Saunders.

———. 1971. Toward the twenty-first century in child health. Address at the dedication of the major addition of the James Whitcomb Riley Hospital for Children, Indianapolis, Ind.

Valliant, G. E., and C. C. McArthur. 1972. Natural history of male psychological health; the adult life cycle from 18-50. Seminars in Psychiatry 4:415-427.

Waldfogel, S., J. C. Coolidge, and P. B. Hahn. 1957. The development, meaning and management of school phobia. American Journal of Orthopsychiatry 27:754-780.

Weed, L. 1971. Medical Records, Medical Education and Patient Care: The Problem-Oriented Record, a Basic Tool. Chicago: Year Book.

PART II

ISSUES THAT DETERMINE THE FRONTIERS AND LIMITS OF THE FIELDS OF PSYCHIATRY

CHAPTER 6

TEMPORAL LOBE EPILEPSY
A Syndrome of
Sensory-Limbic Hyperconnection

David M. Bear, M.D.

INTRODUCTION

> The air was filled with a big noise, and I thought that it had engulfed me. I have really touched God. He came into me myself, yes, God exists, I cried, and I don't remember anything else. You all, healthy people, he said, can't imagine the happiness which we epileptics feel during the second before our attack. I don't know if this felicity lasts for seconds, hours, or months, but believe me, for all the joys that life may bring, I would not exchange this one. . . . Such instants were characterized by a fulguration of the consciousness and by a supreme exaltation of emotional subjectivity. (Dostoevsky, 1935)

This remarkable description from *The Idiot* exhibits features of seizures involving the temporal lobe (Alajouanine, 1963; Ervin, 1967; Williams, 1968, 1969). Specifically, they relate perceptual alteration in two exteroceptive modalities ("big noise," "touched God") to interoceptive sensations of self ("it had engulfed me," "He came into me") in a setting of incandescent affective significance ("for all the joys," "a supreme exaltation of emotional subjectivity"). These phenomenological characteristics, which also appear in reports elicited by direct cerebral electric stimulation (MacLean, 1958; Penfield, 1954a, 1954b, 1955), parallel a basic property of functional neuroanatomy in the temporal lobe: extensive connections from visual, auditory, and somesthetic association cortices to gray matter structures of the limbic system including the amygdala, parahippocampal cortex and hippocampus, and orbital frontal cortex by way of the rostral temporal pole (Whitlock and Nauta, 1956; Gloor, 1960;

Geschwind, 1965; Pandya and Kuypers, 1969; Jones and Mishkin, 1972). This salient feature of structure, reflected in the experience of the ictus, points to a central function of the temporal lobe in attributing visceral or emotional significance to perceived stimuli.

The development of this concept will be central to our analysis of psychological consequences of temporal lobe epilepsy, many of which may be illustrated by further reference to Dostoevsky. There is reason to believe that the opening quotations represent transcriptions of seizures undergone by the author himself (Alajouanine, 1963). And while he suffered repeated temporal lobe seizures, which formed the basis of his many literary descriptions, his interictal personality took on well-known characteristics: deep emotionality, impulsive aggressivity, recurrent depression, mystical religiosity, sense of enhanced personal destiny, heightened moralistic concern over the problem of good and evil, ritualistic obsessionalism culminating in compulsive gambling, and—fortunate in his case—the strong desire to write at length (Alajouanine, 1963; Waxman and Geschwind, 1974).

This discussion supports the view (Gibbs, 1951; Glaser, 1964; Bruens, 1969; Waxman and Geschwind, 1974) that temporal lobe epilepsy is generally associated with progressive changes in personality. Extensive evidence, to be briefly summarized, documents an increased prevalence of particular psychiatric diagnoses such as paranoid schizophrenia in the temporal epileptic population (Davison and Bagley, 1969). Isolated objections that have been raised against these data and prior explanatory hypotheses will be critically discussed in the section "Interictal Psychiatric Diagnoses Associated with Temporal Lobe Epilepsy."

There has been a tendency in the past to limit discussion to such epidemiological correlations between temporal lobe epilepsy and traditional psychiatric diagnoses. However, there is no reason to believe that interictal psychological changes, if present, should correspond precisely to functional psychiatric syndromes described in other contexts where they remain poorly defined. We shall attempt, rather, to analyze specific changes in behavior, emotion, and thought, which are reliably altered in temporal lobe epilepsy as reported by multiple investigators. Eighteen categories have been constructed, and their accuracy in characterizing the interictal syndrome is supported by quantitative results of an ongoing investigation to be briefly reported here. We shall propose a mechanism underlying this constellation of psychological features: modification of affective association (see the section "Characteristics of Interictal Behavior").

A distinct process of attributing emotional valence to perceived objects of intellectual conceptions was first proposed at the turn of the century by Sigmund Freud (1923) in the term "cathexis." We shall attempt to relate this process to the anatomical confluence in the temporal lobe of exteroceptive sensory and limbic modalities (Geschwind, 1965; Jones and Mishkin, 1972). Structural disconnection of sensory and limbic systems resulting in a dissociation of affective qualities from visual or tactile stimuli has been postulated as the basis for experimental and clinical findings in several circumstances, most dramatically the Klüver-Bucy syndrome in monkey, cat, and human (see the section "Sensory Limbic Connection and Disconnection") (Klüver and Bucy, 1939; Schreiner and Kling, 1953; Geschwind, 1965; Terzian and Dalle Ore, 1955; Marlowe et al., 1975).

We shall suggest a contrasting process of sensory limbic hyperconnection, resulting in progressive overinvestment of perception and thought with affective significance, as a unifying mechanism relating diverse psychological changes in patients with longstanding temporal lobe epilepsy. Mechanisms that might lead to such anatomic hyperconnection will be considered in the section "Sensory Limbic Hyperconnection."

INTERICTAL PSYCHIATRIC DIAGNOSES ASSOCIATED WITH TEMPORAL LOBE EPILEPSY

The association of temporal lobe epilepsy (TLE) with interictal psychosis has been supported by clinical observations of neurological and psychiatric investigators in a variety of settings extending from mid-nineteenth century to the present (Davison and Bagley, 1969). Eugen Bleuler, originator of the diagnostic category of schizophrenia, so labeled many temporal epileptic patients, commenting that "epileptiform attacks may appear [in schizophrenia] at any stage of illness. These may remain isolated phenomena or repeat themselves over a period of years" (Bleuler, 1952; see also Rodin et al., 1957; Slater and Beard, 1963).

The quantitative prevalence of psychosis among patients with TLE remains a matter of controversy. Recent figures range from 2 percent (Currie et al., 1971), 25 percent (Hill, 1953a, 1953b), 33 percent (Gibbs, 1948), to 81 percent (Ervin et al., 1955). These discrepancies reflect biases of sampling and divergent criteria of psychosis as well as uncontrolled variation in onset and duration of illness, sex, handedness, and neuropathological lesion, which may correlate with psychosis (Tizard, 1962; Taylor, 1971).

Frequency statistics between poorly defined variables sampled nonrandomly may well be criticized. Yet an abundance of independent evidence (134 accounts reviewed by Davison and Bagley, 1969) compels us to conclude that "an interictal psychosis resembling schizophrenia occurs more often than chance in temporal lobe epilepsy" (Davison & Bagley, 1969). By comparison, the population prevalence of schizophrenia in the United States and the United Kingdom is approximately 0.8 percent (Slater and Beard, 1963; Flor-Henry, 1972).

There is a consensus that psychiatric disturbances including psychosis are more common in an epileptic population than at large (Mignone et al., 1970). The continuing disagreement concerns a specific association between temporal lobe seizures and psychopathology. I should like to discuss some of the objections that have been raised to this conclusion.

It has been noted that many reports of psychopathology among epileptic patients originate from psychiatric centers where selection might inflate the apparent prevalence of psychosis (Tizard, 1962; Stevens, 1966; Mignone et al., 1970). The critical observation from these data, however, is the association of psychopathology specifically with temporal lobe epilepsy, far above its incidence among all the epilepsies (Slater and Beard, 1963; Flor-Henry, 1972). There are certainly grounds for caution in extrapolating from these reports to a population prevalence of psychiatric disturbance in the epileptic population, but the observed correlation of psychopathology with TLE is not thereby invalidated.

Contrary to earlier objections (Stevens, 1966), several series of temporal epileptics evaluated preoperatively in neurosurgical (rather than psychiatric) settings demonstrated striking frequencies of sexual aberration, aggressiveness, and paranoid psychosis (Blumer and Walker, 1967; Blumer, 1970a, 1970b, 1974; Falconer, 1965, 1973; Taylor, 1969, 1971, 1972; Serafetinides, 1965a; Serafetinides and Falconer, 1962; James, 1960). Patients undergoing temporal lobectomy at the National Institutes of Health, a sample described as biased against psychiatric disease (Mignone et al., 1970), suffered a 40 percent incidence of psychiatric disorders prior to surgery (Van Buren et al., 1975).

A well-known study by Guerrant et al. (1962) has been summarized as showing no significant psychological differences between temporal and grand mal epileptics (Stevens, 1966). However, consideration of the nine tabulated psychopathologies[1] reveals that psychomotor patients

[1] From Stevens, 1966:

Psychopathology	Psychomotor	Grand mal
Adhesive	40.5	29.5
Mental slowing	25.0	11.5
Thought disorder	40.5	29.5
Apathy	21.8	11.5
Emotional lability	31.0	19.2
Anxiety	53.0	46.1
Compulsive	18.6	15.4
Withdrawal	53.1	42.4
Impulsive	34.5	34.6

showed higher frequencies on eight. On the ninth trait, impulsivity, the groups showed equal prevalence, which is at variance with many findings of aggressivity specific to TLE (Davidson, 1947; Glaser, 1964; Ervin et al., 1955; Serafetinides, 1965a; Taylor, 1969). Accepting the data as presented, the null hypothesis of no group difference should be rejected, since the probability is only .004 (binomial sign test) that so extreme an asymmetry of outcome is due to chance. Waxman and Geschwind (1974) have also noted that 23 percent of the psychomotor patients in this study (versus 4 percent of epileptic controls) obtained psychotic MMPI (Minnesota Multiphasic Personality Inventory) profiles.

A novel form of objection to the direct association of TLE and psychiatric pathology was proposed by Stevens (1966). The suggestion was made that TLE and psychiatric pathology are indeed correlated but only indirectly, since they are related through the underlying third variable of age. If the probability of psychomotor epilepsy increases with age as does the likelihood of psychiatric hospitalization, an older-aged sample might be expected to show both more TLE and psychiatric illness.

Even if true, such an epidemiological observation could not disprove a direct association. For example, hypertension is more common with advancing age, so are cerebral vascular accidents, and yet they are directly, not indirectly, related. But it is clear that no age group could be selected from a normal population to have a 25 percent, 33 percent, or 80 percent incidence of psychosis. The critical groups to test this hypothesis are age-matched populations. Yet Stevens' psychomotor group had the lowest mean age (35 years) of her contrasted samples with the highest rate of psychiatric hospitalization. Thus, a tendency for TLE and psychiatric hospitalization to increase with age could not account for her data.

A pervasive source of confusion in investigations of interictal psychopathology specific to TLE has been the seemingly reasonable strategy of contrasting "psychomotor" patients with those suffering from "grand mal" or "centrencephalic" seizures. The difficulties here are several. All epileptic groups have typically been quite abnormal (Stevens, 1966; Small et al., 1962; Small et al., 1966; Small and Small, 1967; Mignone et al., 1970). The investigator's methodology then may not be sensitive enough to distinguish the groups by more precise criteria. Since the epileptic "controls" are often abnormal, it has been falsely concluded that the TLE group is not, by comparison, deviant. For example, 29.4 percent of Stevens' grand mal group (1966) had undergone psychiatric hospitalization, which is atypical for a population drawn from a general epilepsy clinic (Gibbs, 1951). This almost makes 31.9 percent hospitalization in the psychomotor group seem normal. Clearly, such frequent psychiatric hospitalization is remarkable.

Further description reveals that the groups were qualitatively distinguishable on the basis of reasons for hospitalization. Schizophrenia, mood disturbance, anxiety, and withdrawal were diagnoses among psychomotor patients; mental slowness and apathy predominated in the grand mal group. Dongier (1959) reached a similar qualitative differentiation of psychomotor from centrencephalic patients, the former suffering longer psychotic episodes with affective disturbance, the latter frequent confusional attacks without progression and accompanied by EEG abnormalities suggestive of petit mal status.

Attempts to differentiate these groups with standard instruments such as the Minnesota Multiphasic Personality Inventory, Rorschach Inkblots, and Reitan Battery have led to equivocal results (Tizard, 1962; Herrington, 1969). This outcome suggests that the relevant psychological variables have not been assessed. Since the Rorschach Test may fail to distinguish schizophrenics from normals (Friedman, 1951) and the Reitan Battery clusters schizophrenia, manic depressive disease, and TLE with "brain damage" (Donnelly et al., 1972), these procedures are inadequate for diagnostic discrimination.

A more fundamental hazard of comparisons across epileptic subgroups is the probability that nontemporal epileptic samples include subjects with temporal lobe involvement. Here the distinction between a focus confined to the temporal lobe and invasion of the temporal lobe by seizure activity at some point in the ictus is relevant. If interictal psychopathology can follow repeated electrical stimulation of limbic structures, clearly it could develop with foci outside the temporal lobes that project to limbic sites (Ajmone-Marsan and Goldhammer, 1973; Ludwig et al., 1975).

There are at least two other ways of conceiving temporal lobe involvement in patients not electrographically identified as temporal epileptics: (1) A cortical focus outside the TL may coexist with a TL focus. Since TL foci are difficult to detect by scalp EEG, the patient may be diagnosed by the more readily detected focus. (2) All sensory association cortices project into the TL, and creation of a new epileptic focus following repeated electrical stimulation has been shown to be characteristic of temporal limbic structures (Morrell, 1959, 1960, 1961; Goddard et al., 1969). Thus, patients with extratemporal foci may subsequently develop secondary TL abnormalities. This effect has been observed following epileptic implants to parietal cortex of monkeys in which learning deficits characteristic of lesions of the amygdala appeared in those animals that developed secondary temporal foci (Stamm and Rosen, 1971).

While not free of such pitfalls, the most convincing group comparisons contrast focal nontemporal with temporal patients. Generally, these contrasts have been dramatic: Vislie and Henriksen (1958),

Juul-Jensen (1964), and Stevens (1966) found a low incidence of psychiatric disorder among focal nontemporal patients. In fact, Stevens reports only one (of twelve) such patients hospitalized for psychosis (versus seventeen out of fifty-four psychomotor patients), and this clearly for a toxic confusional state following anticonvulsant overdose. These comparative data are consistent and constitute control observations for the nonspecific psychological sequelae of "having epilepsy."

Perhaps the greatest difficulty in the study of the TLE psychopathology has resulted from attempting to force-fit traditional psychiatric diagnoses or psychological assessment scales derived from them to interictal psychological descriptions. This would seem to be working backwards. The electrophysiological diagnosis of TLE provides an anatomic reference, in some cases augmented by neuropathological observations (Falconer, 1965). With this foundation secure, more is to be gained scientifically by characterizing the resultant psychological state accurately than by squeezing all observations into the Procrustean bed of schizophrenia. "Procrustean bed" suggests a precision that this psychiatric category lacks; it is often used as a diagnostic wastebasket (see Chapter 2 on acute psychosis). The search for regular features of thought and behavior, which need not correspond to psychopathological labels, leads both to a clearer clinical account and to further testable hypotheses.

Characteristics of an advanced stage of interictal change following TLE emerge from the careful descriptions of Hill (1953a, 1953b), Pond (1957, 1962), Slater and Beard (1963), and Slater and Moran (1969). Slater and Moran presented sixty-nine patients without personality or genetic predisposition to schizophrenia who developed a psychotic state on the average of fourteen years following onset of seizures. The striking features of the group are summarized in order of approximate prevalence in this report and elsewhere. Affective disturbance was "shown by all patients," most frequently a deepening of emotion (Slater and Moran, 1969) and preserved affective intensity (Pond, 1962). Delusional ideas appeared in sixty-seven out of sixty-nine patients, mystical religious conceptions being extremely common. Paranoid feelings and explanatory systems justified a diagnosis of paranoid schizophrenia in forty-six patients. Disorders of thought were frequent, thirty-one patients displaying nonlogical, extraneous, or idiosyncratic associations. Hallucinations occurred in sixty-three patients, typically consisting of formed visual images or conversational phrases experienced with intense emotional significance (e.g., a vision of Christ on the cross in the sky, the voice of God saying, "You will be healed, your tears have been seen"—Slater and Beard, 1963). The quality of high emotional intensity—of images, thoughts, and conceptions shot through with a sense of urgency—is noteworthy in the description of many patients. These features of a state specifically associated with temporal lobe epilepsy have been corroborated by subsequent accounts (Bruens, 1969; Falconer, 1973; Taylor, 1971, 1972; James, 1960; Serafetinides and Falconer, 1962; Glaser, 1964; Dewhurst and Beard, 1970).

This syndrome, which occurs in a small though epidemiologically significant number of patients with longstanding seizures (Slater and Beard, 1963), has prompted many attempts at explanation. Commonly, the psychological pressures of suffering a chronic disease with a socially limiting, embarrassing, unpredictable episodic course are stressed (Horowitz, 1970; Savard and Walker, 1965). Of course, these factors are present but fail to explain the features of the clinical picture above. Such a state is not a regular consequence of focal nontemporal epilepsy, chronic episodic conditions like ulcerative colitis, or progressive neuromuscular diseases (to be discussed below).

The "holistic" notion that cognitive disturbances of time sense and memory, direct sequelae of TL involvement, add to the patient's psychological concerns at the moment to produce the psychiatric picture has been offered (Ferguson et al., 1969; Weinstein, 1959). Again, individual episodes of psychotic confusion may be so explained, but the end stage common to many patients cannot be. An important observation in this regard is that the development of psychosis in TL patients correlates negatively with psychomotor seizure frequency (Flor-Henry, 1969a). Subtle interictal disturbances of time sense and memory have been demonstrated among temporal epileptic patients prior to surgery, but only by careful experimental methods (Milner, 1971b). These cognitive deficits are clearly inadequate to account for the psychiatric syndrome.

A related view (Pond, 1962) explained the psychotic mental state as the end product of patients' attempts to make sense of bizarre psychomotor seizure experiences. However, this proposal is weakened by Pond's own observation (1957) that psychosis emerges as fit frequency decreases, confirmed by Flor-Henry (1969, 1972). No association between qualities of seizure aura, such as the (rare) presence of hallucinations, and probability of psychotic development has been found. As Flor-Henry's (1969a) series demonstrates, many psychotic patients undergo less than one seizure per year.

The abnormal mental state has also been conceptualized as a direct effect of ongoing seizure activity in subcortical limbic structures (Ervin, 1967; Sweet et al., 1968; Ervin et al., 1968; Mark and Ervin, 1970). It is unclear how this activity would differ from that leading to psychomotor seizures, and yet it has been noted that the frequency of psychomotor seizures correlates negatively with psychopathology (Pond, 1957; Flor-Henry, 1969a). In fact, the absence of spiking or even its cessation (forced normalization of the EEG) has been observed during psychotic periods among temporal epileptics (Dongier, 1959; Landolt 1953, 1958). Also making it difficult to support this view is evidence that better convulsant control of seizures fails to improve mental status but, in fact, is said to worsen it (Flor-Henry, 1972; Blumer, 1974).

Epileptic spiking in the amygdala, recorded by depth electrode, has been observed during rage attacks in several patients; at least one patient could be provoked to attack by stimulation of the amygdala (Ervin et al., 1968; Mark and Ervin, 1970). Episodic emotional outbursts can be elicited by stimulation of limbic structures in animals (Grossman, 1963; MacLean, 1958; Mark and Ervin, 1970). Yet immediate expression of emotion or undirected emotional response coexistent with stimulation (the situation of a patient attacking a concrete wall) is different from the development of an organized series of religious ideas, an enduring change in affect, or the regular elaboration of similar delusional patterns among patients over many years. Both phenomena are well established but the former does not explain the latter.

Furthermore, the conclusions of Penfield (Penfield and Jasper, 1954; Penfield, 1954, 1955; Penfield and Roberts, 1959) and others (Van Buren, 1975) who have extensively stimulated limbic structures in the human temporal lobe is that inhibition of emotional activity is a far more common effect than emotional activation. As stimulation of speech cortex leads to arrest rather than utterance, so temporal lobe invasion by seizure or electric current characteristically produces psychoparesis (Penfield, 1955) or disruption of processing. Likewise, an interruption of emotional evaluation—depersonalization, automatism— is statistically much more frequent in psychomotor seizures than strongly felt emotion (Van Buren et al., 1975). Thus, the progressive deepening of affect interictally seems opposite to the most usual ictal effect and probably involves a different mechanism.

These prior explanations are not mutually exclusive, and they may account for distinct aspects of the interictal mental state. However, another type of explanation was presented in general form by Symonds (1962): that the epileptic events are but one manifestation of underlying pathophysiology in the limbic system, which expresses itself through other mechanisms in disturbance of affect and thought. Slater and Beard (1963) had posited underlying brain damage as a factor in their cases. However, Flor-Henry (1969), on reexamination of this series of patients, found no abnormality in neurological or radiological contrast examinations that distinguished psychotic from nonpsychotic epileptics (Flor-Henry, 1969). Symonds (1962) commented that nonepileptic neurological lesions of the temporal lobe do not produce a characteristic "schizophrenic-like" mental state. And a further difficulty in directly implicating the structural lesion that led to seizures is the long delay between its development, most commonly in early or mid childhood (Falconer, 1973), and the eventual psychosis.

These observations are consistent with the hypothesis that an epileptic process involving the limbic system and occurring over a period of time is necessary to produce the psychiatric state, but that progressive changes in limbic structure secondary to seizure activity represent an underlying pathophysiology.

CHARACTERIZATION OF INTERICTAL BEHAVIOR

The account of schizophrenia-like psychosis, developed largely by English neurologists and Kraepelinian psychiatrists, identifies specific dimensions of behavior and thought affected in temporal lobe epilepsy. Convincing arguments were advanced to demonstrate that this clinical state occurs more frequently than the random association of temporal epilepsy with schizophrenia (Slater and Beard, 1963; Slater and Moran, 1969).

However, such a psychotic state is reached in a minority of patients. It seems probable that by tabulating psychiatrically diagnosable pathology—psychosis or behavior disorder—Slater and his colleagues describe an infrequent end stage of the temporal lobe epileptic process. The long mean interval of fourteen years between seizure onset and psychosis (Slater and Moran, 1969) again suggests that schizophrenia, like psychosis, is a late effect of a process that may be analyzed into more elementary psychological changes.

Lacking a descriptive orientation, clinical psychiatrists may fail to attend to nonpathological features of behavior. Yet the tendency to write excessively (Waxman and Geschwind, 1974) or undergo religious conversion (Dewhurst and Beard, 1970) might clarify the nature of interictal change.

To identify changes potentially present in a large number of patients who never become psychotic or at early stages of their psychiatric evolution, I have constructed a list of eighteen behavioral features associated with temporal lobe epilepsy in previous reports or suggested by my clinical experience. These are listed in Table 1 with brief clinical delineation and references. They are not, in general, personality traits defined by standard diagnostic tests, nor do they represent at this stage unique factors isolated by factor analysis. It is unlikely that they all coexist in any one patient. Indeed, I would like to stress the interdependency among them by a grouping that will be developed.

That these are important aspects of thought and behavior among TL epileptics is supported by preliminary results of an ongoing study. Patients have been chosen from five general epilepsy clinics without

TABLE 1 Interictal Characteristics Attributed to Temporal Lobe Epileptics

Group	Characteristics	Clinical observations	Described by
I	Emotionality	Deepening of all emotions; intense affect	Hill, 1953a, 1953b Slater and Beard, 1963; Slater and Moran, 1969 Waxman and Geschwind, 1974 Davison and Bagley, 1969 Glaser, 1964
	Manic tendencies	Euphoria; grandiosity; psychiatric diagnosis: manic-depressive disease	Slater and Beard, 1963 Flor-Henry, 1969a, 1969b Gregoriadis et al., 1971
	Depression	Sadness, suicide; psychiatric diagnosis: depression	Dominion et al., 1963 Glaser, 1964 Slater and Moran, 1969 Williams, 1956
	Humorlessness	Ponderous, sober, overgeneralized serious concern	Glaser, 1964 Geschwind, 1973 Bear and Fedio, 1977
II	Altered sexuality	Hyposexualism, loss of libido; fetishes; transvestism; hypersexual episodes, exhibitionism	Blumer and Walker, 1967 Blumer, 1970a, 1970b, 1974 Gastaut and Collomb, 1954 Davies and Morgenstern, 1960 Mitchell et al., 1954 Hierons, 1971 Hooshmand and Brawley, 1970
	Anger, hostility	Combative, argumentative	Treffert, 1964 Falconer, 1973 Sweet et al., 1968 Taylor, 1969

TABLE 1 (continued) Interictal Characteristics Attributed to Temporal Lobe Epileptics

Group	Characteristics	Clinical observations	Described by
	Aggression	Bad temper, rage attacks; violent crimes, murder	Serafetinides, 1965a Mark and Ervin, 1970 Davidson, 1947 Ervin et al., 1968
IIIa	Religiosity	Deep religious belief; multiple conversions, mystical states	Dewhurst and Beard, 1970 Slater and Beard, 1963 Slater and Moran, 1969 Hill, 1953a
	Nascent philosophical interest	Metaphysical speculation, cosmic concerns, cosmological theories	Waxman and Geschwind, 1974 Slater and Beard, 1963 Glaser, 1964
	Augmented sense of personal destiny	Events personalized; divine guidance attributed to many aspects of patient's life	Slater and Beard, 1963 Glaser, 1964 Bear and Fedio, 1977 Waxman and Geschwind, 1974
	Dependence, passivity	Cosmic helplessness, "at hands of fate"	Blumer, 1974 Slater and Beard, 1963 Bear and Fedio, 1977
	Paranoia	Suspicious, overinclusive; psychiatric diagnosis: paranoid psychosis	Hill, 1953a Pond, 1957, 1962, 1969 Slater and Beard, 1963 Slater and Moran, 1969 Glaser, 1964 Bruens, 1969

IIIb	Moralism	"Law and order"; excessive attention to rules; desire to punish offenders	Mark and Ervin, 1970 Waxman and Geschwind, 1974 Blumer, 1974
	Guilt	Self-recrimination, self-rebuke, litany of faults	Bear and Fedio, 1977 Dominion et al., 1963
IIIc	Obsessionalism	Ritualistic; compulsive and orderly	Bruens, 1969 Waxman and Geschwind, 1974 Blumer, 1974 Glaser, 1964
	Circumstantiality	Loquacious, pedantic; overly detailed, peripheral	Slater and Beard, 1963 Geschwind, 1973 Waxman and Geschwind, 1974
	Viscosity	Cognitively repetitive; emotionally clinging	Blumer, 1974
	Hypergraphia	Keeping extensive diaries, detailed notes; writing autobiography or novel	Waxman and Geschwind, 1974 Blumer, 1974

regard to the existence of prior psychiatric diagnosis or treatment. The principal requirements were electroencephalographic evidence of a temporal lobe focus for more than three years (Gibbs and Gibbs, 1964), history of psychomotor seizures by clinical criteria (Ervin, 1967; Van Buren et al., 1975), absence of additional underlying neurological disease (e.g., tumor), and education level beyond the tenth grade. The sample spans a broad range of socioeconomic, geographical and occupational possibilities. To assess the importance of hemispheric lateralization, only patients with unilateral temporal foci have been selected.

An important qualification is that no patient was (knowingly) tested within seventy-two hours of a seizure. Thus, we have sampled stable interictal characteristics of behavior and thought rather than features of ictal or peri-ictal confusional states.

In one aspect of the study, five questionnaire items, true-false in format, were generated to sample each of the eighteen putative clinical characteristics. Table 2 lists one of these items for each dimension.

Evidence of the utility of these characteristics has emerged from a study of forty-eight subjects: fifteen patients with right (R) and twelve patients with left (L) focal temporal epilepsy, contrasted with twelve normal subjects and nine patients with severe neuromuscular or neuropathic disorders. For each of the eighteen traits, both epileptic mean scores (R and L) exceeded the neurological as well as the normal means. There was a highly significant group effect (two-way analysis of variance, $p < .001$), and epileptics were clearly distinguished from normals or the neurological controls (Scheffé test, $p < .01$) for both comparisons. The group differences were reflected significantly in each of the eighteen characteristics considered separately (one-way analysis of variance, $p < .01$ for eighteen out of eighteen, $p < .001$ for eleven out of eighteen, and epileptics differentiated from nonepileptics (Scheffé test, $p < .01$ for eighteen out of eighteen).

A most intriguing finding is the distinction between left and right focal epileptics, the former demonstrating extreme (verbal) awareness of anger, hostility, and aggression, reflected in high trait scores, the latter denying these tendencies despite dramatic objective documentation of difficulty in these areas. Right focal patients scored highest on an independent measure of defective self-awareness. These observations, consonant with the phenomenon of denial of illness associated with right hemisphere lesions (Weinstein and Kahn, 1955; Gainotti, 1972), will be analyzed elsewhere (Bear and Fedio, 1977).

For our present purposes, the critical conclusion from these results is that features summarized in Table 1 *are* characteristic of temporal lobe epileptics (both right and left focal) unselected by previous

TABLE 2 Sample Items from Behavioral Inventory

Characteristic (from Table 1)	Sample Item (1 of 5)
Emotionality	My emotions have been so powerful that they have caused trouble.
Manic tendency	I have had periods when I felt so full of pep that sleep did not seem necessary for several days.
Depression	I have often felt so bad that I was close to ending my life.
Altered sexuality	Things which never sexually attracted me before have become appealing.
Anger, hostility	Little things make me angrier than they used to.
Aggression	I have a tendency to break things or hurt people when I get angry.
Religiosity	I have had some very unusual religious experiences.
Nascent philosophical interest	I have spent a lot of time thinking about the origins of the world and life.
Dependency, passivity	I feel like a pawn in the hands of others.
Humorlessness	People should think about the point of many jokes more carefully instead of just laughing at them.
Paranoia	People tend to take advantage of me.
Obsessionalism	I have a habit of counting things or memorizing numbers.
Circumstantiality	People sometimes tell me that I have trouble getting to the point because of all the details.
Viscosity	Sometimes I keep at a thing so long that others may lose their patience with me.
Hypergraphia	I write down or copy many things.
Moralism	I would go out of my way to make sure the law is followed.
Guilt	Much of the time I feel as if I have done something wrong or harmful.
Sense of personal destiny	I think that I have a special mission in life.

psychiatric screening. In order to identify a mechanism that might account for the importance of these eighteen features, I will analyze them in terms of three major groupings (Table 1).

Group I—and most particularly emotionality—summarizes the affect intensive changes that are a hallmark of the interictal syndrome. It is characteristic that the affect or feeling tone, independent of the particular emotion involved, is maintained at high intensity. It is often excessive for the situation but qualitatively appropriate, unlike the dissociation of affect from content characteristic of simple schizophrenia. The patients present a sober, somber, humorless intensity, for high affective significance is attributed to virtually every stimulus and situation.

Disorders of mood may seem a special case of maintained high affect, but they have properties that differentiate them from the characteristics below. A mood is maintained independently of and often inappropriately for a particular environment. Euhporia, for example, is projected into the environment and often serves to reorganize perceptual events, rather than being a reaction to these; in fact, euphoria prevents appropriate emotional reactions. Thus, strong affect expressed as mood excess (Table 1, Group I, manic tendencies and depression) differs from cognitive elaboration, often verbal or logical, of specific relationships between stimuli and affect that may culminate in a mystical religious or paranoid system (Group III).

There is reason to suggest that these two forms of reaction may be associated with the right and left hemispheres, respectively. Differences in verbal awareness of emotions between right and left focal patients were mentioned previously as a conclusion of our study; performances of unilateral temporal epileptics on a verbal emotional labeling task are consistent with the distinction (McIntyre, 1975). An association of right hemisphere foci with mood-affective, left with cognitive-paranoid psychoses, has been reported (Flor-Henry, 1969b; Gregoriadis et al., 1971). Also, anesthesia of the nondominant hemisphere may preferentially induce euphoria (Perria et al., 1961; Terzian, 1964); right hemisphere lesions have been selectively associated with disorders of mood and denial of unpleasant aspects of reality (Gainotti, 1972; Weinstein and Kahn, 1955; Galin, 1974). By contrast, the predilection of the left hemisphere may be to develop extensive verbal-cognitive elaboration of intense affect (Bear and Fedio, 1977).

Interictal changes in sexuality and aggression (Group II) have in previous accounts been attributed to quantitative alterations in drive strength (Gastaut and Collomb, 1954; Dongier, 1959; Blumer and Walker, 1967). Hyposexuality as a consequence of an "irritative" epileptic focus in the limbic system (Dongier, 1959) has been viewed as the converse of hypersexuality following ablative lesions (a feature of the Klüver-Bucy Syndrome following bilateral temporal lobectomy). However, change in drive level does not account well for either situation. It is important to distinguish the strength of a drive as measured by frequency of consummatory behavior from the associations of that drive with particular trigger stimuli. We may consider, then, the class of stimuli that elicit sexual responses among temporal epileptics.

In one striking case (Mitchell et al., 1954), "hypersexual" response to a previously neutral stimulus, a safety pin, was accompanied by a drop-off in sexual reaction to the more socially appropriate stimulus, the patient's wife. Accounts of transvestism (Davies and Morgenstern, 1960), lesbianism, exhibitionism, and hypersexualism (Blumer and Walker, 1967; Hooshmand and Brawley, 1970) suggest that the basic process is modification of the class of stimulus objects that elicit sexual responses. Thus, new and often unusual sensory-sexual associations may develop over a period of months or years.

A similar mechanism might account for changes in aggression. It seems established that an immediate effect of amygdaloid seizures in cats is enhanced aggressiveness (Grossman, 1963) and that an amygdaloid seizure may accompany undirected rage attacks in humans (Mark and Ervin, 1970; Sweet et al., 1968). However, the important clinical aggressiveness of temporal lobe epileptics is not such undirected rage but the extension of bad temper into more and more social situations. This represents an increase in the number of stimuli that may initiate the limbic response of anger. The patient's sociocultural background and prior personality are a starting point for this organically induced change and probably continue to modulate its course. Middle-class patients complaining of worsening temper and angry words with their children are far more common than violent psychopaths driven to sadistic acts and murder (Davidson, 1947; Crichton, 1972). The organic process underlying the clinical changes, like those involving sexuality, is the development or extension of associations between stimuli and a limbic response.

A related process underlies the apparently heterogeneous characteristics of Group III. But we must generalize our notions of stimulus and limbic response to speak meaningfully about the process of their association in these cases. For humans, language and abstract concepts have become a principal mode of analysis of the environment. These capacities likely require extensive nonlimbic sensory-sensory associations (i.e., auditory → visual). This is a recent function phylogenetically, and evidence points to a role of the angular gyrus of the dominant parietal lobe in its development (Geschwind, 1965). Since words and concepts are frequently affectively charged, it is probable that polymodal associations, perhaps mediated by the angular gyrus, subsequently link with limbic structures.

While the anatomic projections of this "new" area of parietal association cortex are far from certain in humans, degeneration following parietal lesions in monkeys extended into the superior temporal gyrus, bank of the superior temporal sulcus, and the cingulate gyrus (Pandya and Kuypers, 1969). The temporal structures project to, and the cingulate gyrus is part of, the limbic system (Pandya and Kuypers, 1969; Klingler and Gloor, 1960; Geschwind, 1965).

Words and concepts take on affective significance as commonly as physical objects; word and concepts are stimuli for affective association. The range of affects that may be attributed to such stimuli in human experience is, likewise, broader than the usual reinforcers of animal behavior. Yet limbic association may well account for these subtler associations, since social, maternal, and exploratory, as well as sexual, aggressive, fearful, and appetitive, responses to objects have been disrupted by specifically limbic lesions in animals (Dicks et al., 1969; Franzen and Myers, 1973; Walker et al., 1953; Schwartzbaum et al., 1969; Olds, 1955; Jones and Mishkin, 1972). Of course, some affective qualities elicited by limbic stimulation probably occur uniquely in humans. The visceral sensation of self-reference, so prominent in Dostoevsky's temporal seizure, may form the basis of an "I am" quality (Williams, 1956) that invests experience with a sense of immediate, personalized relevance.

With these implications of "stimulus" and "limbic response," the characteristics of Group III can be viewed as attributions of limbic significance to a broad class of previously neutral stimuli. Subgroup (IIIa) summarizes cognitive reactions. Experiencing all objects and events as shot through with emotional significance engenders a mystically religious world view. If one's immediate actions and thoughts are so cathected, the result may be an augmented sense of personal destiny. Again, a felt significance behind events that others dismiss may form a seedbed for paranoia or confirm the notion that the patient is a passive pawn in the hands of larger forces that structure the world.

Moralism and guilt (subgroup IIIb) have been grouped between cognitive contemplative (IIIa) and overt behavioral (IIIc) responses. Thus, feeling strongly about laws may lead to action in which the patient "takes the law into his (or her) own hands" (hypermoralism). Sensing emotional importance in even the smallest acts, the patient may perform these ritualistically and repetitively (obsessionalism). Since every detail bears the imprimatur of affective significance, many details will be mentioned in the patient's lengthy speech (circumstantiality, viscosity) and will be recorded (hypergraphia).

The concept of affective associations with an enlarging class of stimuli accounts for a superficially heterogeneous set of interictal characteristics. This proposed mechanism is also heuristic in suggesting a function-structure relationship, for we are led to consider anatomic connections within the temporal lobe that might mediate sensory limbic bonds. Identification of such pathways has come largely from the analysis of sensory limbic dissociation through disconnections.

SENSORY-LIMBIC CONNECTION AND DISCONNECTION

Bilateral temporal lobectomy leads to a dramatic syndrome in monkeys described in 1939 by Klüver and Bucy. This syndrome includes: immediate taming—loss of previously acquired fear of humans, handling gloves, nets; "psychic blindness"—inappropriate responses to visualized objects despite intact acuity (visual agnosia); changes in food and sexual preference, which were termed hyperphagia and hypersexuality; and extensive exploration of the environment by sniffing and mouthing, referred to as hypermetamorphosis.

Increases in hunger and sex drives were first stressed as important effects of the temporal lesion. But it is instructive to contrast the behavioral effects above with those following destruction of the ventromedial nucleus (VMN) of the hypothalamus of animals (Marshall et al., 1955; Nisbett, 1972; Singh and Meyer, 1968). While the VMN animals dramatically overconsume their usual laboratory chow, rats and monkeys with temporal lesions maintain a constant weight despite the remarkable inclusion of meat, feces, and metal objects among their dietary preferences (Anand and Brobeck, 1952; Klüver and Bucy, 1939). The VMN animals might be described as appropriately hyperphagic, while those with temporal ablations are inappropriately normophagic. Sexual alterations have been previously analyzed similarly: the effect of temporal lesions is not more (hetero) sexual drive but a loss of specificity among the (visual) stimuli that elicit sexual responses. Thus, the Klüver-Bucy animal will attempt to copulate with members of the same sex or of different species (Klüver and Bucy, 1939; Schreiner and Kling, 1953).

Adaptive regulation of drive requires both control of drive level, based on autonomic and endocrine surveillance of the internal milieu, and the subsequent association of drive with appropriate, exteroceptively perceived stimuli. Hypothalamic and endocrine lesions disrupt the former process. Bilateral temporal lobectomy by contrast, appears to interrupt the latter, dissociating stimuli from drive-related reinforcement values (Weiskrantz, 1956) by anatomically disconnecting sensory association cortices from the limbic system (Geschwind, 1965).

Since most cross-modal associations in animals are sensory-limbic (Burton and Ettlinger, 1960; Ettlinger, 1961; Geschwind, 1965), disruption of such connections renders an animal agnosic or "psychically blind." He fails to connect the fearful or sexual or delicious limbic quality with a visually or tactually discriminated object (Horel,

1971; Keating, 1971). Olfactory and gustatory stimuli have preserved access to the limbic system following temporal lobectomy, so that intense exploration of the environment by sniffing and mouthing may be attempted compensation for the exteroceptive-limbic disconnection.

It has been argued whether increased oral exploration of objects, a prominent feature of bilateral temporal lesions in humans (Poeck, 1969; Marlowe et al., 1975) is similarly compensatory (Geschwind, 1965) or represents regression to an oral stage of development (Poeck, 1969). Both of these descriptions may be correct if early mouthing in infants represents exploration prior to later myelination (Flechsig, 1901) of limbic connections from sensory association cortices.

It is intriguing to speculate that for a cat or monkey, the relation of abstracted properties of a perceived stimulus to the limbic system is the primary or only "meaning" assigned to that stimulus. Entification in the animal may entail, for example, that a complex of visual edges and borders discriminated by units of the inferotemporal visual cortex (Gross et al., 1972) be followed by food or sex or pain, which then defines the "visual object." Similar processes may relate to somesthetic-limbic reification (Deuel et al., 1971; Stamm and Rosen, 1971; Keating, 1971). The loss of limbic association would be, therefore, the loss of all significance of that stimulus for the animal.

For humans (and perhaps language-using chimpanzees), limbic attributes of a visual stimulus do not constitute its only meaning. Nonlimbic cross-modal associations, perhaps mediated by the angular gyrus of the parietal lobe, allow for visual-auditory, visual-tactile, as well as visual-visual, etc., links upon which language builds. Thus, the visual outline of a spoon can call up its feeling to tongue and mouth, outlines of related utensils such as a fork, the noun "spoon." The notion of "what a spoon is" does not depend solely on limbic associations.

A temporal lobectomized human thus would be expected to differ from a monkey in an important regard: the human need not develop a total visual or tactile agnosia. The deficit is specifically a limbic agnosia, a loss of appropriate "emotional behavior" most striking in the presence of persons (parents, fiancée) or objects (food, feces) that formerly elicited it. Such patients have been described as "emotionless in speech," without facial or gestural expression of emotion (amimia), newly and inappropriately homosexual, oral, and with loss of food/nonfood distinctions (Terzian and Dalle Ore, 1955; Pilleri, 1966; Poeck, 1969; Marlowe et al., 1975).[2]

[2] Wernicke's aphasia as well as apraxia was prominent in a patient, recently described, following herpetic encephalitis (Marlowe et al., 1975). These deficits likely signify additional dominant hemisphere involvement posterior to the usual boundaries of surgical temporal lobectomy (Benson and Geschwind, 1973). The more general agnosia of this patient is not characteristic of the Klüver-Bucy syndrome in humans.

The loss of appropriate emotional responses to stimuli following bilateral temporal lobectomy has been reproduced in monkeys by other lesions that act to disconnect sensory from limbic structures. Following crossed ablation of the occipital and the temporal lobe in opposite hemispheres, section of cerebral commissures produces "psychic blindness" (Horel, 1971). Analogous ablation of crossed parietal and temporal lobes leads to a tactile deficit in distinguishing food from a metallic object in the hand contralateral to the parietal lesion; commissurectomy, disconnecting intact parietal and temporal lobes, extends the deficit to both hands (Keating, 1971).

These are situations in which primary sensory cortices have been disconnected from the entire temporal lobe. However, bilateral amygdalectomy leads to seemingly similar dissociation (Weiskrantz, 1956), and unilateral amygdalectomy followed by commissurotomy produces "visual taming" (presumed visual limbic dissociation) confined to the contralateral hemifield (Downer, 1962). Restricted ablation of polar temporal neocortex bilaterally reproduces essential (visual) features of the Klüver-Bucy syndrome (Akert et al., 1961).

These observations have led to attempts to specify particular structures and pathways critical for linking sensory with limbic systems. Anatomic and functional accounts have advanced most with regard to visual limbic associations (Petr et al., 1949; Pribram et al., 1950; Geschwind, 1965; Jones and Mishkin, 1972).

Much evidence now establishes posterior inferior temporal cortex (area TE of Bonin and Bailey, 1947) as a receiving link in the sequential chain extending from retinal ganglion cell via lateral geniculate body to striate and peristriate cortices (Mishkin, 1966, 1972; Gross et al., 1972; Rocha-Miranda et al., 1975). Behavioral experiments have shown the inferotemporal visual cortex (IT) to be critical for complex visual discriminations (Mishkin, 1972). Extracellular recordings have established a strong dependence of IT units on striate input, anatomically relayed through peristriate areas 18 and 19, both ipsilaterally and contralaterally via forebrain commissures (Rocha-Miranda et al., 1975).

Summarizing the subsequent limbic connections of IT in monkeys, Jones and Mishkin (1972) distinguished three destinations: the amygdala by way of ventral cortex of the temporal pole; the fusiform-hippocampal gyrus and hippocampus; and orbital frontal cortex. Among contrasted bilateral ablations of each of these structures, only the temporal pole–amygdala (TPA) removal produced an impairment consistent with difficulty in the formation of visual limbic associations.

The importance of functional linkage between IT and TPA was further documented in experiments with animals with crossed lesions in these structures. Following section of the anterior commissure, which had connected intact IT and TPA interhemispherically, subjects developed an equivalent visual limbic deficit (Sunshine and Mishkin, 1975).

These results are consistent with prior behavioral evidence that visual limbic dissociations of the Klüver-Bucy syndrome follow bilateral amygdalectomy (Weiskrantz, 1956) or temporal pole ablations (Akert et al., 1961) but not entorhinal-hippocampal lesions alone (Iversen, 1969). They demonstrate a dependence of visual limbic associations on a specific pathway extending from peristriate to inferotemporal visual cortex, continuing after probable synapse in the ventral temporal pole, to the amygdala.

It is important to qualify this conclusion. Following bilateral lesions to the pathway, simple stimulus reinforcement learning is still possible. The behavioral deficits described previously often ameliorate over a period of months, again suggesting possible, if slow, visual limbic relearning (Weiskrantz, 1956). Parallel pathways may exist that can take over associative functions, given time and relatively fewer associative demands (Jones and Mishkin, 1972). Other limbic structures (septum, cingulate gyrus) have been implicated in associative learning (McLeary, 1966). Furthermore, ablations of orbital frontal cortex and hippocampus, which were contrasted with TPA removal, did have significant effects on associative reversal learning. The nature of these deficits, however, suggested interference with decision processes following the stage of visual limbic association (Jones and Mishkin, 1972). Thus, further sequential, as well as parallel, processing by other limbic structures is probable.

With these qualifications, the importance of the amygdala in sensory-limbic association is established (for evidence of a role in somesthetic limbic learning, see Stamm and Rosen, 1971). The implication of this specific medial temporal structure may further support the concept of altered sensory limbic connections as an underlying mechanism in temporal lobe epilepsy.

Thus, spiking in this structure has been most associated with psychiatric abnormality among epileptic patients studied by depth electrode (Sweet et al., 1968; Mark and Ervin, 1970). Radio frequency lesion or surgical ablation of the amygdaloid complex (often including the ventral temporal pole) is alleged to produce dramatic amelioration of epileptic psychopathology, particularly aggressive and sexual (Narabayashi et al., 1963; Mark and Ervin, 1970; Flor-Henry, 1974). The amygdala has the lowest threshold for development of altered synaptic connections following repeated electrical stimulation (Goddard et al., 1969), a phenomenon that may provide the basis for sensory limbic hyperconnection (discussed below).

There is, in addition, an epidemiological observation concerning psychosis among surgically treated temporal epileptics that may be clarified by these functional and anatomic considerations. Thus, Falconer (1973) concludes that mesial temporal sclerosis—the most common pathological substrate—rarely leads to psychosis but that "there is some relation between temporal lobe epilepsy, psychosis, and hamartoma that I do not understand." He suggests a possible functional correlation with the neuropathological differences between the lesions—the first sclerosis, gliosis, and the latter, cryptogenic tumor. Again, however, the long delay between the lesion's occurrence and psychological changes makes explanation from direct neuropathological properties of the lesion improbable. Geschwind (1973), drawing on observations of Taylor (1971, 1972), suggests that age of onset (less than 2 years for sclerosis, early teens for hamartomas) may be the variable correlating with psychosis. An association of genetic abnormalities with hamartomas (Razavi, 1974) is also cited.

It is at least as probable and consistent with our analysis that the anatomic difference in location of these lesions is the critical variable. Thus, mesial temporal sclerosis is, by definition, a hippocampal lesion, and this structure has been increasingly identified with memory rather than affect (Douglas, 1967; Iversen, 1969). Hamartomas and the related cryptogenic tumors were most commonly found within or near the amygdaloid nucleus, adjacent to the pathway specifically implicated in sensory-limbic connections.

SENSORY-LIMBIC HYPERCONNECTION

I have considered evidence derived from disconnective lesions that sensory-limbic association is a specific neural process involving a pathway via ventral temporal complex to the amygdala. My analysis of the psychological changes occurring interictally in temporal lobe epilepsy emphasized extensive and progressive investment of stimulus complexes with intense affective significance. It was suggested that this phenomenon be produced anatomically by the formation of new, extensive, and excessive sensory (or polysensory) limbic bonds.

Although it is not possible to establish the existence of such connections directly at the present time, we may consider several mechanisms through which an epileptic process might bring these about. A recent electrophysiological study of striate cortical units holds out the possibility of eventual test of the postulated hyperconnections.

It has been suggested that a functional process strongly associated with the limbic system—learning—could produce new sensory-limbic connections in the presence of an epileptic focus (Geschwind, 1975). As a patient examines his or her "neutral" wristwatch, for example, a limbic epilpetic discharge leads to the feeling of intense fear. Now, in uninvolved association cortex, a spurious, sensory-limbic association has been recorded. Over a long period of time with many such experiences, the patient would build a bizarrely emotionalized concept of the world, which might result in psychosis.

Such learning may well occur, and since conditioned responses extinguish slowly, even one trial pairing of stimulus and limbic response may lead to lasting behavioral consequences (Hilgard, 1956). However, there are some limitations to this view of the process that make it alone an improbable basis for all aspects of the interictal psychological syndrome. The paradigm presumes independence of sensory (stimuli) from limbic (epileptic) events. Thus, we might expect a near random pairing of different emotions with stimulating objects—or, indeed, with the same object at different times. But the clinical picture suggests that patients have emotions appropriate in kind to the stimulus; the pathognomonic changes are in affective intensity and generalization of affect to more and more stimuli. Moreover, patients do not cite episodic experiences of emotion on viewing previously neutral objects. Such sensory-limbic pairings, if they constituted learning trials, would presumably be dramatic emotional experiences themselves.

Distinguished from such functional learning, physiological, or "organic," learning may be considered. As emphasized by Morrell (1959, 1960), the development of a mirror or secondary epileptic focus following prolonged stimulation from the primary epileptic focus, is a type of learning involving the formation of new synaptic connections within the limbic system. In the related phenomenon of kindling, Goddard et al. (1969) has demonstrated that repeated electrical stimulation—with lowest threshold in the amygdala—leads to modification of synaptic connections in a pool of units surrounding the electrode. The study of intrahemispheric effects between two kindling electrodes further supports the possibility of new synaptic interconnections among units repeatedly stimulated.

If such enhanced interconnections among adjacent units are created by epileptic activity, a recent experiment (Ebersole and Levine, 1975) involving striate cortex of cats underlines the possible consequences for information processing in an organized sensory cortex. Ebersole and Levine first identified by extracellular recording a striate cell excited by an appropriately oriented white bar over a limited area of visual space ($2°$); this constitutes the receptive field of a simple cortical cell (Hubel and Wiesel, 1962). By iontophoresis of penicillinate ions, a temporary epileptic focus was created in adjacent striate cortex. Two effects were then noted on the "index" cell: a potentiation of its triggered response to the appropriate bar stimulus (interpreted as a direct effect of penicillin on the cell's membrane) and "new" spike responses to stimuli with differing angular orientations over a wider area of visual space. It was possible to define a receptive field for the epileptic focus: the area of visual space (and range of stimulus orientations) that led to synchronous epileptic spiking grossly recorded from the cortex. Presumably, the broad receptive field of the focus reflected the population of cells in adjacent cortical columns—each with an initially specific angular and retinotopic selectivity—influenced by the penicillin. Because of the orderly topographical mapping with adjacent columns preferring incremental stimulus orientations (Hubel and Wiesel, 1962), this "receptive field of the focus" had the quality of generalization across retinal space and along the stimulus variable of angular orientation.

My interpretation of the effect on the index unit is that its receptive field was generalized from its original selective trigger preference toward the characteristics of the focus's receptive field. It was the intrinsic organization of the cortex affected, then, that determined the nature of the functional generalization.

We do not, of course, know the organizational structure of the ventral temporal pole, the amygdala, or even the inferotemporal visual cortex from which units have been recorded (Gross et al., 1972; Rocha-Miranda et al., 1975). In the latter case, highly abstracted geometric properties of the stimulus, independent of its retinal position, seem the likely basis of structural ordering. Could there be a similar abstraction of affects from primary visceral percepts, leading to a sensory-limbic association cortex in which stimuli are grouped by their associated limbic state?

Although this is speculative, the ability of an epileptic focus to potentiate functional connections among adjacent units and thereby to broaden a gradient of discrimination reflected in underlying cortical structure seems established. For anterior and medial temporal cortex, hyperconnections analogous to those in striate cortex could lead to some form of affective generalization.

The consequences of such enhanced connections, suggested by functional neuroanatomy, may be clearer at this point than their detailed mechanism. Acutely, they could result from facilitation of existing excitatory synaptic organizations or loss of inhibitory effects; chronically, new synaptic organizations may develop around an electric focus (Goddard et al., 1969). These possibilities will become testable electrophysiologically, as receptive fields of temporal units distal to IT become defined.

However, it is currently feasible, with anatomic and behavioral methods, to investigate the importance of enhanced sensory-limbic connections involving the temporal pole and amygdala in producing behavioral changes. Unilateral amygdalectomy in a commissurectomized monkeys leads to the dramatic condition of visual taming confined to the hemifield contralateral to the ablation. Within the ipsilateral field, visual stimuli may initiate activity along an intact pathway between inferotemporal visual cortex, temporal pole, and amygdala (Downer, 1962).

A commissurectomized animal with one epileptic amygdala would be of equal interest. Complete interhemispheric disconnection eliminates the possibility of a mirror focus in the control hemisphere. My hypothesis then, predicts that, over time, hyperconnection confined to the epileptic hemisphere will invest visual stimuli seen through the ipsilateral eye projecting to that hemisphere with enhanced affective significance. Changes in eating, sexuality, and aggression may be compared with "control responses" when only the contralateral eye is uncovered. Associative reversal learning and component processes of emotional response acquisition, generalization, and extinction can be contrasted between the eyes. This allows for comparison of intrahemispheric effects on particular connections (i.e., sensory-limbic hyperconnection) vis-à-vis nonspecific effects of the focus on all emotional behavior. Only hyperconnection would lead to a behavioral differential between the two eyes. To the extent the model is correct, such an animal will not only undergo "personality change" but will develop a split personality, the particular character selected depending on the eye through which the animal views the world.

It would be possible to explore the role of specific connections relating spiking amygdala to temporal pole and inferotemporal visual cortex (IT). Following ablation of right amygdala and left IT in a cross-lesioned animal, the only intact visual limbic association pathway would proceed from right IT to left amygdala (Sunshine and Mishkin, 1975). Following creation of an epileptic focus in this structure, an intact anterior commissure should be required for development of visual limbic hyperconnections.

SUMMARY

Psychological changes in patients with temporal lobe epilepsy are considered. Prior observations of correlated psychiatric diagnoses and objections to these are reviewed. Specific features of behavior and thought, derived from literature and clinical experience, are suggested as a more effective way of characterizing the interictal syndrome; their accuracy is supported by quantitative results of an ongoing study.

Enhanced affective association is proposed as a mechanism underlying these diverse features. I interpret this in light of theoretical and experimental accounts that anatomic connections between sensory and limbic structures are established within the temporal lobe. In contrast to sensory-limbic disconnection, which results in dissociation of stimuli from affective values, it is suggested that the epileptic process effects sensory-limbic hyperconnection, leading to a suffusion of experience with emotional coloration.

BIBLIOGRAPHY

Adey, W. R. 1959. Recent studies of the rhinencephalon in relation to temporal lobe epilepsy and behavior disorders, International Review of Neurobiology 1:1-46.

Ajmone-Marsan, C., and L. Goldhammer. 1973. Clinical ictal patterns and electrographic data in cases of partial seizures of frontal-central-parietal origin. In Epilepsy: Its Phenomena in Man, M. Brazier, ed. New York: Academic Press.

Akert, K., R. A. Gruesen, C. N. Woolsey, and D. R. Meyer. 1961. Kluver-Bucy syndrome in monkeys with neocortical ablations of temporal lobe. Brain 84:480-498.

Alajouanine, T. 1963. Dostoiewski's epilepsy. Brain 86:210-218.

Anand, B. K., and J. R. Brobeck. 1952. Food intake and spontaneous activity of rats with lesions in the amygdaloid nuclei, Journal of Neurophysiology 15:421-429.

Baldwin, M. 1958. Temporal Lobe Epilepsy. Springfield, Ill.: Charles C Thomas.

Baldwin, M., S. A. Lewis, and S. A. Bach. 1959. The effects of lysergic acid after cerebral ablation. Neurology 9:469-474.

Barrett, T. W. 1969. Studies of the function of the amygdaloid complex in macaca mulatta. Neuropsychologia 7:1-12.

Bear, D. and P. Fedio. 1977. Quantitative analysis of interictal behavior in temporal lobe epilepsy. Submitted for publication.

Benson, D. F., and N. Geschwind. 1973. The aphasias and related disturbances. In Clinical Neurology, A. Baker, ed. Hagerstown: Harper & Row.

Beluzzi, J. D., and S. P. Grossman. 1969. Avoidance learning: long lasting deficits after temporal lobe seizure. Science 166:1435-1437.

Bleuler, E. 1952. Dementia Praecox or The Group of Schizophrenias. New York: Interuniversity Press.

Blumer, D. and A. E. Walker. 1967. Sexual behavior in temporal lobe epilepsy, Archives of Neurology 16:37-43.

_____. 1970a. Changes in sexual behavior related to temporal lobe disorder in man. Journal of Sexual Research 6:173-180.

_____. 1970b. Hypersexual episodes in temporal lobe epilepsy. American Journal of Psychiatry 126:1099-1106.

_____. 1974. Organic personality disorder. In Severe Personality Disorders, J. Lion, ed. Baltimore: Williams & Wilkins.

Bonin, G., von, and P. Bailey. 1947. The Neocortex of Macaca mulatta. Urbana: University of Illinois Press.

Bruens, J. H. 1969. Psychoses in epilepsy. In Handbook of Clinical Neurology. Vol. 15. G. Bruyn and P. Vinken, eds. New York: Wiley.

Buchsbaum, M. and P. Fedio. 1970. Hemispheric differences in evoked potentials to verbal and nonverbal stimuli in the left and right visual fields. Physiological Behavior 5:207-210.

Burton, D., and G. Ettlinger, 1960. Crossmodal transfer of training in monkeys. Nature 186:1071.

Corsellis, J. A. N. 1969. Some observations on the pathology of the temporal lobe. British Journal of Psychiatry, Special Publication 4, 31-34.

Crichton, M. 1972. Terminal Man. New York: Knopf.

Currie, S., K. W. G. Heathfield, R. A. Henson, and D. F. Scott. 1971. Clinical course and prognosis of temporal lobe epilepsy, a survey of 666 patients. Brain 94:173-190.

Davidson, G. A. 1947. Psychomotor epilepsy. Canadian Medical Association Journal 56:410-414.

Davies, B. M., and F. S. Morgenstern. 1960. A case of cysticercosis, temporal lobe epilepsy, and transvestism, Journal of Neurology, Neurosurgery and Psychiatry 23:247-249.

Davison, K., and C. Bagley. 1969. Schizophrenia-like psychoses associated with organic disorders of the central nervous system—review of literature. British Journal of Psychiatry (Special Publication) 4:113-184.

DeJong, R. N., H. H. Itabashi, and J. R. Olson. 1969. Memory loss due to hippocampal lesions. Archives of Neurology 20:339-348.

Deuel, R. K., M. Mishkin, and J. Semmes. 1971. Interaction between the hemispheres in unimanual somesthetic learning. Experimental Neurology 30:123-138.

Dewhurst, K., and A. W. Beard. 1970. Sudden religious conversions in temporal lobe epilepsy. British Journal of Psychiatry 117:497-507.

Dicks, D., R. E. Myers, and A. Kling. 1969. Uncus and amygdala lesions: effects on social behavior in the free ranging monkey. Science 165:69-81.

Dominian, J., E. A. Serafetinides, and M. Dewhurst. 1963. A follow-up study of late onset epilepsy: II. Psychiatric and social. British Medical Journal 1:428-435.

Dongier, S. 1959. Statistical study of clinical and EEG manifestations of 536 psychotic episodes occurring in 516 epileptics between clinical seizures. Epilepsia 1:117-142.

Donnelly, E. F., J. K. Dent, D. L. Murphy, and R. J. Mignone. 1972. Comparison of temporal lobe epileptics and affective disorders on the Halstead-Reitan test battery. Journal of Clinical Psychology 28:61-62.

Dostoevsky, F. 1935. The Idiot, C. Garnett, trans. New York: Random House.

Douglas, R. J. 1967. The hippocampus and behavior. Psychological Bulletin 67:416-442.

Douglas, R. J., and K. H. Pribram. 1966. Learning and limbic lesions. Neuropsychologia 4:197-220.

Downer, J. L., de C. 1959. Changes in visually guided behavior following midsagittal division of optic chiasm and corpus callosum in monkey. Brain 82:251-259.

Downer, J. L., de C. 1962. Interhemispheric integration in the visual system. In Interhemispheric Relations and Cerebral Dominance, V. Mountcastle, ed. Baltimore: Johns Hopkins Press.

Eayrs, J. T. 1969. Anatomy of the temporal lobe. British Journal of Psychiatry (Special Publication) 4:3-8.

Ebersole, J., and R. Levine. 1975. Abnormal neuronal responses during the evolution of a penicillin epileptic focus in cat visual cortex. Journal of Neurophysiology 38:250-266.

Egger, M. D., and J. P. Flynn. 1963. Effects of electrical stimulation of amygdala on hypothalamically elicited attack behavior in cats. Journal of Neurophysiology 26:705-720.

Ervin, F. R. 1967. Brain disorders associated with convulsions (epilepsy), In Comprehensive Textbook of Psychiatry, A. M. Freedman and H. I. Kaplan, eds. Baltimore: Williams & Wilkins.

Ervin, F. R., J. Delgado, V. Mark, and W. H. Sweet. 1968. Rage: A Paraepileptic Phenomenon? Talk delivered to American Epileptic Society, November 1968.

Ervin, F. R., A. W. Epstein, and H. E. King. 1955. Behavior of epileptic and nonepileptic patients with temporal spikes. Archives of Neurology and Psychiatry 74:488-497.

Ettlinger, G., E. Iwai, M. Mishkin, and H. E. Rosvold. 1968. Visual discrimination in the monkey following serial ablation of inferotemporal and preoccipital cortex. Journal of Comparative and Physiological Psychology 65:110-117.

Ettlinger, G. 1961. Learning in two sense modalities. Nature 191:308.

Falconer, M. A., E. A. Serafetinides, and J. A. Corsellis. 1964. Etiology and patholgenesis of temporal lobe epilepsy. Archives of Neurology 10:233-248.

Falconer, M. A. 1965. The surgical treatment of temporal lobe epilepsy. Neurochirurgia 8:161-172.

———. 1973. Reversibility by temporal lobe resection of the behavior abnormalities of temporal lobe epilepsy. New England Journal of Medicine 289:451-455.

Fenichel, O. 1945. The Psychoanalytic Theory of Neurosis. New York: W. W. Norton.

Ferguson, S., M. Rayport, R. Gardner, W. Kass, H. Weiner, and M. Reiser. 1969. Similarities in mental content of psychotic states, spontaneous seizures, dreams and responses to brain stimulation in patients with temporal lobe epilepsy. Psychosomatic Medicine 31:479-497.

Fields, W. S., and W. H. Sweet. 1974. The Neurobiology of Violence. St. Louis: Warren Green.

Flechsig, P. 1901. Developmental (myelogenetic) localisation of the cerebral cortex in the human subject. Lancet 2:1027-1029.

Flor-Henry, P. 1969a. Psychosis and temporal lobe epilepsy: a controlled investigation. Epilepsia 10:363-395.

———. 1969b. Schizophrenic-like reactions and affective psychoses associated with temporal lobe epilepsy: etiological factors. American Journal of Psychiatry 126:400-403.

———. 1972. Ictal and interictal psychiatric manifestations in epilepsy: specific or nonspecific? Epilepsia 13:773-783.

———. 1974. Psychosis, neurosis and epilepsy. British Journal of Psychiatry 124:144-150.

Franzen, E. A., and R. E. Myers. 1973. Neutral control of social behavior: prefrontal and anterior temporal cortex. Neuropsychologia 11:141-157.

Freud, S. 1923. The Interpretation of Dreams (1900). A. A. Brill, trans. London: G. Allen and Unwin.

———. 1930. Three Contributions to the Theory of Sex, A. A. Brill, trans. New York: Nervous and Mental Disease Publishing Company.

Friedman, H. 1951. A comparison of a group of hebephrenic and catatonic schizophrenics with two groups of normal adults by means of certain variables of the Rorschach test. Journal of Projective Techniques 15–16:352–360.

Gainotti, G. 1972. Emotional behavior and hemispheric side of the lesion. Cortex 8:41–55.

Galin, D. 1974. Implications for psychiatry of left and right cerebral specialization. Archives of General Psychiatry 31:572–583.

Gastaut, H., and K. Collomb. 1954. Etude du comportement sexual chez les epileptiques psychomoteurs. Annales Medico-Psychologiques 112:657–696.

Geschwind, N. 1965a. Disconnexion syndromes in animals and man, Part I. Brain 88:237–294.

———. 1965b. Disconnexion syndromes in animals and man, Part II. Brain 88:585–644.

———. 1973. Effects of temporal lobe surgery on behavior. New England Journal of Medicine 286:480–481.

———. 1975. Personal communication.

Gibbs, E. L., F. A. Gibbs, and B. Fuster. 1948. Psychomotor epilepsy. Archives of Neurology and Psychiatry 60:331–339.

Gibbs, F. A. 1951. Ictal and nonictal psychiatric disorders in temporal lobe epilepsy. Journal of Nervous and Mental Disorders 113:522–528.

Gibbs, F. A., and E. L. Gibbs. 1964. Atlas of Electroencephalography. Cambridge, Mass.: Addison-Wesley.

Glaser, G. H. 1964. The problem of psychosis in psychomotor temporal lobe epileptics. Epilepsia 5:271–278.

Gloor, P. 1960. Amygdala. In Handbook of Physiology, J. Field, H. W. Magoon, and V. E. Hall, eds. Section I. Vol. 2. Washington, D.C.: American Physiological Society.

Goddard, G. V., D. C. McIntyre, and C. K. Leech. 1969. A permanent change in brain function resulting from daily electrical stimulation. Experimental Neurology 25:295–330.

Gray, J. A. 1972. The structure of the emotions and the limbic system. Ciba Foundation Symposium 8:87–120.

Gregoriadis, A. et al. 1971. A correlation between mental disorders and EEG and AEG findings in temporal lobe epilepsy. Fifth World Congress of Psychiatry, Mexico. Prensa Medica Mexicana 325.

Gross, C. G., D. B. Bender, and C. E. Rocha-Miranda. 1969. Visual receptive fields of neurons in inferotemporal cortex of the monkey, Science 166: 1303–1306.

Gross, C. G., C. E. Rocha-Miranda, and D. B. Bender. 1972. Visual properties of neurons in inferotemporal cortex of the macaque. Journal of Neurophysiology 35:96–111.

Grossman, S. P. 1963. Chemically induced epileptiform seizures in the cat. Science 142:409–411.

Guerrant, J., W. W. Anderson, A. Fischer, M. Weinstein, R. Jaros, and A. Deskins. 1962. Personality in Epilepsy. Springfield, Ill.: Charles C Thomas.

Heath, R. G., R. R. Monroe, and W. A. Michle. 1955. Stimulation of the amygdaloid nucleus in a schizophrenic patient. American Journal of Psychiatry 111:862–863.

Henke, P. G., J. D. Allen, and C. Davison. 1972. Effect of lesions in the amygdala on behavioral contrast. Physiological Behavior 8:173–176.

Herrington, R. N. 1969. The personality in temporal lobe epilepsy. British Journal of Psychiatry (Special Publication) 4:70-76.

Hierons, R. 1971. Impotence in temporal lobe lesions. Journal of Neurovisceral Relations Supplement X:477-481.

Hilgard, E. 1956. Theories of Learning. New York: Appleton-Century-Crofts.

Hill, D. 1953a. Psychiatric disorders of epilepsy. Medical Research 20: 473-475.

———. 1953b. Clinical study and selection of patients in discussion on the surgery of temporal lobe epilepsy. Proceedings of the Royal Society of Medicine 46:965-976.

———. 1962. The schizophrenia-like psychoses of epilepsy—Discussion. Proceedings of the Royal Society of Medicine 55:315.

———. 1970. Aggression: Innate drive or response? Proceedings of the Royal Society of Medicine 63:159-162.

Hoch, G. H. 1943. Clinical and biological interrelations between schizophrenia and epilepsy. American Journal of Psychiatry 99:507-512.

Hommes, O. R., and L. H. H. M. Panhuysen. 1971. Depression and cerebral dominance. Psychiatria, Neurologia et Neurochirurgia 74:259-270.

Hooshmand, H., and B. W. Brawley. 1970. Temporal lobe seizures and exhibitionism. Neurology 19:1119-1124.

Horel, J. A. 1971. Recovery from the behavioral effects of occipital temporal disconnection. Anatomical Record 169:342-343.

Horowitz, M. J. 1970. Psychosocial Function in Epilepsy. Springfield, Ill.: Charles C Thomas.

Hubel, D. H. 1971. Specificity of responses in cells in the visual system. Journal of Psychiatric Research 8:301-307.

Hubel, D. H., and T. N. Wiesel. 1962. Receptive fields, binocular interaction, and functional architecture in the cat's visual cortex. Journal of Physiology (London) 160:106-154.

Hughes, J. R., and R. E. Schlagenhauff. 1961. Electroclinical correlation in temporal lobe epilepsy with emphasis on interareal analysis of the temporal lobe. Electroencephalography and Clinical Neurophysiology 13:333-339.

Iverson, S. 1969. Studies of the temporal lobe in monkeys and baboons. British Journal of Psychiatry (Special Publication) 4:16-30.

James, I. P. 1960. Temporal lobectomy for temporal lobe epilepsy. Journal of Mental Science 106:543-558.

Jasper, H., C. P. Fitzpatrick, and P. Solomon. 1939. Analogies and opposites in schizophrenia and epilepsy: Electrographic and clinical studies. American Journal of Psychiatry 95:835-851.

Jones, B., and M. Mishkin. 1972. Limbic lesions and the problems of stimulus-reinforcement associations. Experimental Neurology 36:362-377.

Juul-Jensen, P. 1964. Epilepsy: a clinical and social analysis of 1020 adult patients with epileptic seizures. Acta Neurologica Scandinavica (Supplement 5) 40:1-148.

Keating, E. G. 1971. Somatosensory deficit produced by parieto temporal disconnection. Anatomical Record 169:353-354.

Klingler, J., and P. Gloor. 1960. The connections of the amygdala and of the anterior temporal cortex in the human brain. Journal of Comparative Neurology 115:333-369.

Kluver, H., and P. C. Bucy. 1939. Preliminary analysis of functions of the temporal lobes in man. Archives of Neurology and Psychiatry 42:979-1000.

Kuypers, G. J. M., M. Szwarcbart, M. Mishkin, and H. E. Rosvold. 1965. Occipitotemporal corticocortical connections in the rhesus monkey. Experimental Neurology 11:245-262.

Landolt, H. 1953. Some clinical electroencephalographic correlations in epileptic psychoses. Electroencephalography and Clinical Neurophysiology 5:121.

_____. 1958. Serial EEG investigations during psychotic episodes in epileptic patients and during schizophrenic attacks. In Lectures on Epilepsy, A. M. Lorentz de Haas, ed. Amsterdam: Elsevier.

Lorentz de Haas, A. M. (Ed.). 1958. Lectures on Epilepsy, Supplement 4, Psychiat. Neurol. Neurochem, Amsterdam: Elsevier Publishing Company.

Ludwig, B., C. Ajmone Marsan, and J. Van Buren, 1975. Cerebral seizures of probable orbito-frontal origin. Epilepsia 16:141-158.

McIntyre, M. 1975. Comparison of Right and Left Focal Temporal Epileptics. Paper read before International Neuropsychology Society Meeting, April 1975.

MacLean, P. D. 1958. Contrasting functions of limbic and neocortical systems of the brain and their relevance to psychophysiological aspects of medicine. American Journal of Medicine 25:611-626.

_____. 1962. New findings relevant to the evaluation of psychosexual functions of the brain. Journal of Nervous and Mental Disorders 135:289-301.

McLeary, R. 1966. Response—modulating functions of the limbic system: initiation and suppression, In Progress in Physiological Psychology. E. Stellar and J. Sprague, eds. New York: Academic Press.

Malamud, M. 1967. Psychiatric disorder with intracranial tumors of limbic system. Archives of Neurology 17:113-123.

Margerison, J. H. and J. A. Corsellis. 1966. Epilepsy and the temporal lobe. Brain 89:499-530.

Mark, V. H., F. R. Ervin, N. Geschwind, P. Solomon, and W. H. Sweet. 1968. The neurology of behavior: Its application to human violence. Medical Opinion Review 4:26-31.

Mark. V. H., and F. R. Ervin. 1970. Violence and the Brain. New York: Harper & Row.

Marlowe, W. B., E. L. Mancall, and J. J. Thomas. 1975. Complete Kluver-Bucy syndrome in man. Cortex 11:53-59.

Marshall, N. B., R. J. Barnett, and J. Mayer. 1955. Hypothalamic lesions in goldthioglucose injected mice. Proceedings of the Society for Experimental Biology and Medicine 90:240-244.

Mathews, C. G., and H. Kove. 1968. MMPI performance in major motor, psychomotor and mixed seizure classification of known and unknown etiology. Epilepsia 9:43-53.

Meier, M. J., and L. A. French. 1965. Changes in MMPI scale scores and an index of psychopathology following unilateral temporal lobectomy for epilepsy. Epilepsia 6:263-273.

Meldrum, B. S., and J. B. Brierley. 1972. Neuronal loss and gliosis in the hippocampus following repetitive epileptic seizures induced in adolescent baboons by allylglycine. Brain Research 48:361-365.

_____. 1973. Prolonged epileptic seizures in primates: Ischemic cell change and its relation to ictal physiological events. Archives of Neurology 28:10-17.

Mignone, R. J., E. F. Donnelly, and D. Sadowsky. 1970. Psychological and neurological comparisons of psychomotor and nonpsychomotor epileptic patients. Epilepsia 11:345-359.

Milner, B. 1971a. Interhemispheric differences in the localization of psychological processes in man. British Medical Bulletin 27:272-277.

_____. 1971b. Memory and the medial temporal regions of the brain. In Biology of Memory, K. H. Pribram and D. E. Broadbent, eds. New York: Academic Press.

_____. 1974. Hemispheric specialization: Scope and limits. In The Neurosciences—Third Study Program, F. Schmitt and F. Worden, eds. Cambridge: MIT Press.

Mirsky, A. F. 1960. Studies of the effects of brain lesions on social behavior in macaca mulatta: Methodological and theoretical considerations. Annals of the New York Academy of Science 85:785-794.

Mishkin, M. 1966. Visual mechanisms beyond the striate cortex. In Frontiers in Physiological Psychology, R. Russell, ed. New York: Academic Press.

_____. 1972. Cortical visual areas and their interactions. In The Brain and Human Behavior, A. G. Karczmar and J. C. Eccles, eds., New York: Springer-Verlag.

Mitchell, W., M. A. Falconer, and D. Hill. 1954. Epilepsy with fetishism relieved by temporal lobectomy. Lancet 2:626-636.

Morrell, F. 1959. Experimental focal epilepsy in animals. Archives of Neurology 1:141-197.

_____. 1960. Secondary epileptogenic lesions. Epilepsia 1:538-560.

_____. 1961. Lasting changes in synaptic organization produced by continuous neuronal bombardment. In Brain Mechanisms and Learning, J. F. Delafresnaye, ed. Springfield, Ill.: Charles C Thomas.

Narabayashi, H., T. Nagao, Y. Saito, M. Yoshida, and M. Nagahata. 1963. Stereotaxic amygdalectomy for behavior disorders. Archives of General Psychiatry 9:11-26.

Nisbett, R. E. 1972. Hunger, obesity and the ventromedial hypothalamus. Psychological Review 79:433-453.

Olds, J. 1955. Physiological mechanisms of reward. In Nebraska Symposium on Motivation, M. Jones, ed. Lincoln, Neb.: University of Nebraska Press.

_____. 1956. Reinforcement mapping in the rat brain. Journal of Comparative and Physiological Psychology 49:281-285.

_____. 1958. Adaptive functions of paleocortical and related structures. In Biological and Biochemical Bases of Behavior, H. Harlow and C. N. Woolsey, eds. Madison: University of Wisconsin Press.

Pandya, D. N., and H. G. J. M. Kuypers. 1969. Cortico-cortical connections in the rhesus monkey. Brain Research 13:13-36.

Papez, J. 1937. A proposed mechanism of emotion. Archives of Neurology and Psychiatry 38:725-743.

Penfield, W. 1954. Studies of the cerebral cortex of man. In Brain Mechanisms and Consciousness. E. Adrian and J. Delafresnaye, eds. Springfield, Ill.: Charles C Thomas.

_____. 1955. The role of the temporal cortex in certain psychical phenomena, 29th Maudsley Lecture. Journal of Mental Science 101:451-465.

Penfield, W., and H. Jasper. 1954. Epilepsy and the Functional Anatomy of the Human Brain. Boston: Little, Brown.

Penfield, W., and L. Roberts. 1959. Speech and Brain Mechanisms. Princeton: Princeton University Press.

Perria, L., G. Rossidini, and G. F. Rossi. 1961. Determination of side of cerebral dominance with amobarbital. Archives of Neurology 4:173-181.

Petr, R., L. B. Holden, and J. Jirout. 1949. The efferent intercortical connections of the superficial cortex of the temporal lobe (macaca mulatta). Journal of Neuropathology and Experimental Neurology 8:100-103.

Pilleri, G. 1966. The Kluver-Bucy syndrome in man. Psychiatrica et Neurologia (Basel) 152:65-103.

Poeck, K. 1969. Pathophysiology of emotional disorders associated with brain damage. In Handbook of Clinical Neurology, G. Bruyn and P. Vinken, eds. New York: Wiley.

Pond, D. A. 1957. Psychiatric aspects of epilepsy. Journal of the Indian Medical Profession 3:1441-1451.

_____. 1962. The schizophrenia-like psychoses of epilepsy—discussion. Proceedings of the Royal Society of Medicine 55:316.

_____. 1969. Epilepsy and personality disorders. In Handbook of Clinical Neurology, G. Bruyn and P. Vinken, eds. New York: Wiley.

Poirier, L. J. 1952. Anatomical and experimental studies on the temporal pole of the macaque. Journal of Comparative Neurology 96:208-248.

Pribram, J. H., M. Lennox, and R. H. Dunsmore. 1950. Some connections of the orbito-fronto-temporal limbic and hippocampal areas of macaca mulatta. Journal of Neurophysiology 13:127-135.

Razavi, L. 1974. Cytogenic and somatic variation in the neurobiology of violence. In The Neurobiology of Violence: Proceedings of the Houston Neurological Symposium, W. S. Fields and W. H. Sweet, eds. Springfield, Ill.: Charles C Thomas.

Rieman, G. 1953. The effectiveness of Rorschach elements in the discrimination between neurotic and ambulatory schizophrenic subjects. Journal of Consulting Psychology 17:25-31.

Roberts, D. R. 1963. Schizophrenia and the brain. Journal of Neuropsychiatry, 5:71-79.

Rocha-Miranda, C. E., D. B. Bender, C. G. Gross, and M. Mishkin. 1975. Visual activation of neurons in inferotemporal cortex depends on striate cortex and forebrain commissures. Journal of Neurophysiology 38:475-491.

Rodin, E., R. N. Dejong, R. W. Waggoner, and B. K. Bagchi. 1957. Relationship between certain forms of psychomotor epilepsy and schizophrenia. Archives of Neurology and Psychiatry 77:449-463.

Rosvold, H. E., A. F. Mirsky, and K. H. Pribram. 1954. Influence of amygdalectomy on social behavior in monkeys. Journal of Comparative and Physiological Psychology 47:173-178.

Savard, R., and E. Walker. 1965. Changes in social functioning after surgical treatment for temporal lobe epilepsy. Social Work 10:87-95.

Schaltenbrand, G., H. Spuler, W. Wahren, and A. Wilhelmi. 1973. Vegetative and emotional reactions during electrical stimulation of deep structures of the brain during stereotactic procedures. Zeitschrift für Neurologie 205:91-113.

Schreiner, L., and A. Kling. 1953. Behavioral changes following rhinencephalic injury in cat. Journal of Neurophysiology 16:643-659.

Schwartzbaum, J. S. 1960. Changes in reinforcing properties of stimuli following ablations of the amygdaloid complex in monkeys. Journal of Comparative Physiology 53:388-395.

Schwartzbaum, J. S., R. E. Bownes, and L. Holdstock. 1969. Visual exploration in the monkey following ablation of the amygdaloid complex. Journal of Comparative and Physiological Psychology 57:453-458.

Serafetinides, E. A. 1965a. Aggressiveness in temporal lobe epileptics and its relation to cerebral dysfunction and environmental factors. Epilepsia 6:33-42.

———. 1965b. The significance of the temporal lobes and hemispheric dominance in the production of the LSD-25 symptomatology in man. Neuropsychologia 3:69-79.

Serafetinides, E. A., and M. A. Falconer. 1962. The effects of temporal lobectomy in epileptic patients with psychosis. Journal of Mental Science 108:584-593.

Sherrington, C. 1947. The Integrative Action of the Nervous System. Cambridge: Cambridge University Press.

Simpson, J. A. 1969. Clinical neurology of temporal lobe disorders. British Journal of Psychiatry, (Special Publication) 4:42-48.

Singh, D., and D. R. Meyer. 1968. Eating and drinking by rats with lesions of the septum and the ventromedial hypothalamus. Journal of Comparative and Physiological Psychology 65:163-166.

———. 1972. Preference for mode of obtaining reinforcement in rats with lesions of septal or ventromedial hypothalamic area. Journal of Comparative and Physiological Psychology 80:259-268.

Slater, E. 1969. The schizophrenia-like illnesses of epilepsy. British Journal of Psychiatry (Special Publication) 4:77-81.

Slater, E., and A. W. Beard. 1963. Schizophrenia-like psychoses of epilepsy. British Journal of Psychiatry 109:95-150.

Slater, E., and P. A. P. Moran. 1969. The schizophrenic-like psychoses of epilepsy: relations between ages of onset. British Journal of Psychiatry 115:599-600.

Small, J. G., V. Millstein, and J. R. Stevens. 1962. Are psychomotor epileptics different? Archives of Neurology 7:187-194.

Small, J. G., and I. F. Small. 1967. A controlled study of mental disorders associated with epilepsy. Journal of Advances in Biological Psychiatry 9:171-181.

Small, J. G., I. F. Small, and M. P. Hayden. 1966. Further psychiatric investigations of patients with temporal and nontemporal lobe epilepsy. American Journal of Psychiatry 123:303-310.

Smythies, J. R. 1969. The behavioral physiology of temporal lobes. British Journal of Psychiatry, (Special Publication) 4:9-15.

Sperry, R. W. 1968. Hemisphere deconnection and unity in conscious experience. American Psychology 23:723-733.

———. 1973. Lateral specialization of cerebral functions in the surgically separated hemispheres. In Psychophysiology of Thinking, F. J. McGuigan and R. A. Schoonover, eds. New York and London: Academic Press.

Stamm, J. S. and J. H. Pribram. 1961. Effects of epileptogenic lesions of inferotemporal cortex on learning and retention in monkeys. Journal of Comparative and Physiological Psychology 54:614-618.

Stamm, J. S. and M. Knight. 1963. Learning of visual tasks by monkeys with epileptogenic implants in temporal cortex. Journal of Comparative Physiology and Psychology 56:254-260.

Stamm, J. S., and A. Warren. 1961. Learning and retention by monkeys with epileptogenic implants in posterior parietal cortex. Epilepsia 2:229-242.

Stamm, J. S., and S. C. Rosen. 1971. Learning of somesthetic discrimination and reversal tasks by monkeys with epileptogenic implants in antero-medial temporal cortex. Neuropsychologia 9:185-194.

Stepien, L. S., J. P. Cordeau, and T. Rasmussen. 1960. The effect of temporal lobe and hippocampal lesions on auditory and visual recent memory in monkeys. Brain 83:470-489.

Stevens, J. R. 1959. Emotional activation of the EEG in patients with convulsive disorders. Journal of Nervous and Mental Disorders 128:339-351.

_____. 1966. Psychiatric implications of psychomotor epilepsy. Archives of General Psychiatry 14:461-471.

_____. 1973. Psychomotor epilepsy and schizophrenia: A common anatomy? In Epilepsy—Its Phenomena in Man. M. Brazier, ed. New York: Academic Press.

Stevens, J. R., V. M. Milstein, and S. Goldstein. 1972. Psychometric test performance in psychomotor epilepsy. Archives of General Psychiatry 26:532-538.

Sunshine, J., and M. Mishkin. 1975. A visual-limbic pathway serving visual associative functions in rhesus monkeys. Federation Proceedings 34:440.

Sweet, W. H., F. Ervin, and V. H. Mark. 1968. The relationship of violent behavior to focal cerebral disease. In Aggressive Behavior, S. Garattini and E. B. Sigg, eds. Amsterdam, Milan: Excerpta Medica.

Symonds, C. 1969. Disease of mind and disorder of brain. British Medical Journal 1:1-5.

_____. 1962. The schizophrenia-like psychoses of epilepsy. Proceedings of the Royal Society of Medicine 55:314-315.

Taylor, D. C. 1969. Aggression and epilepsy. Journal of Psychosomatic Research 13:229-236.

_____. 1971. Ontogenesis of chronic epileptic psychoses: a reanalysis, Psychological Medicine 1:247-253.

_____. 1972. Mental state and temporal lobe epilepsy: a correlative account of 100 patients treated surgically. Epilepsia 13:727-765.

Taylor, D. C., and C. Ounsted. 1971. Biological mechanisms influencing the outcome of seizures in response to fever. Epilepsia 12:33-45.

Terzian, H. 1964. Behavioral and EEG effects of intracarotid sodium amytal injections. Acta Neurochirurgia 12:230-240.

Terzian, H., and G. Dalle Ore. 1955. Syndrome of Kluver and Bucy reproduced in man by bi-lateral removal of temporal lobes. Neurology 5:373-380.

Tizard, B. 1962. The personality of epileptics: a discussion of the evidence. Psychological Bulletin 59:196-210.

Torrey, E. G., and M. P. Peterson. 1974. Schizophrenia and the limbic system. Lancet 2:942-946.

Treffert, D. A. 1969. The psychiatric patients with an EEG temporal lobe focus. American Journal of Psychiatry 120:765-771.

Ursin, H. 1960. The temporal lobe substrate of fear and anger. Acta Psychiatrica et Neurologica Scandinavica 35:378-396.

Van Buren, J. M. 1975. Personal communication.

Van Buren, J. M., C. Ajmone-Marsan, N. Mutsuga, and D. Sadowsky. 1975. Surgery of temporal lobe epilepsy. *In* Advances in Neurology. Vol. 8. D. Purpura, J. Peury, and R. Walter eds. New York: Raven Press.

Vislie, H., and G. F. Henrikson. 1958. Psychic disturbances in epileptics. *In* Lectures in Epilepsy, L. de Haas, ed. Amsterdam: Elsevier.

Walker, A. E., A. F. Thomas, and J. D. McQueen. 1953. Behavior and the temporal rhinencephalon in the monkey. Bulletin of the Johns Hopkins Hospital 93:65-93.

Walker, A. E. 1973. Man and his temporal lobes. Surgical Neurology 1:69-79.

Waxman, S. G. and N. Geschwind. 1974. Hypergraphia in temporal lobe epilepsy. Neurology 24:629-636.

Weinstein, E. A. 1959. Relationships among seizures, psychosis and personality factors. American Journal of Psychiatry 116:124-126.

Weinstein, E. A., and R. L. Kahn. 1955. Denial of illness. Springfield, Ill.: Charles C Thomas.

Weiskrantz, L. 1956. Behavioral changes associated with ablation of the amygdaloid complex in monkeys. Journal of Comparative Physiological Psychology 49:381-391.

Whitlock, D. G., and W. J. H. Nauta. 1956. Subcortical projections from temporal neocortex in macaca mulatta. Journal of Comparative Anatomy 106:183-212.

Williams, D. 1956. The structure of emotions reflected in epileptic experience. Brain 79:28-67.

———. 1968. Man's temporal lobe. Brain 91:639-654.

———. 1969. Temporal lobe syndromes. *In* Handbook of Clinical Neurology. G. Bruyn and P. Vinken, eds. Vol. 2. New York: Wiley.

Wilson, W. P. and B. Nashold. 1972. The neurophysiology of affect. Diseases of the Nervous System 33:13-19.

Wittenborn, J. R., and J. D. Holzberg. 1951. The Rorschach and descriptive diagnosis. Journal of Consulting Psychology 15:460-463.

Yde, A., L. Edel, and A. Feurbye. 1941. On the relation between schizophrenia, epilepsy and induced convulsions. Acta Psychiatrica 16:325-388.

CHAPTER 7

EXPLANATORY MODELS IN PSYCHOHISTORY

Anastasia Kucharski, M.D.

PREFACE

This chapter attempts to answer some questions I have been asking for several years. As an undergraduate, I wrote a psychohistorical thesis, and I did additional historical research on it with professional historians after graduation. I noticed through that later experience that I had begun to question the relevance of psychological theories to the actual information gathered from the research. I also became more aware of the critical and skeptical stance of historians toward psychohistory.

During medical school and residency training, I was able to look back at my historical training to get a better understanding of the viewpoint of historians. One factor that helped me was the realization that biography is very much like a case history, except that a biography lacks a clinical formulation formally set apart. The formulation itself suggests a critical difference between history and case reporting. Adding a formulation, even if it were integrated into the body of the text, would somehow change the fundamental character of historical reporting. The explanatory models that have been used in psychohistory and that are elaborated in this chapter indicate the virtues and problems encountered in making this integration.

As psychoanalytic theory was elaborated and accepted, many hoped that its concepts and methodology could be extended to the social sciences and used also in art and literary criticism. However, applied psychoanalysis invited controversy, for the appropriateness of its extension was questioned. In the social sciences, for instance, critics suggested that a psychological reductionism was implicit in the application of psychoanalytic theory to sociology, anthropology, and history. On the other hand, in literature and art, the purpose of the psychoanalytic extension appeared ambiguous. Theoretically, an artistic production was equivalent to any other action or behavior, and so was an expression of intrapsychic processes. Thus, the content of a novel was a guide to the psychological conflicts of its author. Linking art somehow to neurosis ultimately led to questions about the meaning of art and its relationship to social systems that could not be answered (Jones, 1974; Phillips, 1957).

Even before the issue of applied psychoanalysis appeared, historians had debated whether history was an art, a science, or some unique combination. Thus, the later controversies about psychological reductionism and the connections between an event and the participants' intrapsychic processes were especially relevant. Moreover, when psychoanalytic theory was first noticed by historians, its application to psychohistory helped to encourage additional speculation about the nature of history and the methods historians used to explain an event. In researching history, writers using psychological concepts also developed different methods. As we look at the models of psychohistorical explanation then, one goal will be to understand the controversial implications of applied psychoanalysis.

Psychohistory is an interdisciplinary field in which historical characters or events are looked at from a psychological point of view. As a discipline related to history, psychohistory is subject to historiographers' critiques about methodology. For example, is its method compatible with a standard historical explanation for events? There is no clear-cut answer, for the explanatory model in psychohistory, or the way in which a topic is looked at, can be descriptive, analogical, or deductive. Thus, psychohistorians are interested not only in what took place, but also in how and why it did, whereas in standard history, the basic explanatory model is descriptive.

In the descriptive model, events are arranged in a temporal sequence and linked together by a common theme. Since description is fundamental to all history, the descriptive model provides a common bond for historians and psychohistorians. However, a psychological theme distinguishes psychohistory from other historical writing that relies on the descriptive approach. As Dray (1959) has noted, the historians' problem is "to discover *what it really was* that happened, by offering an explanation of the form, 'It was a so-and-so.' " Dray added that "it is a matter of the synthesis rather than the analysis of what is to be explained." Hence, historical explanation is "explanation by means of a general concept rather than a general law." Dray's example was the "social revolution" that took place in late-eighteenth-century England. His evidence for the "revolution" was that communications were improved, land was enclosed, and factory production had begun. Hence, through the use of general themes, historians have been interpreting social events, behavior, and personalities in a way they found most appropriate.

The application of the descriptive model creates little disagreement between historians and psychohistorians. In contrast, the analogical model, which has a different goal, that of understanding how something took place, arouses controversy. The analogical model is generally considered to be the prototype of psychohistorical explanation (Meyer, 1971). At first glance this model appears quite similar to the descriptive one, for it requires a straightforward account of what happened, not only for the event under investigation, but also for similar events earlier in the subject's life. Then these two sets of events are related by means of a theoretical construct. This model differs from both the descriptive and deductive models in that the events connected by the theoretical concept need not be temporally close together. They rarely are, since the later events are usually looked at in terms of their relationship to childhood events. This method, then, is especially suitable for biographies and case studies. As Hughes (1964) considers the connection between history and psychoanalysis as obvious, and indeed asserts that "psychoanalysis is history or possibly biography," he is simultaneously limiting history and expanding it as he looks to recent employers of the analogical model such as Erikson and Lifton for "guideposts for pursuing an old task."

Comparative biographical techniques such as Lifton's (1962) suggest the third and final model, the deductive, in which themes or theoretical constructs are not as important to the model as the theory or general law that the subject matter is, or can be, used to verify. With this approach, there seems to be a shift in emphasis from the subject matter to the theory itself.

For the deductive model, an event is explained when it becomes an example of a rule that states that given the presence of certain initial conditions, the subsequent event or the *explicandum* will occur. Hempel (1959) suggested that such covering laws were implicit in history. For example, Nathan Hale was executed after he spied on the British. The covering law for this event, however, seemed of the order of a commonplace or tautology. Hempel was urged to identify these laws, and he was asked whether the precedents were necessary or sufficient for the subsequent event to happen. Hempel modified his view to say that history had "explanation sketches" that had to be filled out (Gardiner, 1961; Hempel, 1966).

Hempel was also open to the criticism that he was not writing history when he sought laws, because it seemed he was changing the focus away from the historical events. Oakeshott (1933) wrote that "the moment historical facts are regarded as instances of general laws, history is disavowed, for this method transforms an historical way of investigating past events into a scientific one." Also, Elton (1967) described studying history for its own sake as characteristic of twentieth-century historians, for whom facts and events (and people) must be individual and particular: like other entities of a similar kind, but not entirely identical with them.

Others who have looked at the three models of psychohistorical explanation stress the resemblance to the way mainstream historians write about their subject. My reason for emphasizing these differences between psychohistory and other history is that they provide a starting point for speculating about why psychohistory has remained as controversial as it was early in the century. At that time Lamprecht was urging people to be interested in the "collective psychology of the past" (Barnes, 1919), while Robinson, speaking before the American Historical Association, encouraged his audience to make use of the developments in psychology (Garrity, 1954). Fifty years later, Langer urged the association to be more interested in psychoanalytical concepts (Langer, 1958; Mazlish, 1971).

Langer's advice did not go unheeded. Demos (1970) relied on concepts like "orality" to describe the tortures seventeenth-century witches were said to inflict—for example, biting, pinching, and pricking. He used "oral aggression" as a theme for the era. Seizures children had after being bitten by witches allowed them to engage in a "considerable amount of direct aggression." Presumably, the children acted out a severe inner conflict in "this little model of aggression attempted and inhibited" (Demos, 1970). Demos suggested that those who might make charges of witchcraft might have had disturbances that could be traced to the oral stage. In line with his descriptive approach, however, Demos merely speculated with this suggestion. Hence, he does not explain who found witches and why witches were prosecuted; instead, he provides a means of synthesizing what happened during this period in New England.

Demos was writing in the descriptive style of psychohistory practiced by writers like Hitschmann (1956). Although the subtitle of his book *Great Men* is *Psychoanalytic Studies*, and he asserted his indebtedness to Freud, Hitschmann described his subjects in terms of character types such as the "exception" and the "demonic," and commented that interest in "pathographies" had declined over the preceding fifty years. Hunter and Macalpine's study (1968) of George III's psychosis provides some information about why interest declined. When referring to the claim that George's psychotic episodes were symptomatic of porphyria rather than manic depressive illness, Brooke emphasized that this new diagnosis was all-important for the historian, as subsequent history of late-eighteenth-century

England would not have to account for a king with a "mentally unstable and weak personality." Events like the American Revolution and George III's marriage would not have to be interpreted through the explanatory theme of George's mental status, which was considered none too healthy between episodes. Instead, he had a definable and self-limited disease (Brooke, 1968).

Meanwhile Freud's speculations about the derivations of all manner of cultural achievements were described as "crawling like a snail over all that is comely in life and art" (Garrity, 1954). Critics questioned the use of Freudian theory in literature (Abbot, 1931; Whilby, 1924). A host of biographies published after World War I that were method-ologically based on Freud's studies of Leonardo da Vinci (1957), Dostoevsky (1961a), and Moses (1964) aroused similar criticism.

Freud (1961a) asserted that Dostoevsky's violent murderous charac-ters reflected "similar tendencies in human souls," including Dosto-evsky's. Freud then related Dostoevsky's novels to the author's neurotic conflicts and his seizures. He asserted that Dostoevsky threw away the chance of becoming a teacher and liberator of humanity; he was con-demned "to this failure by his neurosis," which was hysteria. Acknowl-edging that "it cannot be strictly proved that Dostoevsky's seizures were of the affective type," Freud still held that Dostoevsky's hysteria had manifested itself through his grand mal seizures. The seizures began when Dostoevsky was eighteen, the same year his father was murdered. A father is also murdered in *The Brothers Karamazov.* In his novels, Dostoevsky expressed what he had repressed in his life: his hatred of his father, based on unconscious castration fears. When his fantasies about his father's death became reality, he had seizures and later wrote violent novels about parricide, for he continued to wish for his father's death and to fear what would happen to him for having this wish.

Returning to the three forms of psychohistorical explanation, the descriptive, analogical, and deductive, we can see that Freud is explaining how something took place by setting up a model in which a crucial life event is linked to subsequent behavior by means of theoretical constructs, in this case castration fear. His explanation is analogical.

However, the significant task for the historian is to find out what happened. The historian would be interested in discovering Dosto-evsky's attitude toward his father, the history relevant to his seizure disorder, including reports of early head trauma, and the events that took place at the time of the father's death. The historian would be trying to determine what happened and would use an abstraction or concept as a theme to synthesize the events. Hence, critical reactions to works like "Dostoevsky and Parricide" tend to conclude that Freud's explanation is at best premature, based as it is on incomplete information.

Freud used the analogical model in "A Seventeenth-Century Demonological Neurosis" (1961b) in which he proposed that the devil was a father substitute. Mourning the death of his father, the character discussed in this article made a pact with the devil to give him his soul in order to relieve his depression. The man then came to have the same relationship with the devil as he had had with his lost father. Freud found he could explain these cases because he considered states of demonic possession and ecstasy to be manifestations of hysteria with "the same content as the neuroses of today" (Freud, 1974b).

Freudian theory has been used to explain the sources of other literary works and the formulation of some disastrous foreign policies. Greenacre (1971) thought Jonathan Swift's Meniere's disease was associated with a strong homosexual conflict. She noted that Swift thought his disease came from eating stone fruit in the Temple Garden. Greenacre also found Swift's *Meditations Upon a Broomstick* to be as important as the stone fruit story in showing a homosexual conflict because of its symbolic title.

Binion (1969) used the analogical model when he wrote on Leopold III of Belgium and his policy toward Hitler during the 1930s. Binion asserted that Leopold's policy of Belgian neutrality toward Hitler, beginning in October 1936, was a "disguised way" of relieving his unconsciously guilt-ridden role in the death of his wife in an auto accident in which he was driving. Astrid, a very popular queen, was the symbol of Belgium, which Leopold could also destroy by giving it up to the Germans. Binion assumed that if Astrid could symbolize Belgium, then Belgium could symbolize Astrid, who inadvertently died by means of Leopold. The role of Astrid as a symbol is important to Binion, who is concerned about explaining how the king's policy arose. He does not explain why this particular association occurred at this particular time.

Binion added that in his (Leopold's) inflexible attitude, Leopold was also identifying with his father and predecessor, Albert I, who kept Belgium neutral during World War I. According to a court attendant, while mountain climbing after Albert's death, Leopold took on the "serenity and prudence that had characterized his father," and at his coronation declared that his "most ardent desire" was to follow the path his father had so clear-sightedly traced (Binion, 1969). Facing a different external situation, Leopold nevertheless kept Belgium neutral until the country was overrun by the Germans.

After setting forth what happened and elaborating on how the policy was carried out, Binion commented on the theoretical implications of his method. For Binion, the king's policy from 1936 to 1940 was not only integral to the prehistory of World War II but was also a "clear-cut example of how even in history great effects can follow from small causes." He added that in his theory, adult thought and conflict came from infantile motives transferred to actual situations. Binion is concerned with the transfer in the sense that he notices similarities and symbols, and so is not trying to deduce why the particular policy was put into effect.

Binion admitted that his point of view did not conform to the idea that "big events are causally related among themselves to the exclusion of little events." This idea now "pervades historical writing" and has done so since Hegel (1944) formulated the idea in the nineteenth century (Binion, 1969).

In referring to Hegel, Binion is confounding two quite divergent schools of historical writing and thinking. Contemporary historians tend to concentrate on important events while adding less important facts to elaborate their description. However, Hegel speculated on why the events are related. His dialectical theory of history suggests a historical law (Hegel, 1944).

In terms of methods and goals, Hegel's most important successor is Erikson, whose *Young Man Luther* (1958) combines the Freudian model with a social theory. Erikson bridges the gap between "la grand histoire" and "la petite histoire" (Binion, 1969) by using the concepts of identity and ideology as connecting points between Luther's Oedipal conflicts and his later religious career.

Fifteen years after its publication, Eriskon described the model in *Young Man Luther* as a social theory. He claimed that the great man is the person with a particular life history who can resolve his own identity by resolving that of others at the same time. By doing this for his community, he becomes a leader and thus becomes great in the opinion of others (Lifton, 1974). Erikson, therefore, is suggesting that this particular great man is a necessary, if not sufficient, precondition for the revolution or major social event that would follow.

An important feature of writing in the deductive model is to have a theme or topic that the subject matter can illustrate. Thus, in *Young Man Luther*, Erikson concentrates on identity formation as a contributing factor in the development of religious ideology. In *Gandhi's Truth*, he is interested in the origins of militant nonviolence (Erikson, 1969). Somewhat paradoxically, despite his recognition as a leading psychohistorian, Erikson pays attention only to universal themes.

His followers tend to use his theories and Freud's analogical model in their writings. For example, Brodie (1974) heavily emphasizes the personal parts of Jefferson's life. She referred to Jefferson's conflict over being involved in a revolution as having something to do with his seemingly hostile relationship with his mother: "The destruction of political liberty in the Massachusetts colony set off the time bomb that had long been ticking in Jefferson's heart." She noted that Erikson had concluded that "the matter of indulgences set off the time bomb which had been ticking in Luther's heart."

Although Brodie found Jefferson's conflict to be centered in his mother, she later compared Jefferson's *Summary View* to the *Ninety-Five Theses* Luther hung on the cathedral door. She regarded them both as personal statements directed at paternal figures. The two authors are "communicating tremendous rage, part of which, as Erik Erikson has demonstrated brilliantly, should have been directed at other, more distant people" (Brodie, 1974).

Erikson and other psychohistorians have an approach to explanation that sets their work apart from standard history. As a result, their publications are seldom reviewed in history journals. The neglect of *Young Man Luther*, for example, in history journals arose not from an unfamiliarity with the concept of identity crisis but because of differences in purpose and method. The differences are illuminated in Spitz's recent review (1973) of *Young Man Luther*.

Praising *Luther* as superior to all attempts at a posthumous psychoanalysis, Spitz compared Erikson's approach to that of Preserved Smith who wrote on Luther in 1913. Spitz pointed out that Smith "delivered a primer of 'Freudian' observations with the demon, repressed elementary sexual life, harsh home discipline, preoccupation with concupiscence and depressions." Spitz preferred Erikson's generalization that "the characteristics of Luther's theological advance can be compared to certain steps in psychological maturation which every man must take."

Spitz then showed that Hans Luther was "not harsh, drunken or tyrannical" as Erikson assumed, but rather was pious, stern, and ambitious for himself and for his son. Spitz is attempting to undermine the basic assumptions with which Erikson explained Luther's "fit in the choir," which took place when he was saying his first Mass before his father. Like Dostoevsky's seizures, Luther's fit is explained by Erikson as the expression of unconscious conflict directed at the religious father who symbolized the tyrannical father watching his son.

Instead of directly criticizing Erikson's model, Spitz is trying to determine what happened by sorting out all the information he can about the characters. He notes that the "fit" was first mentioned by an enemy of Luther some forty years after its presumed occurrence, a fact that casts suspicion on the event and certainly undermines its drama. Spitz preferred "fear of demonic possession" to a vocational "identity crisis" as a reason for Luther's alleged reaction, as the former would be more consistent with sixteenth-century thinking. Spitz is thus relying on the standard sort of historical explanation in which a concept is used to synthesize what is described.

Spitz appreciated Erikson's "ring of truth" but went on to use the concepts of psychology in the way historians have used them since Thucydides. He described Luther as having a cyclothymic personality and suggested his religious troubles were a conflict between "secular ambition and ascetic religiosity, the latter winning over the former and his father's wishes." Spitz emphasized Luther's motives in terms of "even though" and not "because of" his father's ambitions. In comparison to Freud and Erikson, Spitz is using a more limited and descriptive concept of explanation that would be consistent with the traditional method of historical explanation in which the purpose is to clarify what took place.

I have attempted through various illustrations to compare the methods of psychohistory and history in order to suggest some reasons for the difficulty of integrating psychohistory into mainstream history. The literature of psychohistory has examples that can be put into each of the categories, descriptive, analogical, and deductive. The descriptive model, fundamental to mainstream history and also to the case study, has been used since Thucydides, because historians have always used behavioral and psychological terms to describe their characters clearly. Hence, as in Demos' and Spitz's papers, the descriptive model provides a means of expanding the use of psychological concepts in historical writing without changing the fundamental nature of history, and emphasizes the uniqueness of the event. This emphasis, which suggests the implicit unreproducibility of historical events through the discipline of history, reminds me of Jaspers' attempt to understand a patient by looking for the meaningful connections in the patient's life, in order to obtain theoretical explanations or summaries to aid the clinician's understanding (Jaspers, 1963). Such enterprise, however, is clearly separable from description, and Jaspers makes no claim for its validity. When historians enter the realm of theory building, as in the analogical and deductive models, they may appear less interested in the individual and may not be writing history. Such was the case with Freud. Furthermore, Erikson's statements on social theory make explicit the covering laws Hempel, the historian, tried to find in history, and these statements appear more forceful than his descriptive accounts.

Several problems have, therefore, come up from looking at explanatory models of psychohistory. Grasping what psychohistory is becomes more difficult as its models of explanation are delineated. Unlike psychology and history, which Elton, for one, believes are particular disciplines with their own methods and subject matter, psychohistory uses methods and models frequently difficult to distinguish from its parent disciplines and topics that are not particularly its own as well. Hence, psychohistory as currently practiced can be described as an attempt, not altogether explicit, to amalgamate psychological concepts, and psychoanalytic, historical, and scientific methods of explanation.

By analyzing the models of psychohistory, the similarity of historical writing to the psychiatric case study also seems clearer, since for both fields, it is important to obtain a decent history for careful assessment. What distinguishes history from the case study is the attempt at theoretical understanding of the latter through a formulation. For the historian, there has been a greater interest in remaining close to the historical events and a greater skepticism about deductive and analogical constructions of historical phenomena. For the psychiatrist, there has been an equally great interest in providing not only the facts but also a framework to enable practitioner and patient to understand their meaning.

REFERENCES

Abbot, W. 1931. Some new history and historians. Massachusetts Historical Society Proceedings 64:285-293.

Barnes, H. E. 1919. Psychology and history: some reasons for predicting their more active cooperation in the future. American Journal of Psychology 30:337-376.

Binion, R. 1969. Repeat performance: a psychohistorical study of Leopold III and Belgian neutrality. History and Theory 7:213-260.

Brodie, F. 1974. Thomas Jefferson. New York: Norton.

Brooke, J. 1968. Historical implications of Porphyria. British Medical Journal 1:109-111.

Demos, J. 1970. Underlying themes in witchcraft of seventeenth century New England. American Historical Review 75:1311-1326.

Dray, W. 1959. "Explaining what" in history. In Theories of History, P. Gardiner, ed. New York: The Free Press.

Elton, G. 1967. The Practice of History. London: Sydney University Press.

Erikson, E. 1958. Young Man Luther. New York: Norton

_____. 1969. Gandhi's Truth. New York: Basic Books.

Freud, S. 1957. Leonardo da Vinci and a memory of his childhood (1910). In Standard Edition, Complete Psychological Works of Sigmund Freud, Vol. 11. J. Strachey, ed. London: Hogarth Press, pp. 57-137.

_____. 1961a. Dostoevsky and parricide (1928). In Standard Edition, Complete Psychological Works of Sigmund Freud, Vol. 21. J. Strachey, Ed. London: Hogarth Press, pp. 173-194.

_____. 1961b. A seventeenth century demonological neurosis (1923). In Standard Edition, Complete Psychological Works of Sigmund Freud, Vol. 19. J. Strachey, ed. London: Hogarth Press, pp. 67-108.

_____. 1964. Moses and monotheism: three essays (1935). In Standard Edition, Complete Psychological Works of Sigmund Freud, Vol. 23. J. Strachey, ed. London: Hogarth Press, pp. 1-137.

Gardiner, P. 1961. The Nature of Historical Explanation. New York: Oxford University Press.

Garrity, J. 1954. Interrelation of psychology and biography. Psychological Bulletin 51:569-582.

Greenacre, P. 1971. Emotional Growth. Vol. II. New York: International Universities Press.

Hegel, G. 1944. The Philosophy of History. New York: Wiley.

Hempel, C. 1959. The function of general laws in history. In Theories of History, P. Gardiner, ed. New York: The Free Press.

———. 1966. Philosophy of Natural Science. Englewood Cliffs, N.J.: Prentice-Hall.

Hitschmann, E. 1956. Great Men. New York: International Universities Press.

Hughes, H. 1964. History as Art and as Science. New York: Harper & Row.

Hunter, R. and I. MacAlpine. 1968. The insanity of George III: a classic case of porphyria. In Porphyria: A Royal Malady. M. Ware, ed. London: British Medical Association, pp. 1-16.

Jaspers, K. 1963. General Psychopathology. Manchester, England: Manchester University Press.

Jones, E. 1974. Psycho-Myth, Psycho-History. New York: Stonehill.

Langer, W. 1958. The next assignment. American Historical Review 63: 283-304.

Lifton, R. 1962. Thought Reform and the Psychology of Totalism. London: Victor Gollancz.

———. 1974. Explorations in Psychohistory. New York: Simon and Schuster.

Mazlish, B. 1971. Psychoanalysis and History. New York: Grosset & Dunlap.

Meyer, D. 1971. A review of Young Man Luther. In Psychoanalysis and History, B. Mazlish, ed. New York: Grosset & Dunlap.

Oakeshott, M. 1933. Experience and Its Modes. London: Cambridge University Press.

Phillips, W. 1957. Art and Psychoanalysis. New York: Criterion.

Spitz, L. 1973. Psychohistory and the case of Young Man Luther. In Historical Interpretation and Religious Biography, D. Capps, ed. Berkeley, Calif.: University of California Press.

Whilby, C. 1924. Indiscretions of biography. English Review 39:769-772.

PART III

ISSUES THAT PROVIDE NOVEL AND SIGNIFICANT PERSPECTIVES IN THE FIELDS OF PSYCHIATRY

CHAPTER 8

PATIENTS' SUBJECTIVE EXPERIENCES OF PSYCHIATRIC HOSPITALIZATION

Miriam Sonn, R.N., Ph.D.

You were doubtless a pretty intolerable character when the maniacal condition came on and you were bossing the universe. Not only ordinary tact but a genius for diplomacy must have been needed for avoiding rows with you; but you certainly were wrongly treated nevertheless. . . . Your report is full of instructiveness for doctors and attendants alike.

—from a letter from William James to Clifford Beers after James had read Beers' manuscript, *A Mind That Found Itself.*

How do patients hospitalized for psychiatric problems view and evaluate their experiences of hospitalization? Practitioners of psychiatry and those engaged in research in psychiatry, though vitally interested in the treatment process and in determining which variables are effective and ineffective in the course of that process, have tended to neglect the patients themselves as a source of information and feedback. This chapter attempts to understand that neglect and to begin to remedy it by dipping into the existing literature on patients' subjective experiences of psychiatric hospitalization and by drawing together some of the thoughts and feelings expressed by patients. It also suggests that such information and feedback be encouraged and collected in a systematic way during and after the course of hospitalization for mental illness.

REASONS FOR NEGLECTING TO LISTEN TO PATIENTS

What has kept psychiatrists from treading on this promising terrain and from asking those who have gone through such illnesses what it was like? Part of the answer may lie in the kind of carefully trained suspiciousness bred into psychiatric trainees that makes them take very little that is said at face value. Every verbal utterance of the patient is grist for the interpretive mill. This can make it difficult for straightforward exchanges of information to take place.

A second factor that makes simply listening to what patients have to say a difficult matter is based on general social attitudes toward mental illness. In our society, psychosis has been viewed as a condition of invalidation, of loss of control and responsibility. The result is that something said by one who is or who has been hospitalized for psychiatric reasons is invalidated.

Although the discussion here is limited to the problems concerning hospitalization for mental illness, it should be said that patients with medical problems tend to encounter the same treatment at the hands of staff as do people hospitalized for psychiatric problems (Lipowski and Stewart, 1973). Their opinions about treatment and care are rarely solicited, and are usually discounted when offered. The fact of their sickness or disability tends to invalidate all the other parts of themselves that may be functioning quite adequately.

Closely related to this invalidation of the whole person because of a partial disablement is the fact that psychiatry has, in the main, aligned itself with the medical world and with the community of the physical sciences. It has tended to see patients as objects to be studied, as data for analysis. As data, patients are not expected to talk back in a way that no longer defines them as data. They are allowed to talk in order to exhibit their psychopathology and to be helped with that, but they are hardly to be listened to for any other purpose.

These factors that limit listening to patients have also suggested why psychiatrists are reluctant to use patients as informants or as co-investigators in the treatment process. Psychiatrists might also choose more actively not to listen to patients. After all, listening to patients with an openness and hearing from them things one has not already planned to hear and to fit into some gridlike pattern of psychopathology is hard work. It can be hard on the ego as well. There are styles of therapy and styles of listening just as there are styles of relating to the world. One variable of style is the degree of openness to the unexpected and uncontrollable that one is willing to let in cognitively and emotionally. Safety and comfort lie in predictability and containment. This is brought home vividly in Sechehaye's *Autobiography of a Schizophrenic Girl* (1951). There the analyst repeatedly confronts her own ignorance and periodic failures in trying to treat the severely ill Renee. Sechehaye flounders often but always tries to listen carefully to what her patient says she needs. Sechehaye lets Renee flow through her life instead of trying to confine her to fifty-minute hours and office couches. This is a strenuous business both practically and psychologically. Many therapists would not choose to work with patients in a way that would leave them so open to the patients' invasiveness or to their own self-doubts.

There are, then, functions for the therapist in *not* listening to patients as whole people who have many parts to them, some in good order and others not. These functions can be seen especially clearly on inpatient units where psychiatric residents are being trained. I work on such a unit where residents come through for six-month periods. In the interests of training, patients' cases may be over-simplified to be used as illustrations of various mental disorders that the residents have been reading about. In addition to this tendency to squeeze the patient into a mold for didactic purposes, there is the issue of confidence for the young doctor. Those responsible for the training of residents want to instill the residents with a sense of confidence in their abilities to diagnose and treat patients despite their lack of knowledge and experience. Oversimplification is again called upon to save the fledglings from being overwhelmed by their ignorance.

ARGUMENTS FOR LISTENING TO PATIENTS

I have noted that there are a variety of barriers to listening to and hearing what patients have to say about psychiatric hospitalization. On the other hand, why *should* we listen to them? What have they to offer to those working in the field? Answering these questions forces us to recognize psychiatry and its residential treatment centers as social systems and as organizations with goals. There is a tendency on the part of members of all organizations to see less and less of the broad features of their enterprise as they become more immersed in its daily workings. Over time, goals may be lost sight of and the organization may shift to exist for the sake of existing rather than to satisfy the needs for which it was originally created. One problem facing organizations, then, is how to build in some means of ensuring renewal and growth and thus preventing stagnation. Criticism is needed and may come from a source external to the organization or from within. Until recently, outside criticism of professionals was rare. The scientific community, with psychiatry as one representative, had made itself esoteric and mysterious enough to convince most outsiders that only an initiate could evaluate its workings. The luxury of psychiatric insulation from outside pressures is fast disappearing as intrusions from lawyers and laypersons become more frequent. Internal criticism and evaluation have little influence in the fields of

psychiatry, a review of psychotherapy research, for instance, underlines the ambiguity and inconsistency of findings concerning what
works and what does not (Meltzoff and Kornreich, 1970). Yet
psychiatry fails to implement constructive changes in line with this
criticism.

The limitations of our present knowledge call for a certain
humility and a sensitivity to what patients are being put through
during their hospitalization. Indeed, patients may be in a good
position to provide some of this needed internal criticism. They
become members of the system for a briefer time than staff on
short-term units and so are not subject to the same kind of blurring
of vision that longtime members of organizations tend to develop.
They are, however, hardly objective observers, yet they do offer a
perspective very different from that of staff, a perspective that may
complement a rather one-sided view of what staff sees as taking
place.

In trying to deepen our perspectives on the treatment we offer, we
should not underestimate the complexity of the inpatient psychiatric
unit. It may be too much to expect that every psychiatrist working
on an inpatient service be a sociologist, but he or she can at least be
aware of the complexity of the setting, so as not to deny certain
obvious social realities affecting process and outcome.

In a comparison of mental hospitals to resorts, Benjamin and
Dorothea Braginsky (1973) draw attention to some of the factors
besides intrapsychic mechanisms and individual psychopathology that
frequently determine what really goes on in a mental hospital. They
do this by going directly to the patients and asking them what they
see and want. They find that the mental hospital is frequently the
only alternative available to lower-income people who cannot or do
not want to survive in mainstream society. Patients indicated to them
that they wanted a comfortable, enjoyable, nondemanding milieu in
the hospital. Depending on what they wanted, patients were quite
capable of subverting the therapeutic efforts of staff. They were able
to exploit their symptoms and tailor their general performance before
the doctors to get what they wanted—for example, avoidance of a
locked ward or avoidance of discharge.

Braginsky and Braginsky (1973) account for a certain naiveté on
the part of many psychiatrists in understanding and treating their
patients by positing a conceptual wall between doctors and patients.
This wall, they say, is made up of a variety of theoretical models that
distort an accurate picture of what is happening. They mention three
models of mental illness—the medical model, the behavioral model,
and the imprisonment model. In all of these models, the patient is
seen as a victim—someone in whom and to whom things happen.
Braginsky and Braginsky insist that patients have far more volitional

control over their condition and over the outcome of their treatment than is suspected by most practitioners of psychiatry.

Probably the largest contribution to the tendency in psychiatry to overlook the complex forces operating on an inpatient setting is the model of the dyadic relationship between doctor and patient. Much of the theoretical writing to which psychiatrists are exposed in their training centers on the individual—his or her intrapsychic workings themselves and their relationship to the therapist. In order for psychiatrists to be able to take into account some of the issues raised by the Braginskys, they would have to at least be exposed to other models and perspectives that focus more on other features of the treatment environment.

WHO HAS LISTENED TO PATIENTS

Having said that there would be value in looking at the process of psychiatric hospitalization as it affects patients as people, that this process must be viewed in broad perspective to encompass the complexity of that experience, and that psychiatrists have generally not done this, we must now ask if anyone else has done so. Apart from the patients who have written of their experiences and the existiential therapists whose basic approach centers on trying to understand the patient's point of view but who are not often found in hospital settings, there are two groups that have busied themselves with mental illness from the patient's perspective. One includes writers of novels and plays, film makers, and a few psychiatrists. The other is comprised of social scientists. Both groups have influenced the development of some of the current models of mental illness. The first group has tended to present views and characters that romanticize mental illness. The second group has described hospitals and wards as social systems and has tended to characterize patients as little different from normals. This second view slips easily into that expressed by Szasz as the myth of mental illness.

De Broca in *King of Hearts* is one representative of the romanticizing group. The film is about a French town deserted by its folk because it is expected to be blown up by the Germans. The only inhabitants remaining are the patients in the insane asylum who leave the institution and take over the town for themselves. The hero of the film is a Scottish soldier sent in to find the explosives and prevent the town's destruction. At the end of the film, the hero succeeds, the townspeople return, the patients go back to the asylum, and the hero *chooses* to enter the asylum as a statement about the insanity of society and the greater humanity of the insane.

Günter Grass in *The Tin Drum* (1961) places his hero in a mental institution from which base he operates business and artistic dealings with great skill and success. Grass describes him as a 3-year-old who decided not to grow up, ostensibly because he took a long look at the world and at his society, in particular, and said a big "no."

Ronald Harwood's patients in *The Girl in Melanie Klein* (1969) comment on their views of therapy and mental illness:

> We do not welcome change. We want our lives to continue as they always have done: serene and beautiful and unmolested!

Elsewhere they say:

> The dreadful truth would have to be faced: he was determined to cure us.

The patients watch the director of their institution on television with a young girl. In telling of how he cured her of seeing the Virgin Mary, she says:

> They're so terribly clever now. In days gone by they might have cured Beethoven of his Fifth Symphony.

Ken Kesey in *One Flew Over the Cuckoo's Nest* (1962) depicts the patients on a psychiatric ward in rich colors and with depth and attractiveness. Staff, on the other hand, are described in two-dimensional terms and as being petty, mean, and blundering. Patients are, again, the misunderstood and heroic figures in a bland society that seeks to stifle individuality and unconventionality.

R. D. Laing in *The Politics of Experience* (1967) and in his other writings has been very influential in glamorizing the psychotic experience. One comes away from his work with the sense that going crazy is an exciting opportunity for growth and development, rather than a weakness or an illness that needs rapid curing. Analogies have been drawn by him and by some of his followers to the drug experience, particularly to experiences with LSD. Some have even described mental patients as prophets who are telling it "like it is" better than anyone else in the society. What is sometimes ignored in differentiating the two experiences is that taking a drug usually involves a conscious choice and can be prepared for in a variety of ways. Psychosis is rarely sought and is far less easily controlled and guided. On the other hand, it should not be underestimated how beneficial the Laingian view can be in the restoration of morale and a decent self-image to the person who has undergone or is experiencing psychosis.

The contributions of the second group, the social scientists, have focused mainly on the mental hospital and on the psychiatric unit as a small society and as a social system. Using a social framework, certain facts become obvious that could easily go ignored if only a psychological model is used. Goffman (1961) is the outstanding figure in bringing to life the various sectors of the social system of the mental hospital. He describes a patient culture as well as a staff culture and classifies mental hospitals along with many other nonpsychiatric institutions as sharing characteristics that have little to do with their manifest goals. In reading his work, one can at times forget that he is describing a mental hospital at all. Stanton and Schwartz drew attention in an earlier work, *The Mental Hospital* (1955), to an important aspect of ward life—the unanticipated consequences of staff interaction on patient behavior.

There is an implication in much of the work of the social scientists that there is little difference between the patient society and the "normal" society. Since roles, norms, and expectations can be described for patients' behavior, the patients are apparently functioning as normally as anyone else. This implicit assumption needs to be examined carefully to determine its accuracy in some areas and its distortion in others.

On the side of accuracy, it should be noted that it was only recently that the independent effects of hospitalization or institutionalization were recognized. Before this, the behavior of patients in mental institutions had been seen as the product of their illnesses rather than as the outcome of incarceration, herding, isolation from the outside world, and depersonalization. This newer realization has stimulated a good part of the efforts to get long-term patients out of mental hospitals and back into the community.

On the other hand, the fact that patterns of interaction and behavior can be found in any setting does not suggest that the patterns of individual functioning are normal. In other words, the fact that a sociologist can describe something called a patient society does not mean that the individuals involved are capable of functioning in a normal setting. The normal society may involve substantially greater pressures, and less structure, and fewer supports than mental health institutions.

Another point that should be made is that many of the kinds of observations described thus far have been made in long-term settings where the factor of sheer amount of time spent in the institution tends to outweigh all other factors of care and treatment. Also, size of institution is an important factor. Long-term psychiatric care has for centuries taken place in large institutions where all the features of giant bureaucracies have recognizable counterparts. These observations are pertinent in evaluating short-term inpatient units of limited size as well; however, they do not deserve the major importance that they assume in large institutions for chronic care.

WHAT PATIENTS SAY

What do patients say? What are their views of and feelings about psychotherapy and other forms of treatment during hospitalization? How do they see and evaluate their therapists? What is the hospital environment like for them? How do they view their own disturbance, in particular, and mental illness, in general? The answers patients give to these questions often reveal their criticisms and recommendations. Historically, the sources of information have been mainly auto-biographical writings of ex-mental patients. I will add contributions from informal talks I have had with patients and ex-patients on the ward where I work. A future source of such data in the form of a follow-up study of patients is now in the planning stage. This will include interviewing patients toward the end of hospitalization and six months later about their views of the experience of hospitalization.

PATIENTS' VIEWS ON PSYCHOTHERAPY

One pervasive theme underlying what patients say it is like to experience talk therapy in the hospital might be called "therapy as vivisection." Doctors are seen as butterfly chasers, specimen collectors who love to name things and discover things but who do not know what to do with their treasures once they find them:

> I wish I could put a bell on him [the doctor]—so I would be aware when he starts probing around in the crooks and crannies of my crooked brain, hunting for phobias. He can do nothing when he finds them, so what is the use of hunting? Phobias are sensitive little critters—and it's like having a boil lanced, to have them probed into. He cannot cure them. All he does is go prowling around among them, knocking them over. . . . After he has found it [a phobia], he does not know what to do with it. All he has in proof of his discovery is a long-handled word to paste in his album. And I wish—that I had the genius to take some of the smug self-complacency out of him. . . . I know now how rabbits and guinea pigs feel when they are vivisected. Vivisection is painful. (Jefferson, 1947)

The process is described by patients as being painful without necessarily being helpful:

> The thought of having to bare my very soul again is by no means pleasant to me. . . . I don't like to be dissected as a pathological subject. I don't want to say more than is necessary and then only to those I trust absolutely. (Boisen, 1960)

Patients describe themselves as entering the hospital with a sense of hopefulness mixed with vulnerability and helplessness. They are willing to do anything if it will help, but it is at considerable expense that they open themselves up to the probings of psychiatry. Gradually, in many cases, their hopefulness turns to disillusionment and anger. Mary Cecil (1956) returns home after hospitalization with little more understanding of what went wrong for her than before she entered treatment. At home, she curses herself "for the dutiful pouring out of tawdry secrets which had been told before to more constructive friends." The question that recurs again and again is, What happens to all the information collected and extracted from patients during hospitalization? Patients speculate a good deal about this, and in the absence of direct responses from the collectors, they draw their own conclusions, not always the most flattering to the institution:

> We go into hospital with hope and confidence. Alternating with the usual bouts of despair we see ourselves emerging on the other side of the nightmare new and purged personalities. With what ardour we fill up the questionnaires, struggle through intelligence tests, hand in our paintings, and pour out our histories. And it is all swallowed up into the bowels of the organisation and never heard of again. More cynical patients assure one it is used for statistics and research. (Cecil, 1956)

After they have done all this work of exposing their innards, patients find themselves dismissed and on their own:

> The morass of matter pulled out of one's mind for airing is left to the patient to put back as best he can. (Cecil, 1956)

This was written by a patient who was followed in outpatient therapy after discharge from the hospital, but whose after-care did not, apparently, offer her the reassurance or explanations she was seeking.

At times, verbal probing into patients' minds and motives seems to take on, for patients, an almost inquisitional flavor, as seen in Stefan's account. The patient's wife visits him after talking with his psychiatrist in the hospital. She reports that the doctor thinks Stefan may be hiding something. Stefan replies:

> "Hiding something?" I was trembling with rage. "How the hell can I hide anything? With all these idiot nurses and attendants running around jotting down everything a man says or does. A guy can't piss without having someone recording the time and whether he looks relieved when he comes out of the john. What the hell am I hiding? I've poured out my guts to G. and now M. . . . It's none of their damn business, but I've told them everything because I thought it would help me get well. But it hasn't. It doesn't make any difference. . . . Go on down there and tell M that I'll

cooperate. Tell 'em that I'll admit to anything. Tell him that anything he
wants me to admit, I'll admit about my past." (Stefan, 1966)

Sometimes even more frightening to patients than what will be
done to them is what will not be done to and for them. Many
patients entering the hospital are entering a system that is entirely
new to them. They have fears and expectations. Among these is the
expectation that they will receive relief from their immediate
suffering and some clarity and understanding with which to fortify
themselves when they leave. What they sometimes come away with,
instead, is confusion and contradiction. Cecil describes how she
contributes to her own ignorance by trying to be a "good patient."
Nothing is explained to her of her therapy, and she follows the other
patients around and does not ask questions in order to show how
calm and rational she is. Much more disturbing to her is when she is
told, rather abruptly, by her new doctor that she can leave the
hospital. She had thought there would be a comprehensive sorting
out process, that she would hear the reasons for the breakdown and
be given armor before going out again. She asks the new doctor her
stock questions and receives completely contradictory replies to those
of the other doctors and says:

I planted these contradictions with the others already flowering in the
herbaceous border of my mind. (Cecil, 1956)

WHAT PATIENTS WANT OF PSYCHIATRISTS
AND OTHER STAFF

With a variety of complaints and a smattering of compliments
about psychiatric personnel, patients return again and again to the
issue of how much or how little the doctors and others understand
their plight, their feelings, and their needs. Closely connected to the
issue of understanding is that of the degree and kind of distance staff
put between themselves and patients. The images painted by patients
of doctors resemble that of the butterfly chaser mentioned earlier
who cannot see or hear the person behind the presenting symptoms.
Several examples will help to describe some of patients' feelings.

Patients kick and scream and fight when they aren't sure the doctor can
see them. It's a most terrifying feeling to realize that the doctor can't see
the real you, that he can't understand what you feel and that he's just
going ahead with his own ideas. . . . I had to make an uproar to see if the
doctor would respond to me, not just his own ideas. (In Hayward and
Taylor, 1956)

Beyond wanting a fundamental recognition of themselves as people, patients want their doctor or nurse to sympathize with their problems with control. They frequently run into a singular lack of appreciation for their strenuous efforts to keep from exploding and tearing the place apart. A poignant account of this comes from the eloquent and explosive Lara Jefferson. Lara feels that a demon-like being inside her is gathering momentum and may burst out. She asks the nurse to tie her down. The nurse refuses several times. Lara says:

> They were going to make me control that which there was no holding. (Jefferson, 1947)

She struggles for control but knows she cannot last. She knows she has to do something to convince the nurse before it is too late. Finally, after Lara hurls as many verbal threats as she can, the nurse ties her down.

> When I was tied down securely and could relax my hold upon myself all my shame flowed out in a wild flood of tears. They were partly tears of vexation that I should have been such a coward. That I had not had the courage to do the things I had such an urge to do—but more, they were tears of relief that I had not done them. Mostly, they were tears of rage and confusion at the necessity for the whole unspeakable thing. . . . The doctor came in and spoke to me. . . . He chided and ridiculed me for giving up so easily. (Jefferson, 1947)

The lack of empathy and human understanding that patients sometimes feel in the presence of their therapists and caretakers is described in yet another way by a schizophrenic girl during a psychotic period:

> It seemed to me that most of the nurses were like marionettes on a string, with no personalities of their own, being manipulated by powerful forces outside themselves. I saw them as under the influences of hypnotic suggestion. They were, I thought, in the control of others whose minds were more powerful than theirs. (Anonymous, 1955)

It is difficult to say how much of this description can be brushed off as a product of psychopathological distortion and how much of it involves the patient discerning an unbecoming reality in some of the interpersonal encounters between nurse and patient.

Patients often report feeling a distance between themselves and their therapists when they try to ask questions about what is happening to them, what their treatment consists of, and so forth:

> After a fortnight in a sort of reception ward, I complained to the doctor

that nothing was being done. "Ah, but we're doing a great deal for you." I almost believed him, but wasn't that far gone. I'd learned it was a waste of time asking questions. Psychiatrists thrive on their air of mystery. (Cecil, 1956)

Patients may go to great lengths to establish some sort of closeness with their doctors. What frequently emerges is a double-edged relationship. On the one hand, patients try to learn all about their doctors from whatever minute cues they can lay their hands on, and, on the other hand, they ridicule and put down their doctors in a number of ways, at least in the telling. For example:

The new doctor waxed very excited about ink-blots. In fact the extravagance of what I saw in them was only surpassed by the extravagance of his interpretations, some of which haunt me to this day. But he was so well-meaning, and I felt he had such a thin time of it from the Rebel, that I was always polite and agreed with anything he said. Then his face lit up and he was happy. (Cecil, 1956)

This example, which takes place at an individual level, is repeated many times as patients tell each other and the reader what one must do to succeed in the patient-staff system. A strong note of bitterness resounds that is at times only barely camouflaged with humor. The most bitter of these patient pronouncements are also among the earliest historically and may reflect the great desperation of patients who had to prove they were not insane in order to be released from the mental institution rather than leave their caretakers with the burden of proof of their insanity.

The question, then, lies between the power of the patient to endure and the power of the quack to break his spirit. (Perceval, 1840)

Davidson describes the circularity of some of the reasoning used to describe patients' behavior in the hospital:

Some time after this, it struck me that it was dangerous to make any reference or quotation in such a place, for you run the risk of being considered as imagining yourself to be the author or character referred to. On the other hand, you must not keep quite silent and refuse to answer questions, or you are melancholy, perhaps suicidal, or even homicidal. If you talk, you are talkative and excitable; if you pay no attention to what is going on round you, you are sinking into idiocy; if you carefully look about you and take an interest in everything, you are inquisitive and meddlesome; if you sit still, you are comatose; if you take much exercise and feel happy in spite of your surroundings, you are unduly elated; and if you whistle or sing, you are marked down as a candidate for a violent ward. If, however, you don't show to a marked extent any of the above symptoms of insanity, which the attendants are told to watch for, you are a practically hopeless case, needing the most careful watching, for you are a patient determinedly and wickedly insane and maniacally cunning that you are able to successfully conceal your insanity. (Davidson, 1912)

A more succinct but vitriolic statement of this kind is made by Custance:

Why, then, have the doctors changed their minds about me? Why do they think I am sane? The answer is quite simple. Yielding to the persuasion of my wife, I agreed to crawl to the doctors—to say nothing of any grievances I may have, and to give the impression that I am quite satisfied with my own treatment. (Custance, 1952)

Cecil, on the other hand, usually manages to inject some humor into any subject, however painful:

We were all to pass before a committee. . . . There was a shrewd peaceable North Countryman who'd say behind his pipe: "Ah just tells 'em what they want to hear." So when my turn came, I was gay and witty, made jokes against myself, denied all my notions, told the watchful quartet how clever they were and exalted shock treatment to the skies. (Cecil, 1956)

The verdict—off shock.

Although patient accounts contain far more criticism of hospital staff than acclaim for them, they do occasionally point to strengths and approved behavior on the part of those tending them. These positive points are the counterparts of what has come earlier in this chapter. Patients feel good and grateful when they are understood and when they are treated with respect. Boisen offers one example of gratitude for respect shown to him as a person:

During the day I was visited by a certain Dr. Klopp, who was said to be a distinguished physician from another state. He had heard that I had some important ideas about saving people. He was very much interested in this problem and he wondered if I would be willing to tell him about them. I rather liked Dr. Klopp's looks, but I replied that I had rather not talk. He immediately went away. This raised my opinion of him greatly and made me think that I had made a mistake. (Boisen, 1960)

Sechehaye presents a more complicated and subtle example of the therapist's success in listening to and understanding her patient's needs and of the patient's appreciation for her efforts:

I was glad that Mama changed her method at the end of the first year of analysis. In the beginning, she analyzed everything I said, my fear, my guilt. . . . From these sessions I went home more unhappy, more blameworthy, more isolated than ever, without any contact, alone in my own unreal world. But after Mama sat down beside me, talked to me in the third person and especially seemed to understand without looking for causes at all, how relieved I was! She alone could break through the unreal wall that hemmed me in; she alone kept me in some contact with life. (Sechehaye, 1951)

HOSPITAL ENVIRONMENT

Apart from the obvious elements that constitute psychiatric hospitalization—the treatments offered and the people who administer them—there are features of being in the hospital that, though not a part of the formal definition of what takes place, figure largely, nonetheless, in an assessment of the hospitalization experience. It has been noted earlier, in the discussion of who has paid attention to patients' perspectives, that social scientists have interested themselves in this area. Here, mention is limited to the features of the situation of hospitalization that patients bring up spontaneously. In listening to patients on a small, well-staffed psychiatric unit in a modern general hospital, I found the comments to be hardly different from many of those made by Clifford Beers in 1908. The deprivation of liberty, the restrictions on movement and activities are time-honored discomforts noted again and again by patients. Time is said to hang heavy, and patients feel that they spend most of their time waiting around. During Beers' hospitalization, he sent many memos to the director of the hospital with complaints and suggestions regarding these problems. The issue of time and waiting is one that staff can be quite insensitive to when they have busy schedules. Sometimes only the lower-echelon personnel, such as the aides, have any appreciation for what it means to spend approximately sixteen hours a day confined to a small area with few activities and fewer substantial contacts with staff and to watch staff go busily and importantly about their tasks.

One other feature of the environment that patients frequently refer to is the set of implicit rules by which their behavior is judged. Thus, patients are frustrated, feeling that there lies somewhere a book of rules to which they are denied access but whose clout they feel when they break one of them. Davidson expressed a frustration that many patients continue to express today:

I then continued to the doctor that insanity was not confined to the patients, for to impress upon a man the necessity for observing all the rules of a place, and then to tell him there were not rules or, if there were, to refuse him a copy of them, was not sensible. (Davidson, 1912)

MEANING OF MENTAL ILLNESS

Thus far, the issues that have been presented from the patients' viewpoint have reflected the fairly visible and concrete forces that confront them once they enter the hospital. The next issue concerns the less concrete and more symbolic effects that we create for patients, regardless of our intent, as they pass through our hands. A few medical examples will remind the reader how powerful the meaning of an event can be as compared to its actual magnitude and force. Obviously, the meaning for the individual of contracting venereal disease or cancer, or of being pregnant, cannot be subsumed by the sheer medical definition of the treatment and outcome. Some of the crucial variables operating to determine these meanings are social and cultural. With respect to mental illness as well, as much as we might like to confine ourselves to studying and working with the medical "facts" and the intrapsychic and interpersonal dynamics, we cannot do so and claim to have come near to understanding what has actually happened to a particular patient.

There is a substantial literature on the stigma of mental illness and hospitalization, labeling theory and deviance in relation to mental illness, and cross-cultural studies of mental illness. This literature has been used by various groups to strengthen their arguments for or against one or another model of mental illness. For present purposes, I prefer not to impose any more conceptual and theoretical suprastructures on the data than seem really necessary. Instead, I will let the patients reflect on the meanings for them of their hospitalization and their illness and on the ways in which these meanings clash with or match the meanings offered by staff.

McCall expresses a view that, although not a popular one among patients who have been aggressive enough and prolific enough to write of their experiences, may well represent a view common to the majority of patients.

> I knew by this time that my mind was affected and, to me, this was *shameful*. It was a bitter disgrace that must be concealed if possible.... If some part of my body had been misbehaving, I would have gone immediately to the best specialist available. But because my brain was the offender I could not bring myself to enlist aid from any source. (McCall, 1947)

This view of mental illness as something to be hidden and to feel ashamed of can be contrasted with a more rebellious tone expressed in most other writings. Some patients are angry with the doctors and other staff who do not treat the psychosis as anything of value to be explored and understood but who, instead, want to suppress it as rapidly as possible, In different ways, patients are saying that the psychotic experience is a very important experience in their lives that they do not want to negate or deny. Boisen, for example, insists that all his abnormal experiences began under the same conditions that characterized his creative mental activity. He complains that "those in control are industriously engaged in suppressing the symptoms which might lead to recovery." He goes on:

> This kind of sanity which has to be preserved by sticking close to camp and washing dishes for the rest of my life is not worth preserving. . . . especially when I feel that the particular territory in which I lost my way is of greatest interest and importance. I want to explore and map that territory. (Boisen, 1960)

It seems particularly difficult for those with manic depressive illness to reject their experiences, as Custance indicates:

> I have not the slightest intention of returning to "sanity" if that means rejecting my own inner experiences. . . . Only if I accept my experiences, my manic consciousness, in toto and resolutely adapt them to "reality" does it seem to me that there is any hope of a permanent cure. (Custance, 1952)

Krim goes farther than any by describing his psychotic break as a choice he made:

> When I was considered out of my mind during my original upward thrust into the sheer ecstasy of 100% uninhibitedness, I was aware of the daringness of my every move; it represented at heart an existential choice rather than a mindless discharge. It could not be tolerated by society, and I was punished for it. . . . I was trying to close this distance between Me and Thou, between the mind and externality, that I was instinctively attempting when I cut loose with my natural suffocating self in 1955. . . . The imagination of living human beings, not dead gods, must be openly embodied if there is to be some rational connection between what people actually are and what they are permitted to show. (Krim, 1964)

DISCUSSION

I would like to review briefly what patients have said and to offer some comments regarding these statements. First, patients have described psychotherapy during hospitalization as painful and intrusive and not often helpful. There are two factors to be noted here that offer possible explanations for this complaint. One is that patients entering the hospital have not usually sat down calmly and contracted with a therapist to engage in psychotherapy. Admission to the hospital is usually preceded by a crisis. The element of choice is largely eliminated as the nature of the process of hospitalization dictates other priorities. There are, furthermore, many people who do not believe in talking out problems. It is easy to forget how much is presupposed in the phenomenon of seeking office psychiatric help, how much education is needed to arrive at that point, how for most such help is a luxury. We are not dealing with the same group of people when we speak of the hospital population.

A second factor is that the nature of inpatient psychotherapy differs from that of outpatient therapy, especially on a short-term unit. What is called psychotherapy may actually amount to little more than serial mental status examinations and explorations of history and present abilities, in order to make clearer the diagnosis and prognosis of the case. The doctor may, in fact, feel that he or she is doing a great deal for the patient, but the patient may feel that he or she is doing all the giving and not getting anything in return. Since we do not always make clear the distinction for ourselves or for patients between our giving and taking, it is no wonder that patients are often confused and disgruntled.

Second, patients complain that they often leave the hospital with no clearer sense of what went wrong, or is still wrong, than when they entered. We need to think through how much of this comes from the fact that we often do not have the answers, and that we do not always communicate what we have found as carefully to patients as to our colleagues. On a service where the teaching of residents is a top priority, case conferences may be unusually informative, and yet precious little information gets passed on to the patients being discussed.

Third, about their therapists, patients say in many ways that they want a human relationship with them. They want to be seen, to be understood, and to be cared for. They often feel that staff minimize patients' difficulties, that they do not treat them with respect. They seem to expect a great deal from doctors, and the bitterness of the attacks on them probably results from the doctors' failure to meet these high expectations rather than from an objective view of serious abuse. The intensity of the accusations, however, should not allow us to dismiss the charges completely or write them off as issues of transference. The conditions of hospitalization plus the mystique surrounding psychiatry and hospital care promote the regression of patients and the most unrealistic expectations of what they will get from their doctors and from the hospital. On the one hand, patients may want magic and a godlike creature to cure or transform them. On the other hand, they may simply be asking for an understanding friend who will be patient and kind to them. In their eagerness to be professional and scientific, psychiatrists and other health professionals sometimes overlook these simple facts that reflect a basic need of patients in any kind of care.

Perhaps to respond to this need seems too small and undramatic a role to play. If one truly listens to what patients say, however, one hears that they often put up with the antics, pet methods, and theories of their therapists in order to be with them. One young schizophrenic patient said to her doctor:

> There was such a tremendous difference between you and your words. You seemed so wonderful, but your words were so horrible. (In Hayward and Taylor, 1956)

Fourth, regarding the hospital environment, little has been said here or elsewhere. This seems to be an area ripe for eliciting patient opinion and evaluation. In informally discussing the environment with patients, I have found that there is clearly less concern for this issue than for those previously discussed. In answering my questions, patients tend to respond reflectively and without great intensity, whereas with other issues they show much greater anxiety.

The final issue raised above—that of the patient's views of illness and of its meaning—is perhaps the most fascinating, the trickiest, and the issue that may also highlight one of the chief limitations of the data presented here and in the literature. The search for some higher, philosophical meaning in one's misfortune can be very appealing and morale raising. Viktor Frankl's logotherapy writings speak eloquently for the human need to discover meaning in life in psychological adversity. Some great thinkers, including Freud, have been intrigued by this concern and have written of creativity and the unconscious, of the relationship between the creative and the psychotic processes. It is quite another question whether this intellectual fascination characterizes the patient population.

Here we come to the question of how representative the sample of patients in the literature is of the larger group of those hospitalized for mental illness. Patients with the ability and motivation to write essays and books are hardly a random sample of the population. At least, we cannot assume that they constitute a random sample without some sort of independent investigation of a more randomly chosen selection of people. It would be interesting to know in what ways they are similar to and different from other patients.

Studies are needed to pursue just these questions in a more systematic and inclusive way. They must take into account the nature of the psychiatric setting, the patient population, and the interview situation. This last matter presents methodological difficulties. Patients may be polite and passive in responding to questions. However, the data from the literature consists mainly of negative statements about therapy and hospitalization. It is not clear whether this negative orientation has developed because those who have had negative experiences are more likely to write than are those who have had more benign experiences or whether this negativism represents the views of most patients. Perhaps, with other oppressed groups and incipient social movements, the early period of consciousness raising tends to focus on the bitterness and the oppression rather than on the benefits accruing to the position and status involved.

As I mentioned earlier, a follow-up study of patients on a small psychiatric unit in a general hospital is in its early stages of planning and execution. It includes an interview with patients, concerning their experiences and evaluation of hospitalization and of treatment modalities, the help expected and received or not received, the negative and positive aspects of care, and their general criticisms and suggestions. I hope that this area of inquiry will develop beyond the initial contributions of a few speaking for the many. The complexities of treating patients in a residential setting call for all the perspectives and input that can be obtained. Patients' views represent one of the most potentially valuable sources of information available. This source waits to be tapped.

REFERENCES

Anonymous. 1955. Autobiography of a schizophrenic experience. Journal of Abnormal and Social Psychology 51:677–689.

Beers, C. 1908. A Mind That Found Itself. New York: Longmans-Green.

Boisen, A. 1960. Out of the Depths. New York: Harper & Brothers.

Braginsky, B., and D. Braginsky. 1973. Mental hospitals and resorts. Psychology Today. March:22 et seq.

Cecil, M. 1956. Through the looking glass. In The Inner World of Mental Illness, B. Kaplan, ed. Harper & Row, pp. 18–29.

Custance, J. 1952. The universe of bliss and the universe of horror: a description of a manic-depressive psychosis. Reprinted from Wisdom, Madness and Folly. New York: Farrar, Straus and Cudahy. In The Inner World of Mental Illness, B. Kaplan, Ed. Harper & Row, pp. 43–61.

Davidson, D. 1912. Remembrances of a Religio-Maniac. Stratford-on-Avon, England: Shakespeare Press.

Goffman, E. 1961. Asylums. New York: Anchor Books.

Grass, G. 1961. The Tin Drum. New York: Pantheon Books.

Harwood, R. 1969. The Girl in Melanie Klein. New York: Holt, Rinehart, and Winston.

Hayward, M. A., and J. E. Taylor. 1956. A schizophrenic patient describes the action of intensive psychotherapy. Psychiatric Quarterly 30:211-247.

Jefferson, L. 1947. These Are My Sisters. Tulsa, Okla.: Vickers.

Kesey, K. 1962. One Flew Over the Cuckoo's Nest. New York: New American Library.

Krim, S. 1964. The insanity bit. Reprinted from Views of a Nearsighted

Cannoneer. New York: Excelsior Press. *In* The Inner World of Mental Illness, B. Kaplan, ed. Harper & Row, pp. 62–79.

Laing, R. D. 1967. The Politics of Experience. New York: Ballantine Books.

Lipowski, Z. J., and A. Stewart. 1973. Illness as subjective experience. International Journal of Psychiatry in Medicine 4(2):155–171.

McCall, L. 1947. Between Us and the Dark. Philadelphia: Lippincott.

Meltzoff, J., and M. Kornreich. 1970. Research in Psychotherapy. New York: Atherton Press.

Perceval, J. 1840. Narrative of the treatment experienced by a gentleman during a state of mental derangement. Reprinted from book of same title. London: Effingham Wilson. *In* The Inner World of Mental Illness, B. Kaplan, ed. Harper & Row, pp. 235–253.

Sechehaye, M. 1951. Autobiography of a Schizophrenic Girl. New York: Grune & Stratton.

Stanton, A., and M. Schwartz. 1955. The Mental Hospital. New York: Basic Books.

Stefan, G. 1966. In Search of Sanity. The Journal of a Schizophrenic. New York: University Books.

CHAPTER 9

THE FATHERS
(NOT THE MOTHERS)
Their Importance and
Influence with Infants and
Young Children

Felton Earls, M.D.

In 1927, Malinowski observed that the Tobrianders placed major significance on psychological fatherhood but managed only a naive view of biological paternity. In our own very different society, it would be useful to enlighten our naive view of psychological paternity given our scientifically splendid view of biological paternity. A more encompassing cross-cultural survey of fathering, if available, would no doubt disclose various degrees of paternal investment during infancy and early childhood, determined by a complex interaction of biological (sex and fertility patterns) and sociocultural (economic and mythological) conditions.

The physical needs of infants for nourishment and affection appear to be so obviously provided by mothers that Western psychology has been able to comfortably ignore the relationship of fathers to infants. If there has been reason to consider this relationship, it has derived from the extent that fathers provide a supportive environment generally, and contribute to a good marriage specifically. Interaction between fathers and children is usually regarded as accessory to maternal behavior and responsibility.

PURPOSE OF THIS REVIEW

This review focuses on the psychopathological impact of paternal behavior on infants and young children. Three developmental periods

From *Psychiatry*, 1976, *39*, 209-226. Copyright © 1976 by The William Alanson White Psychiatric Foundation, Inc. Reprinted by special permission of The William White Psychiatric Foundation, Inc., and the author.

are surveyed in relation to what is known of paternal behavior and its influences on the child: pregnancy, infancy, and childhood.

Throughout this review, we must appreciate that influences may be bidirectional (i.e., father affecting child as well as child affecting father) and that behavior problems in children are usually determined by the coexistence of several factors. The objective here, however, is to examine the father-child relationship specifically as one possible early determinant of behavior deviance in children. Because the literature is sparse, it is necessary to carefully examine manifestations of paternal and child behavioral deviance as they may influence each other.

To develop clearer concepts and more precise methods of examining the father-child relationship in the prevention and treatment of behavior disorders in children is the objective of this chapter, more than an interest in clarifying the facts. While prevention of mental disorders is a sufficient reason to gather more information on the contribution of fathers to early child rearing, we should also note that families with young children constitute one of the major burdens of mental health services (Rosen et al., 1964). It must also be appreciated that ignoring, or minimizing, the importance and influence of fathers may not only pose a barrier to effective treatment, but may even intensify the stress of a young family.

OVERVIEW OF LITERATURE

In *The Analysis of a Phobia in a Five Year Old Boy*, Freud (1955) established the notion that a form of sexual rivalry existed between a father and his son over the mother's affection. The resulting fear of his father developed by "little Hans," in this case, was hidden behind a symbolic screen cleverly penetrated by Freud. Embellishing this case with classical significance, as Freud did, promoted its appreciation as a universal phenomenon occurring specifically around the age of 5 and serving as a critical stage in the maturation toward healthy adult adjustment. The strength of this example continues to provide the basis for a prevalent belief that the "Oedipal period" marks the first clearly defined significant interaction of fathers with their sons. The relationship of fathers to their daughters is much less clearly conceptualized in psychoanalytic theory.

Beginning with the mental hygiene movement and large-scale sociological study projects at the turn of the century (Burt, 1925; Healy and Bronner, 1936), both of which were concerned with overcoming rising rates of juvenile delinquency, many social and familial factors have been examined for their etiological significance in the genesis of antisocial behavior, among them the paternal relationship. Given the multiple factor approach used in most of this research, the paternal relationship is difficult to separate from other factors and the strength of its association with delinquency is not always striking. Nevertheless, there is a convincing body of literature indicating that "broken" homes, absent or deviant fathers, and maternal deprivation lie near the origins of such conduct (Burt, 1925; Healy and Bronner, 1936; Glueck and Glueck, 1950; Bowlby, 1944; Andry, 1960; West and Farrington, 1973).

The dominant theme emerging from this literature that is the concern of this chapter is paternal absence. After several decades of using the concept of paternal absence as an explanatory variable in research on delinquency, it is becoming clear that it is a complex phenomenon (Herzog and Sudia, 1969). We might reasonably assume, for instance, that paternal absence for socially acceptable reasons, such as for military service or employment or that following death, has different consequences on family life than paternal absence for socially unacceptable reasons, such as for desertion or imprisonment. A further problem is the association between social and economic deprivation and paternal absence. It seems necessary to appreciate that this phenomenon becomes embedded in the complex social processes that sustain poverty. Men who have only limited opportunity to achieve and maintain a sense of high self-regard may be in symbolic absence even if they are physically present in the family.

The sociological literature has not dealt sufficiently with conditions less extreme than total absence of the father, and has thus implied that it takes this level of family insult to produce emotional repercussions in children. Yet it is clear that a range of outcomes exists when fathers are present. One of the more provocative studies linking paternal influence to mental illness is that of Paffenbarger and Asnes (1966), who investigated suicide in a college population. Among a variety of familial, physical, sociocultural, and psychological factors studied, paternal lack of attention and death emerged as striking correlates of suicide, and were certainly of more apparent impact than maternal factors. They noted that paternal lack of attention assumed a prominent role in the backgrounds of male suicides especially, and that in at least one form was linked to high professional status of fathers.

In what represents possibly the only study linking a father's personality to a defined behavior syndrome of early childhood, Eisenberg (1957) showed that fathers of children with infantile autism were unusually cold, detached, and obsessive compared to a control group. Since more recent work has tended to support an organic basis for infantile autism, current interest in psychological correlates has dwindled (Rutter, 1971). It seems entirely reasonable to suspect that the manner in which a man approaches and organizes his role as father has sustaining consequences for the relationship he establishes with his child. This fact, in turn, must influence the behavioral adjustment of the child. That this relationship may vary from one child to the next for a single father, depending on social circumstances, is clearly documented in *Father Relations in War-Born Children* (Stolz, 1954).

It should be clear from research of the past fifty years that attempts to use personality characteristics as indicators of parental deprivation are as harmful and unjustified as those ill-fated excursions into "maternal deprivation." A more satisfactory approach might be to explore the effect of paternal illness on the health and behavior of children. The most compelling research in this area is found in epidemiological surveys of family health. The work of Buck and Laughton (1959) in a prepaid medical practice in Canada, and that of Kellner (1963) in a British community, indicated that the health of mothers but not fathers was associated with behavior disturbances in children. However, Hare and Shaw's study (1965) in a London community provides the following summary statement:

> Each type of behavior disorder in children is significantly commoner when the father had neurosis, but there is no association between behavior disorder and neurosis in the mother.

Several sources of bias contribute to the contrasting results of these studies. However, Hare and Shaw's study had more subjects and appears to have been done more carefully. This investigation adds a new dimension to the sociological studies on delinquency, and to the work of Paffenbarger and Asnes on suicide in young adults, by suggesting that paternal factors must be considered to have possible etiological significance for a range of behavior disturbances in children.

Another kind of epidemiological approach is provided in the longitudinal and generational studies of Lee Robins (1966). Convincing evidence was generated that children seen in a child guidance clinic for conduct disorders tend to remain antisocial into adulthood. Further, having an antisocial father increases the likelihood that the male child will continue such behavior into adulthood. Robins has made more recent research contributions by providing some validation that this is indeed an intergeneration effect (Robins et al., 1975).

A final general comment on the literature concerns what may well be a gradual abandonment in child development research of the exclusive interest in the mother-child relationship. Among the many books that signal this vanguard movement, Henry Biller's *Father, Child and Sex Role* (1971) provides the most succinct and well organized summary of past research. *Father Power*, a more recent book by Biller and Meredith (1975), presents a clear psychological and sociological perspective on fathering, intended as much for fathers as for the professionals who are concerned or who care for them.

CONCEPTION AND PREGNANCY

Since the father's biological influence begins with conception, the examination of forms of behavioral deviance in the offspring, especially when such disturbances are known to exist in the father, must logically focus on characteristics determined by genetic and sex-linked transmission. Recent studies using Danish population and psychiatric registers have proven useful in this regard because they are based on well-documented material and acceptable scientific design. Examining the prevalence of mental illness in the biological and adoptive families of adopted schizophrenics, Kety et al. (1968) noted that in the biological families of the index cases:

> More than half of the schizophrenic spectrum disorders were found in paternally related half-siblings with whom the index cases should have had in common not even an *in utero* environment but only some genetic overlap.

Schulsinger (1972), comparing the prevalence of sociopathy in the biological and adoptive parents of offspring with the same diagnosis, found that the biological fathers were five times more prone to sociopathic behavior than adoptive fathers. Consideration was given to the age of separation from biological parents and to the birth experience. Neither factor changed the evidence for heritability. More recently, studies have appeared using the same registers showing that sons of alcoholics separated from their parents and reared by foster parents were four times more likely to develop alcoholism than were controls (Goodwin et al., 1974). There is evidence that the fathers of boys diagnosed as hyperactive have an excess of alcoholism and sociopathy compared to those of nonhyperactive boys, and that hyperactivity may itself be an early manifestation of later school underachievement and delinquency (Cantwell, 1972; Weiss et al., 1971). Detecting hyperactivity in young boys may provide an opportunity to study father-child interaction that will better account for environment variables capable of explaining such deviance. Even more useful would be to follow a cohort of young children during early development who are born to alcoholic or sociopathic fathers.

A potential mistake in the interpretation of such data is to assume that behavior, a phenotypic character, equals genotype. Whatever the physiological basis of schizophrenic disorders, alcoholism, or antisocial behavior, be it stress intolerance, decreased physiological threshold to alcohol, or impulsivity, it seems that the environment must exert a critical effect in producing clinical forms of deviance. To delineate this effect, it would be interesting to know what environmental factors protected the sons of alcoholics in the

Danish studies who did not go on to manifest this same behavior in adulthood.

Evidence of a somewhat different variety suggests that aberration of sex chromosomes in the form of multiple Y-chromosomes in males is linked to criminal behavior of the aggressive "episodic dyscontrol" type (Casey et al., 1966; Nielsen et al., 1968). It is now possible to diagnose such aberrations at birth and follow their carriers' behavioral development over time, attempting to parcel out effects of the environment from those presumed to be of genetic origin. At the present time, evidence for a relationship between socially aggressive behavior and genotype is weak, however, which leads us to doubt its value as a developmental hypothesis.

Turning to psychological features of conceptions and pregnancy, we note that the only period in early development considered a potential hardship or harm to a father is pregnancy, and perhaps the neonatal period. In an early paper, Zilboorg (1931), examining cases of depression in new fathers, suggested that a hostile dependent personality was the major underlying risk factor. His interpretation of this depressive phenomenon was that the pregnancy experience revived in his patients an unconscious hatred of their own fathers. At the same time, many of these men felt intensely jealous of their new offspring. Although Zilboorg's study requires replication, other evidence suggests that hostile dependency is a common experience in the onset of depressive episodes as well as psychosis. The most thorough study in this area contrasted twenty-eight expectant fathers hospitalized for psychotic disorders with a control group (Towne and Afterman, 1955). Symptoms of hostility and rivalry predominated in the acute clinical picture surrounding admission to the hospital. As the illness resolved, the fathers' dependency needs became paramount and the focus of after-care psychotherapy. This study receives a degree of partial replication in other, more anecdotal studies (Curtis, 1955; Freeman, 1951; Wainwright, 1966; Bucove, 1964; Jarvis, 1962; Retterstol, 1968; Lacoursiere, 1972).

In another study, unreplicated in the literature, Hartman and Nicolay (1966) showed that expectant fathers appearing in a court psychiatric clinic are more frequently charged with crimes of sexual deviancy than are nonexpectant married men of similar age and background. The most common deviancy was exhibitionism, but instances of pedophilia and rape accounted for more than a third of the cases.

More evidence of adverse paternal experience during pregnancy is provided by the "couvade" phenomenon. Originally, "couvade" was described in anthropology to depict the male ritualization of labor pain by certain preindustrial groups (Frazer, 1928). Anthropologists have hypothesized that the degree to which this phenomenon is prevalent in a particular society gives evidence of the strength of maternal influences over masculine behavior into adulthood (Bacon et al., 1963). Only recently has it been shown that the "couvade" occurs in Western, "civilized" societies in nonritualized, but symptomatic form. Trethowan and Conlon (1965) and Trethowan (1968), in a survey of expectant fathers, found that 11 percent exhibited somatic symptoms, mainly loss of appetite, nausea, and toothache, that appeared directly related to pregnancy. The symptoms appear to peak in the third month of pregnancy and again toward the termination of pregnancy. The question left unanswered by this work is whether these symptoms are justifiably considered as a reflection of a father's anxiety about pregnancy.

Evidence, however meager, demonstrates that a variety of psychopathological manifestations may be associated with a father's adjustment during pregnancy (see Table 1). What is not provided by any of these studies, and is obviously crucial to ascertain, is how these situations affect the subsequent father-child relationship. Such behavioral disturbance in the father may be an early sign of continuing difficulty in the father-child relationship, with resultant behavior deviance in the child. This is reasonable, but not demonstrated.

A man's response to his wife's pregnancy may reveal a pattern of personality disturbance that is relatively nonspecific to a variety of stressful situations. With the emergence of new social patterns of family life and paternal responsibility, requiring a higher degree of male sensitivity and involvement than has been customary in this century, men may be expected to show more signs of stress related to paternity than the literature reflects to date.

INFANCY

John Bowlby (1969) elevated the "attachment phenomenon" to a position of supreme importance in early emotional development when he suggested its pervasive influence throughout the life cycle. Sketching the basis for good maternal care, as well as for maternal deprivation, Bowlby's work provides a theoretical, biological framework for the mother-infant affectional tie. The implication that arouses greatest suspicion in Bowlby's argument is the insistence that the mother-infant bond is by instinct an exclusive one. In recent years, this insistence about mother-infant exclusiveness has been challenged. Schaeffer and Emerson (1964), in their monograph on social attachment, give evidence for multiple, primary paternal as well as primary maternal, attachments. By eighteen months, one third of their sample were mainly attached to their fathers. Kotelchuck (1972) provides a replication of Schaeffer's findings, indicating that there is a

TABLE 1 Review of Twelve Articles on Paternal Psychopathology During Pregnancy

Reference	No. of cases	Diagnoses	Comment
Asch and Rubin, 1974	1	Acute psychotic reactions	Discusses four variations of postpartum reactions: mother, grandmother, post-adoption, and father.
Bucove, 1964	3	Paranoid schizophrenia (postpartum psychosis)	Only one case discussed in some detail.
Curtis, 1955	55	Various diagnoses grouped according to severity of symptoms	Interesting use of projective tests to categorize level of disturbance in fathers. "Expectant fatherhood brings out Oedipal situation."
Freeman, 1951	6	5-Psychosomatic (abdominal pain) 1-Paranoid psychosis	Emphasis on feelings of hate, envy, and jealousy in patients unable to find "normal" outlet.
Hartman and Nicolay, 1966	91	Exhibitionism, pedophilia, rape; sexual deviancy	Demonstrate $p < .01$ difference in excess of sexually deviant crimes in psychiatric court sample over a control group.
Jarvis, 1962	4	Depression, paranoid psychosis	Some indication of the progress made by two fathers in psychoanalytic psychotherapy.

Lacoursiere, 1972	4	Depression, paranoid psychosis	Reviews literature—notes no prospective studies done; dynamics speculated are due to disruption of dependency needs and sibling rivalry.
Retterstol, 1968	4	Paranoid psychosis	Compares 2 percent incidence of postpartum psychosis in males (4 out of 169) with 7 percent incidence in females.
Towne and Afterman, 1955	28	Acute psychotic reactions	Cases distinguished by anger and hostility, often associated with threats of violence; infantile behavior.
Trethowan and Conlon, 1965	36	Psychosomatic manifestations	Nausea, loss of appetite and toothache are most prevalent symptoms occurring in 11 percent of general population sample of 327 men during their wive's pregnancies.
Wainwright, 1966	10	Depression, suicidal ideas common, paranoid psychosis	Six dynamics discussed to reveal hidden meaning of symptoms. Drug dependence, homosexuality, promiscuity, cancer phobia seen as symptomatic.
Zilboorg, 1931	30	Psychotic depression	Complex and intricate intrepretations of behavior. Cases of postpartum depression in women also discussed.

parallelism between paternal and maternal attachment, qualitatively defined on the basis of the strength of protest following separation from parents. Both paternal and maternal bonds are dependent on the amount of interacting and caretaking given by the parent. These bonds also share a similar time course over the first two years of the infant's life. An interesting finding in Kotelchuck's work, also observed in a study by Spelke et al. (1970), is that highly interacting fathers had children low in "protest behavior" following their separation, though the same infants showed strong "proximity seeking" in the father's presence. Paternal feeding was related to the amount of spontaneous play the child would engage in on entering a laboratory setting simulating a natural home environment. These studies are unique in that psychological interviews of both parents were accomplished, along with direct observation of parent-child interaction.

In a study of eight 9-month-old infants, less meticulously carried out, Pedersen and Robson (1969) defined "attachment" behavior on the basis of greeting responses rather than responses aroused by separation from a parent. They found that fathers were more frequently attached to male infants. Paternal attachment was associated with the amount of caretaking, the strength of emotional investment, and the amount of stimulating play the father involved himself in with the infant. By appreciating the bilateral nature of the attachment phenomenon, Pedersen and Robson found that the majority of infants, regardless of their sex, exhibited attachment to their fathers.

These studies, although employing different definitions of the same phenomenon, reach a similar conclusion: paternal attachment does exist and is related to the quality of interaction between the father and child. Kotelchuck's and Spelke's studies provide important additional information that paternal attachment may influence the child's behavior in specific ways (for instance, relationship between paternal feeding and amount of spontaneous play engaged in by the infant). The notion that maternal behavior is instinctual and specific, or that paternal behavior is organized by a different biological drive system, is at present untestable. But judging from observed and reported behavior, there is little evidence to support such a distinction in attachment behavior. There is currently no information available on whether paternal attachment influences behavioral adjustment in the child. In this regard, it is clear that the use of the term "paternal deprivation," linking defective parenting with poor behavior adjustment as it does, is as unwarranted and ill advised as is the use of the term "maternal deprivation."

Evidence is available from work with subhuman primates that paternal care of infants is recognizable in a variety of species. Itani

(1959), one of the first to systematically observe the wild Japanese macaques, remarks in a charming descriptive study of this species:

> With respect to the beginning of paternal care, a very interesting phenomenon was observed. The female who was delivered of a baby first that year was Au; this was on May 11. On May 12, the next day, four subleader males simultaneously showed the first paternal care shown that year. It was clear that Au's delivery stimulated them, but at the same time we felt that there might exist a sort of sense of rivalry.

Paternal care demonstrated by these monkeys was usually directed to 1- or 2-year-old infants, not newborns, and only during the breeding season. It consisted of hugging, grooming, carrying, and protecting the infants. Itani remarked on the notable reduction in aggressiveness and marked tolerance shown by paternal monkeys. Mitchell (1969), in a review of paternal care in the primate literature, finds that New World male monkeys are quite caring toward their young. By contrast, rhesus varieties appear unresponsive to infants. This makes the recent laboratory work by Gomber and Mitchell (1974) all the more intriguing. Following the surrogate rearing studies of Harlow and Harlow (1969), Gomber and Mitchell allowed male rhesus monkeys to exclusively "raise" infants, and noted a gradual reduction of adult male aggressive, threatening behavior over the first few months and an increase in mutual grooming and nonthreatening rough-and-tumble play between adult male and infant. By the infant's seventh month, a time when proximity-seeking behavior between mother and infant rhesus is decreasing, the paternal-infant bond appears to be strengthening. These results are roughly consistent with Schaeffer's (but not Kotelchuck's) work showing that attachment to fathers was a more progressive event over the infant's first two years compared to maternal attachment.

If, indeed, there is a specific biological organization to paternity, it would be important to identify factors that encourage or frustrate its expression. Greenberg and Morris (1974) have provided a unique descriptive study of father's response to their offspring immediately after birth. In a condition he calls "engrossment," a group of men are described who express a strong sense of closeness and delight at the sight of their newborn. He did not find that "engrossment" was related to the father's presence at delivery. The question remains, however, whether participation in the delivery, or visual or tactile contact with the infant immediately after delivery, elicits attachment behavior in fathers. There is a compelling body of data from animal studies suggesting that there exists a "critical period" for mothers immediately following birth of their infants during which only tactile contact elicits "attachment" (Leifer, et al., 1972). Research on this phenomenon has been extended in humans only to the mother-infant relationship.

In a rare psychoanalytically oriented paper on the early father-child relationship, Burlingham (1973) acknowledges what she regards as a fundamental difference in paternal care:

> Maternal care is more gentle, soothing, and comforting while paternal involvement is more active, exciting, stimulating, and occasionally also arouses discomfort and anxiety. With regard to maternal care the infant is above all a passive recipient, while paternal care is more likely to produce active reactions in the child.

Whether such comments are the result of different biological organizations of parental behavior or stereotyped sex roles is not known.

The flexibility of male parental behavior is being challenged by the changing social structure of parenthood. It may be possible to answer questions concerning the specific nature of parental bonding in the near future by observing infants reared under different family and marital situations. As is commonplace in the social sciences, methodological problems abound, and must be painstakingly worked out before such efforts are productive of definitive conclusions.

EARLY CHILDHOOD PERIOD

It is important to note the increase in paternal attachment during the second year, since this is also a time when social training and behavioral control become prime concerns of child rearing. It may be that fathers exhibiting attachment during infancy are the ones observed to be most effective with their children during this period of primary socialization.

A group of studies supervised by Lois Stolz (Stolz, 1954) and published in a book entitled *Father Relations of War-Born Children* is a useful beginning to the analysis of this supposition. Two small samples of families with young children living in a university community were studied intensively, using a variety of interview techniques with parents and play techniques with children. In all cases, the children were the first born to their families. The crucial difference between the two groups was the father's absence for military service during the first year of the child's life in one group, and the father's presence throughout this period in the control group. All fathers had been resettled with their families for a period of years at the time of the study. This collection of studies emphasizes the difficulty that the fathers and their children continued to experience years after the fathers' return. Fathers felt that their war-born offspring were different and difficult children, and that these children did not share temperamental qualities with them. This was in marked distinction to the better relations perceived to exist between the fathers and their second children born after the father's return. Several fathers went so far as to call their war-born sons "sissies." The war-born children were also seen to be less socially acceptable to their peers than were other children and to manifest "stronger underlying feelings of aggression," although *overt* manifestations of aggression were not observed in these children. Stolz surmised that the war-born children's stronger feelings of hostility may have resulted from the rather severe punitiveness initiated by fathers toward them on their return. Father presence in the intervening years, she further conjectures, may have been responsible for the child's degree of behavioral control over hostile feelings. These interesting findings point clearly to the importance of fathers early in the child's environment and the continuing difficulty that can follow a socially acceptable period of paternal absence. A complicating factor in this regard is that maternal response styles may be altered by paternal absence or paternal disregard. If paternal absence continues to be a fruitful area of research, it would be important to carefully follow compensatory maternal behavior during the period of absence. Another problem unexplored in this study is how the particular experience of being separated for military purposes influenced the father's family relations on his return. It would be important in future work to compare a father's absence for socially condoned reasons, such as for military service or employment, with paternal absence for socially unacceptable reasons, such as for imprisonment.

When the father is present throughout the first years of the child's life, qualitative differences in paternal behavior influence the young child's adjustment. In his classic study, *Maternal Overprotectiveness*, David Levy (1943) provides the following description of the fathers:

> [They] had to deal with mothers who monopolized the child. Their rather ready adjustment to that situation is not difficult to understand, in view of our typical cultural pattern of family life. These fathers appear, however, readily adapted to such complete surrender of the paternal role by virtue of their generally submissive traits. . . . In contrast with their responsible and aggressive wives, they may be described as responsible and submissive.

From a vast literature of child rearing, the studies of Becker et al. (1962) and Baumrind (Baumrind and Black, 1967; Baumrind, 1971) are most impressive. Becker, interviewing parents separately, found that factors such as hostility, physical punishment, and strictness in fathers were related to agressiveness in boys and withdrawal in girls. He noted the possibility that this paternal effect in girls may have only become manifest in the presence of a submissive mother who provided an appropriate model for the girl's behavior.

In a subsequent paper, Becker and Krug (1965) argued convincingly that one of the basic strategies used in assessing the influence of parental behavior on a child's socialization (Parent Attitude Research Inventory) elicited highly biased remarks from parents, giving it an uncertain relationship to actual parent behavior. Many of the recommendations that Becker made in reference to parent-child interaction studies were incorporated in the research of Baumrind. Baumrind and her co-workers have combined interviews with parents, observations in the home of the interaction between parents and child, and social observation of the child in nursery school, in arriving at descriptive categories of patterns of parental authority and their effect on the social competence of children. Emerging from her data is a picture of "authoritative," in contrast to "authoritarian," or "permissive" parents. Such parents use rational authority, which seems to preserve a sense of autonomy in the child. The children of such parents appear friendly, engaging, confident, and competent in the nursery school class. Baumrind does not attribute this result to either parent, but rather implies that the parental effects are shared and horizontal.

Given a classification of the parents' shared authority patterns, however, particular characteristics in the behavior of the children do emerge on the basis of sex differences. For instance, the variable "paternal consistent discipline" is related to autonomous, imaginative, and confident behavior in boys, while in girls it is related to conforming, dependable behavior. The horizontal nature of parenting implied by Baumrind may be an effect of marriage, but it also may be a bias inherent in the choice of her population (a highly educated university community) or her methods. Quality of marriage should be an independent factor separated for research purposes from specific parent-child interactions, since clinical (Oleinick et al., 1966) and epidemiological (Stevenson and Richman, 1976) studies demonstrate that a poor quality marriage is often associated with behavioral deviance in children. The strength of Baumrind's results, however, add significantly to the literature, by demonstrating that parental restrictiveness and warmth combined with interaction that preserves the child's sense of autonomy underlie the most competent and confident behavior in boys. The fact that girls are stable and competent but less exuberant and more conforming than boys given this pattern of parenting may represent, as Baumrind suggests, a more implicit and subtle cultural patterning of expected sex differences in behavior. Again, the importance of these studies is that they provide a clear model for conceptualizing and organizing observational data around early parent-child interaction.

Still remaining, however, is the relatively uncharted domain of the father-child relationship. Examining such factors as employment, cognitive and affective styles, mental health, and quality of marriage from the paternal perspective would enlarge our appreciation of fathering. For instance, it has been noted that lower-class fathers are more rigid and domineering than middle-class fathers (Baumrind and Black, 1967) and that this may induce more disturbed aggressiveness in boys. One must wonder how this all too stereotyped notion would fare under rigorous analysis. It has also been suggested that a strong and intimate paternal relationship prevents creativity in boys (Emmerich, 1959). Several studies have indicated that lax, rather than restrictive, paternal control is more common in the experiences of juvenile delinquents (Burt, 1925; McCord and McCord, 1959). Nagging or irritability in fathers (Glueck and Glueck, 1950), relatively recent immigration with preservation of "Old World" ethnic traditions in fathers (Eron et al., 1961), and increased physical punishment used by fathers (McCord et al., 1963) have all been shown to be related to antisocial aggressiveness in children.

Another variable for consideration in relation to salient features of the father-child relationship in early childhood is early sex-role development. It has already been pointed out that differences in the behavior of boys and girls may arise as a consequence of the pattern of parental authority. The concept of psychosexual development, although implicit in the acquisition of social competence, may be thought of as a parallel, independent phenomenon. It is generally agreed that "sex-typed" or sex-appropriate behavior is acquired by a child's fourth year (Kagan, 1964), although projective techniques, which have been the most frequent measures used to determine this, are generally not considered methodologically sound.

Perhaps the most forceful argument that sex-role learning is critically determined quite early in the child's life comes from the study of pseudohermaphrodites, individuals born with ambiguous genitalia (Hampson, 1965). Attempts to reassign sex on the basis that the parents or physician assigned the wrong sex at birth are usually unsuccessful unless the change is made before the child is 2 years old. Mussen (1969) has pointed out that theories of how children acquire sex-specific behavior far outweigh available evidence accumulated from systematic studies. The varieties of theoretical frameworks (social-learning, Oedipal, developmental identification, cognitive developmental) employed in such studies often belie real differences in approach. Different theoretical persuasions, however, may have a profound effect on how one observes, organizes, and interprets data. The two extreme constructs of whether a child identifies with a father out of fear of castration or out of love and affection for him persuade one to think very differently about the same father-child relationship.

Separation from fathers during early life seems to have a more discernible effect on boys by producing more affectionate, more agreeable, and less aggressive behavior than in father-present boys (Stolz, 1954; Sears et al., 1946; Bach, 1946; Hetherington, 1966; Lynn and Sawrey, 1959; Tiller, 1961). Further evidence suggests that such boys have more difficulty establishing peer relations and may be prone to developing compensatory or exaggerated masculine behavior in adolescence (Mussen and Distler, 1960). A study completed years ago found that aggressive criminal behavior in boys in one context could be associated with passive and effeminate behavior in another context (MacDonald, 1938). The 10- to 13-year-old boys examined all had unsatisfactory relationships with their fathers; their mothers were characterized as rejecting and punitive. When these passive boys were forced into masculine roles, often by peers, they became anxious and fearful of homosexual urges. A dynamic interpretation was used to explain their episodic aggressive behavior as an attempt to cope with this flood of illicit feelings. It is not clear whether such a behavior pattern is common among boys with conduct disorders, since replication of this study cannot be found, or whether such interpretations are at all accurate. But we know less about determinants of effeminate behavior in boys, and even less about homosexuality.

There is data that suggests that fathers perceived as "powerful" and nurturant frequently have children rated in nursery school as high in "masculinity" (Mussen and Distler, 1959). Such a description is reminiscent of Baumrind's description (1971) of the "authoritative" parent.

A concern that homosexuality, particularly in men, may be related to the quality of fathering is confounded by the confusion between effeminate behavior and sex preferences. Effeminate behavior in boys is sometimes thought to be related to domineering or overprotective mothers or to hostile, aloof fathers, but there is nothing conclusive in the literature regarding this. Johnson (1963) has pointed out that fathers may be crucial to the appropriate sex orientation of girls and boys alike, based on the extent to which their interactions carry demands for "instrumentality" (competitiveness, success, etc.) in behavior. In her view, the nuclear family ideally represents different role specifications for mothers and fathers. Mothers are responsible for "expressivity" (responding to others with tenderness, love, caring so as to please) and fathers for "instrumentality." If fathers choose to demand and reward instrumental behavior in girls, girls adopt a masculine orientation, just as boys do. Such a narrow view of family life and sexual roles may be either a gross simplification or a serious distortion of the variability in human behavior.

Finally, we should note that paternal involvement also carries consequences for cognitive development in early childhood. Radin (1973) has demonstrated a strong association between the degree of paternal nurturance shown toward 4-year-old boys and their relatively high cognitive performance at school age. This exploratory study needs to be extended to larger groups and replicated. One finding of great interest is that the effect of paternal nurturance on the cognitive performance of boys was unrelated to social class differences.

DELAYED EFFECTS OF EARLY PATERNAL INFLUENCE

Whatever influence fathers have on infants and young children must also be viewed from the standpoint of a possible delay of effect. This is especially important in relation to psychopathology in childhood, since most children seen clinically have already reached school age. The most difficult problem in considering delayed effects of paternal deprivation is "clinical threshold." At what age, for what problems, and with what parental frustrations and expectations do children arrive at the doors of a clinic or a juvenile court? There is a suggestion, for instance, that death of a father in early life does not result in manifest emotional problems in the child until adolescence, while separation from a father due to marital discord may be expected to produce greatest disturbance at the time of separation, even if this occurs early in the child's life. Wolfenstein (1966) has hypothesized that adolescence constitutes the necessary developmental stage in which to mourn loss of a parent. Adolescents with schizophrenia (Wahl, 1954), depression (Beck et al., 1963), and medical illness (Seligman et al., 1974), compared to healthy peers, experience a similar frequency of parental loss; however, the former groups' losses occur earlier in life. In these studies, paternal loss exceeded maternal ones. It must be conceded that these findings may simply be artifactual—indicating that men are more at risk of death, especially sudden death, than are women, but some effort to control for this was made in the study by Beck. In a large retrospective study of children suffering loss of a parent, Gregory (1965) found that delinquency was much more frequent in boys who had lost a father through separation or divorce, and only somewhat more frequent when the loss was through death. This study, combined with that of Paffenbarger and Asnes (1966), represents an impressive body of findings that parental loss or deprivation is an important contributing factor to later maladjustment, especially for boys. Other work, however, has not supported the notion that death of the same-sexed parent predisposes the child to later maladjustment (Gibson, 1969; Rutter, 1971; Rutter, 1972), thus suggesting that a healthy adjustment in the remaining parent is sufficient to protect the child, regardless of the sex of that parent.

Although there is impressive evidence that the origins of conduct disorder may date back to a very young age (McCord and McCord, 1959), a study by Anderson (1968) suggests that a later age may be more crucial. In contrasting paternal absence among delinquent and nondelinquent boys, Anderson noted that the rate of father substitution between the ages of 4 and 7 years was much higher for nondelinquent boys with similar social situations than for delinquent boys. Father absence after the age of 4, but particularly after age 12, was related to arrest for the delinquent youths. Undisclosed by such a study, of course, is the nature of the father-child relationship before the separation took place. Rutter's analysis (1971) suggests that for marital conflict, the preceding disruption may be at least as difficult for the child as the separation itself.

A study by McCord et al. (1963) showed that if father absence occurred after the age of 6 years, the child was more likely to exhibit a "feminine aggressive pattern," implying that paternal absence before that age did not result in such a deviant pattern. "Feminine aggressive pattern" was not defined in the paper, but such a description would most likely fit comfortably into the Oedipal theory, suggesting a "sensitive period" in the development of sex-appropriate behavior and behavioral control. Of course, it may be that sexually inappropriate behavior had been present in these children since the preschool years and that with the greater peer contact and demands for more appropriate sexual behavior of school, the deviant pattern had become more disturbing.

Findings from cognitive studies suggest that early father absence in males is associated with a pattern of scores on the SAT more typical of females (Nelson and Maccoby, 1966; Carlsmith, 1964). The notion that one's cognitive style is dependent on sexual identification that can be reflected in performance on standardized tests or by perceptual measures (Barclay and Cusumano, 1967) has been supported by a large and not very convincing body of literature. Much recent work, extensively reviewed by Maccoby and Jacklin (1974), suggests, however, that this notion should be abandoned.

THERAPEUTIC INTERVENTION

Since the purpose of this chapter is to help orient and encourage a more active concern for fathers in the prevention and treatment of behavioral problems in children, this final section will deal with such considerations. The reason that antenatal care facilities, well baby clinics, day care centers, and nursery schools are female dominated must be related to the obvious stereotypes of maternal responsibility and maternal concern expected of women. While there is a recognizable trend toward males being more involved in their wives' pregnancy, especially among the middle class, it seems fair to say that the rearing of infants and young children is still considered primarily a feminine concern. This point of view is expressed in scholarly literature by such statements as the following, from Hoffman (1963) in a review article on child rearing:

> Perhaps it is only after the child has attained a relatively advanced level of cognitive maturity that the father's discipline can have an important effect despite his absence most of the day from the child's immediate life space.

In all fairness, it should be said that this statement is more than a decade old, and specifically related to discipline as one form of interaction between a father and his child. Do the attitudes of men and women generally support such a view as culturally appropriate in the 1970s? Appreciating the social and cultural change of the past quarter-century, the question can be put another way: How fast and in what direction are the attitudes of the sexes changing in regard to parental responsibility? Daring to generalize, one might say that as women demand greater opportunity in the work force, men become more disgruntled with what work and occupational roles have come to represent for them. Both men and women are seeking a more complete and enriched life in technologically advanced societies. Sociologists' growing interest in and awareness of the predicament of men in contemporary society have been admirably reviewed by Pleck and Sawyer (1974). We might expect that men will, of their own accord, seek more responsibility in infant and child care. At the same time, health professionals must achieve a greater awareness of men's roles in the lives of their families and children.

There are several areas of difficulty where intervention techniques should include and utilize the resources of fathers. One area is the investigation of how families adapt to illness, separation, or death of mothers. An exploratory study by Merrill (1969), reporting the response of fathers and their families to hospitalization of a schizophrenic mother, deserves particular mention. The following excerpt from that study provides some interesting commentary:

> During the mother's fluctuations between her usual and the symptomatic behavior, the children were constantly aligning and shifting their positions in favor of one parent or the other on various family issues. They eventually aligned themselves with the father and his more consistent and protective position. The alignment of the children with the fathers, along with the children's efforts to maintain some degree of usual family life, represented a reorganization of the family which excluded the mothers from family relationships to a considerable degree. . . . Discussions with the majority of husbands. . . . showed an unusually high degree of time and effort had been devoted to coping with the illness during the grossly

disruptive period prior to hospitalization. These husbands seemed extra-
ordinarily capable and willing to shoulder care of home and children in
addition to maintaining their jobs during the time their wives were ill.

Whether this pattern persists for less overt forms of behavior deviance
in mothers or for illness of mothers generally has been dealt with
very unsatisfactorily in the literature.

The effect of divorce of parents on the subsequent father-child
relationship is another area of special concern in child psychiatry.
The often enforced isolation of fathers from their children may lead
to feelings of abandonment in the children. The difficult and
complex task of studying the effects of divorce stress on children has
received little systematic study. Two studies in the recent literature
provide evidence that the persistence of quarreling and disagreement
in the post-divorce period places the child at particular risk of
developing emotional problems (McDermott, 1970; Westman et al.,
1970). Since it appears that about 25 percent of marriages result in
divorce in the United States (which does not include the number of
permanent separations and desertions), involving millions of children,
more than half of whom are very young, further study of this
problem is mandatory (Anthony, 1974). Of particular interest and
value would be the greater coordination of the social work, legal, and
psychiatric professions in research activity, as well as treatment.

If more were known about the attitudes of fathers toward their
young children, more rational strategies of intervention could be
developed. Gardner's paper of 1943 was searchingly done, but offers
little of relevance today. An interesting approach to the study of
attitudes is provided in a study by Fein (1974), who interviewed
fathers before and after the birth of their first child. What is most
interesting about the findings reported is the range of attitudes and
the varieties of emotional adjustments expressed by this group of
fathers. This study, taken with studies mentioned above that
demonstrate the existence of paternal attachment, should be used to
examine social and job policy implications for working fathers
(Terkel, 1974).

Some attention has been given to the establishment of group
meetings with fathers within the context of child guidance centers
(e.g., Beron, 1944; Strean, 1962; Grunebaum and Strean, 1964). By
far the most provocative of these papers is that of Tuck (1971), who
worked in a black community in Chicago. Over a period of years, he
traced the difficult and uncertain beginning of a group to its
subsequent strong impact on the community. An important aspect of
this change was the expressed need of the men to move away from
the traditional work of talking psychotherapy to a position of
assuming a more active interface with their environment. These

fathers saw their role not as confined to a discussion of their feelings (which were often ones of powerlessness and hopelessness) but as somehow to create a better community in which to rear their children.

Much of family therapy must found in discovering how to get fathers involved in treatment. A paper by Bell et al. (1961) deserves particular mention because it makes a successful attempt to understand the resistance of fathers to engage themselves in therapy sessions. In describing four stages of this resistance, the authors point to the existence of different values and expectations between middle-class therapists and working-class fathers as the fundamental source of difficulty. They advise that rather than assume disinterest or unmitigated resistance on the part of the fathers, therapists should make understanding and resolving these differences objectives of therapy encounters with fathers.

An extreme case of what can happen by neglecting fathers in casework was reported in a review of twenty-nine cases of fatal infant battering, caused by fathers. In each case, the child was less than 5 years old and was the stimulus of the father's attack. The murders were never instrumental, nonbiological fathers were not more violent than biological fathers, and in only 25 percent of the cases were work and child care roles reversed between the father and mother. Although 75 percent of the men are reported to have had a history of personality disorder, in many ways the most important finding was that in the majority of cases, the fathers gave warnings of their intent to harm the child, revealing their decreasing abilities to cope. Presumably because caseworkers and others had not established a rapport with the fathers, their warnings were appreciated only after the violence had taken place.

Instead of speculating on what the difficulties of getting fathers involved in preventive health practices are, when there is so little knowledge and experience to be shared, it is advisable to take an affirmative and active point of view. Fathers may not elect to attend clinics with their wives, view pregnancies, feed their infants, or play with them, at least not according to the design of a therapist. A variety of alternatives must remain open for father participation in the several institutions that attend to the needs of children, however. Providing a common, permissive, and supportive environment in which men can be respected in their roles as fathers should do much to enhance the effectiveness of preventive mental health measures, not just for the men involved, but for their wives and children.

SUMMARY AND CONCLUSIONS

An unwieldy literature, too often dependent on methodologically poor and unreplicated work, has been reviewed to support the proposition that fathers are important to young children. The corollary proposition that uninvested or absent fathers may be involved in the genesis of psychopathology in young children has only been approximately demonstrated. Psychopathology is poorly defined in early childhood for the majority of conditions, merging with purely developmental problems at one extreme and family and social disorganization at another. Even with these limitations, the main point should be clear: we do share an ignorance about fathers. Perhaps the impassioned apologias of Josselyn (1956) and Nash (1965) that we take account of paternity in research and clinical work are just beginning to find an audience.

In the interest of further research, five variables have been discussed that bear on the importance of the father-child relationship in early childhood: genetic sex-linked transmission, paternal behavior during pregnancy, paternal attachment, paternal discipline, and paternal influences on the adoption of sex-typed behavior by the child. Each of these requires considerable refinement in terms of definition, measurement, and follow-up study. We need to know not just more about the specific nature of fathering in early development, its limits and tolerances, but also more about the effect of paternal investment on family organization. It seems important to know whether men must necessarily make compromises in their wider social and work roles in order to enjoy an increased investment with their young children.

Though scientifically conducted research may contribute to a relaxation of prejudices and stereotypes, it is obvious that much of the work will be done outside the domain of scientific study. Clinicians and policy administrators must come to appreciate and respect the father as a significant and indispensible person in the child's early experience.

We could speculate that the neglect and omission of fathers in the work of psychiatry and the social sciences reflect powerful social bonds with patriarchy that allow it a degree of immunity from investigation. But the social order, at least of contemporary American society, is changing fast in ways that depart critically from traditional patriarchy. The inclusion of fathering in the interests of research and practice should help define and enhance the experience of witnessing this fundamental social process.

REFERENCES

Anderson, R. E. 1968. Where's Dad? Paternal deprivation and delinquency. Archives of General Psychiatry 18:649.

Andry, R. G. 1960. Delinquency and Parental Pathology. London: Methuen.

Anthony, E. J. 1974. Children at risk from divorce: a review. *In* The Child in His Family, E. J. Anthony, ed. Vol. III.

Asch, S., and L. Rubin, 1974. Post-partum reactions: some unrecognized variations. American Journal of Psychiatry 131:870-874.

Bach, G. R. 1946. Father fantasies and father-typing in father separated children. Child Development 17:63-80.

Bacon, H. K., I. Child, and H. Barry. 1963. A cross-cultural study of correlates of crime. Journal of Abnormal and Social Psychology 66:291-300.

Barclay, A. and D. Cusumano. 1967. Father absence, cross-sex identity and field dependence in male adolescents. Child Development 38:243-250.

Baumrind, D. 1971. Current patterns of parental authority. Developmental Psychology 4(Suppl.):1-103.

Baumrind, D., and A. Black. 1967. Socialization practices associated with dimensions of competence in preschool boys and girls. Child Development 38:291-327.

Beck, A., B. Sethi, and R. Tuthill. 1963. Childhood bereavement and adult depression. Archives of General Psychiatry 9:295-302.

Becker, W. C., and R. S. Krug. 1965. The parent attitude research instrument—a research review. Child Development 36:329-365.

Becker, W. C., D. Peterson, Z. Luria, D. Shoemaker, and L. Hellmer. 1962. Relations of factors derived from parent interview ratings to behavior problems in five year olds. Child Development 33:509-535.

Bell, N., A. Trieschman, and E. Vogel. 1961. A sociocultural analysis of the resistances of working class fathers treated in a child psychiatric clinic. American Journal of Orthopsychiatry 31:388-405.

Beron, L. 1944. Fathers as clients of a child guidance clinic. Smith College Studies of Social Work 14:351-366.

Biller, H. 1971. Father, Child and Sex Roles: Paternal Determinants of Personality Development. Lexington, Mass.: Heath.

Biller, H., and D. Meredith. 1975. Father Power. New York: David McKay.

Bowlby, J. 1946. Forty-Four Juvenile Thieves: Their Character and Home-Life. London: Ballière, Tindall, and Cox.

――――. 1969. Attachment and Loss. New York: Basic Books.

Buck, C., and K. Laughton. 1959. Family patterns of illness: the effect of psychoneurosis in the parent upon illness in the child. Acta Psychiatrica et Neurologica Scandinavica 34:165-175.

Bucove, A. 1964. Postpartum psychoses in the male. Bulletin of the New York Academy of Medicine 40:961-971.

Burlingham, D. 1973. The preoedipal infant-father relationship. Psychoanalytic Study of the Child 28:23-47.

Burt, C. 1925. The Young Delinquent. London: University of London Press.

Cantwell, D. P. 1972. Psychiatric illness in families of hyperactive children. Archives of General Psychiatry 27:414-417.

Casey, M. D., C. Blank, D. Street, L. Segall, J. McDougall, P. McGrath, and J. Skinner. 1966. YY chromosomes and antisocial behavior. Lancet 2:859-860.

Carlsmith, L. 1964. Effect of early father absence on scholastic aptitude. Harvard Educational Review 34:3-21.

Curtis, J. C. 1955. A psychiatric study of 55 expectant fathers. U.S. Armed Forces Medical Journal 6:937-950.

Eisenberg, L. 1957. The fathers of autistic children. American Journal of Orthopsychiatry 27:715-724.

Emmerich, W. 1959. Parental identification in young children. Genetic Psychology Monographs 60:257-308.

Eron, L. D., T. Banta, L. Valdev, and J. Laulicht. 1961. Comparison of data obtained from mothers and fathers on child rearing practices and their relation to child aggression. Child Development 32:457-472.

Fein, R. 1974. Men's experiences before and after the birth of a first child: an exploratory study. Doctoral dissertation, Harvard University.

Frazer, J. G. 1928. The Golden Bough: A Study in Magic and Religion. New York: Macmillan.

Freeman, T. 1951. Pregnancy as a precipitant of mental illness in men. British Journal of Medical Psychology 24:49-54.

Freud, S. 1955. Analysis of a phobia in a five year old boy (1909). In Standard Edition, Vol. 10. J. Strachey, ed. London: Hogarth Press, pp. 1-147.

Gardner, L. P. 1943. A survey of the attitudes and activities of fathers. Journal of Genetic Psychology 63:15-53.

Gibson, H. B. 1969. Early delinquency in relation to broken homes. Journal of Child Psychology and Psychiatry 10:195-204.

Glueck, S., and E. T. Glueck. 1950. Unraveling Juvenile Delinquency. New York: The Commonwealth Fund.

Gomber, J., and G. Mitchell. 1974. Preliminary report on adult male isolation-reared rhesus monkey caged with infants. Developmental Psychology 10:298.

Goodwin, D. W., F. Schulsinger, N. Miller, L. Hermansen, G. Winokur, and S. Guze. 1974. Drinking problems in adopted and nonadopted sons of alcoholics. Archives of General Psychiatry 31:164-169.

Greenberg, M. and N. Morris. 1974. Engrossment: the newborn's impact upon the father. American Journal of Orthopsychiatry 44(4):520-531.

Gregory, I. 1965. Anterospective data following childhood loss of a parent. Archives of General Psychiatry 13:110-119.

Grunebaum, H. U., and H. S. Strean. 1964. Some considerations of the therapeutic neglect of fathers in child guidance. Journal of Child Psychology and Psychiatry 5:241-249.

Hampson, J. 1965. Determinants of psychosexual orientation. In Sex and Behavior, F. A. Beach, ed. New York: Wiley.

Hare, E. H., and G. K. Shaw. 1965. A study of family health: (2) A comparison of the health of fathers, mothers and children. British Journal of Psychiatry 111:467.

Harlow, H. F., and M. K. Harlow. 1965. The affectional systems. In Behavior of Nonhuman Primates, A. Schrier et al., eds. New York: Academic Press.

Harlow, H., and M. K. Harlow. 1969. Effects of various mother-infant relationships on rhesus monkey behaviors. In Determinant of Infant Behavior, B. M. Foss, ed. Vol. 4. London: Methuen.

Hartman, A. A., and R. C. Nicolay. 1966. Sexually deviant behavior in expectant fathers. Journal of Abnormal Psychology 71:232-234.

Healy, W., and A. Bronner. 1936. A New Light on Delinquency. New Haven, Conn.: Yale University Press.

Herzog, E., and C. E. Sudia. 1969. Fatherless homes: a review of research. *In* Annual Progress in Child Psychiatry and Child Development, S. Chess and A. Thomas, eds. New York: Brunner-Mazel.

Hetherington, M. 1966. Effects of paternal absence on sex-typed behaviors in Negro and white pre-adolescent males. Journal of Personality and Social Psychology 4:87-91.

Hoffman, M. L. 1963. Child rearing practices and moral development: generalizations from empirical research. Child Development 34:295-318.

Itani, J. 1959. Paternal care in the wild Japanese monkey, Macaca fuscata. Journal of Primates 2:61-93.

Jarvis, W. 1962. Some effects of pregnancy and childbirth on men. Journal of the American Psychoanalytic Association 10:689-700.

Johnson, M. 1963. Sex role learning in the nuclear family. Child Development 34:319-334.

Josselyn, I. M. 1956. Cultural forces, motherliness and fatherliness. American Journal of Orthopsychiatry 26:264-271.

Kagan, J. 1964. Acquisition and significance of sex-typing and sex role identity. *In* Review of Child Development Research, M. L. Hoffman and L. W. Hoffman, eds. Vol. 1. New York: Russell Sage Foundation.

Kellner, R. 1963. Family Ill-Health: An Investigation in General Practice. London: Tavistock.

Kety, S., D. Rosenthal, P. Wender, and F. Schulsinger. 1968. The types and prevalence of mental illness in the biological and adoptive families of adopted schizophrenics. Journal of Psychiatric Research 6(Suppl):345-362.

Kotelchuck, M. 1972. The nature of a child's tie to his father. Doctoral dissertation, Harvard University.

Lacoursiere, R. 1972. Fatherhood and mental illness: a review and new material. Psychiatric Quarterly 46:109-124.

Leifer, A. D., P. H. Leiderman, C. R. Barnett, and J. A. Williams. 1972. Effects of mother-infant separation on maternal attachment behavior. Child Development 43:1203-1218.

Levy, D. 1943. Maternal Overprotection. New York: Columbia University Press.

Lynn, D., and W. C. Sawrey. 1959. The effects of father absence on Norwegian boys and girls. Journal of Abnormal and Social Psychology 59:258-262.

McCord, J., W. McCord, and A. Howard. 1963. Family interaction as antecedent to the direction of male aggresiveness. Journal of Abnormal and Social Psychology 66:239-242.

McCord, W., J. McCord, and I. Zola. 1959. Origins of Crime. New York: Columbia University Press.

Maccoby, E., and C. Jacklin. 1974. The Psychology of Sex Differences. Stanford, Calif.: Stanford University Press.

McDermott, J. 1970. Divorce and its psychiatric sequelae in children. Archives of General Psychiatry 23:421-427.

MacDonald, M. W. 1938. Criminally aggressive behavior in passive, effeminate boys. American Journal of Orthopsychiatry 8:70-78.

Malinowski, B. 1927. The Father in Primitive Psychology. New York: Norton.

Merrill, G. 1969. How fathers manage when wives are hospitalized for schizophrenia: an exploratory study. Social Psychiatry 4(1):26–32.

Mitchell, G. 1969. Paternalistic behavior in primates. Psychological Bulletin 71:399–417.

Mussen, P. H. 1969. Early sex role development. In Handbook of Socialization Theory and Research, D. A. Goslin, ed. Chicago: Rand McNally.

Mussen, P., and L. Distler. 1959. Maculinity, identification, and father-son relationships. Journal of Abnormal and Social Psychology 59:350–356.

————. 1960. Child rearing antecedents of masculine identification in kindergarten boys. Child Development 31:89–100.

Nash, J. 1965. The father in contemporary culture and current psychological literature. Child Development 36:261–297.

Nelson, E., and E. Maccoby. 1966. The relationship between social development and differential abilities on the Scholastic Aptitude Test. Merrill Palmer Quarterly 12:269–284.

Nielsen, J., T. Tsuboi, G. Stürup, and D. Romano. 1968. XYY chromosomal constitution in criminal psychopaths. Lancet 2:576–577.

Oleinick, M., A. Bahn, L. Eisenberg, and A. Lilienfeld. 1966. Early socialization experiences and intrafamilial environment. Archives of General Psychiatry 15:344–353.

Paffenbarger, R. S., and D. P. Asnes. 1966. Chronic disease in former college students: III. Precursors of suicide in early and middle life. American Journal of Public Health 56:1026–1036.

Pedersen, F. A., and K. S. Robson. 1969. Father participation in infancy. American Journal of Orthopsychiatry 39:466–472.

Pleck, J., and J. Sawyer, eds. 1974. Men and Masculinity. New York: Prentice-Hall Spectrum Books.

Radin, N. 1973. Observed paternal behaviors as antecedents of intellectual functioning in young boys. Developmental Psychology 8:369–376.

Retterstol, N. 1968. Paranoid psychosis associated with impending or newly established fatherhood. Acta Psychiatrica Scandinavica 44:51–61.

Robins, L. 1966. Deviant Children Grown-up. Baltimore: Williams & Wilkins.

Robins, L., P. West, and B. Herjanic. 1975. Arrests and delinquency in two generations: a study of black urban families and their children. Journal of Child Psychology and Psychiatry 16:125–140.

Rosen, B. M., A. Bahn, and M. Kramer. 1964. Demographic and diagnostic characteristics of psychiatric clinic outpatients in the U.S.A., 1961. American Journal of Orthopsychiatry 34:455–468.

Rutter, M. 1971. Parent-child separation: psychological effects on the children. Journal of Child Psychology and Psychiatry 12:233–260.

Rutter, M. 1972. Maternal Deprivation Reassessed. Harmondsworth, England: Penguin Books.

Schaeffer, H. R., and P. E. Emerson. 1964. The development of social attachments in infancy. Monographs of the Society for Research in Child Development 29(3, Serial No. 94):1–77.

Schulsinger, F. 1972. Psychopathy: heredity, environment. In Life History Research in Psychopathology, Vol. 2. M. Roff et al., eds. Minneapolis, Minn.: University of Minnesota Press.

Sears, R. R., M. Pintler, and P. Sears. 1946. Effect of father separation on preschool children's doll play aggression. Child Development 17:219-243.

Seligman, R., G. Gleser, J. Rauh, and L. Harris. 1974. The effect of earlier parental loss in adolescence. Archives of General Psychiatry 31:475-479.

Spelke, E., P. Zelaso, J. Kagan, and M. Kotelchuck. 1970. Father interaction and separation protest. Development Psychology 9:83-90.

Stevenson, J. E., and N. Richman. 1976. Personal communication.

Stolz, L., 1954. Father Relations of War-Born Children. Stanford, Calif.: Stanford University Press.

Strean, H. S. 1962. A means of involving fathers in family treatment. American Journal of Orthopsychiatry 32:719-725.

Terkel, S. 1974. Working. New York: Avon Books.

Tiller, P. O. 1961. Father Separation and Adolescence. Oslo, Norway: Institute for Social Research.

Towne, R. D., and J. Afterman. 1955. Psychosis in males related to parenthood. Bulletin of the Menninger Clinic 19:19-26.

Trethowan, W. H. 1968. The couvade syndrome—some further observations. Journal of Psychosomatic Research 12:107-115.

Trethowan, W. H., and M. F. Conlon. 1965. The couvade syndrome. British Journal of Psychiatry 111:57-66.

Tuck, S. 1971. Working with black fathers. American Journal of Orthopsychiatry 41:465-472.

Wahl, C. W. 1954. Some antecedent factors in the family histories of 392 schizophrenics. American Journal of Psychiatry 110:668-676.

Wainwright, W. M. 1966. Fatherhood as a precipitant of mental illness. American Journal of Psychiatry 123:40-44.

Weiss, G., K. Minde, J. Werry, V. Douglas, and E. Nemeth. 1971. Studies on the hyperactive child. VIII. Five year follow-up. Archives of General Psychiatry 24:409-414.

West, D. J., and D. P. Farrington. 1973. Who Becomes Delinquent? Second Report of the Cambridge Study on Delinquent Development. London: Heineman.

Westman, J. E., D. Cline, W. Swift, and D. Kramer. 1970. The role of child psychiatry in divorce. Archives of General Psychiatry 23:416-420.

Wolfenstein, M. 1966. How is mourning possible? Psychoanalytic Study of the Child 21:93-123.

Zilboorg, G. 1931. Depressive reactions to parenthood. American Journal of Psychiatry 10:927-962.

CHAPTER 10

MIDDLEHOMES
An Introduction to Residence and Developmental Needs

Gordon P. Harper, M.D.

INTRODUCTION

Because Western thought, at least since the Renaissance, has been concerned with culture and with the ways it is passed from generation to generation, and because at least since the mid-nineteenth century it has been widely assumed that the relationships among people are both a critical part of such transmission and subject to rational study, a continuing scholarly and popular interest in those relationships is understandable. More puzzling is how infrequently, in this century, such interest has been focused not just on the relationships, but also on where they take place. Where are we to live? With whom? Where are children to be raised? Where shall "dependent" adults live? What groups of relatives (or nonrelatives), in what situations, "go well" together?

A century ago, these questions stimulated lively discussion and considerable practical effort. Owens, Fouriere, Brook Farm, and Oneida are some of the personal and place names associated with nineteenth-century movements, religious and secular, utopian and reformist, that sought to express their visions of a better society in communal living arrangements (Kanter, 1972). Even at the turn of the century, the new Department of Social Ethics at Harvard collected and left behind in glass display cases photographs of tenements and street playgrounds as part of their recognition that where people lived had much to do with how they lived.

This chapter is based on research supported by a grant from The Commonwealth Fund.

Shortly after that department was founded, however, a rapid expansion of knowledge and of investigative tools for understanding the *relationships* among people coincided with a post-Victorian conservative redefinition of the family as the "right" place for people to live, with the twin results that the major social manipulations of residence in this century ("public housing") have been assumed to deal with those outside the mainstream of American Society, and that academic and popular interest in human relationships has slipped back from the *where* of life toward the *how*. At some point the Department of Social Ethics ceased to be and a Department of Social Relations appeared. And the pictures of tenements moved to an upper floor, out of the way.

There are still times, to be sure, when the interaction between residence and relationships occupies attention. Examples include the work of Spitz (1946) and Bowlby (1950) on the effects of raising infants in institutions, the contemporary discussion of day care and women's employment, periodic exposés of nursing homes, the faddish dissection of the warts and the glories of the nuclear family, and the frequent descriptions of the contemporary enthusiasm for communal living (Kanter, 1973). But these are generally related to special circumstances, such as the condition of orphanhood, or of old age without family, or the decay of the family in the American 1960s, or the search for a countervailing culture in the special malaise of the Vietnam-time.

The lack of a general discussion seems to reflect an underlying assumption that "normal" people in "normal" times live in families and that "families" means (unless some special cultural, familial, or personal fate intervenes) the nuclear family of origin or procreation. An insinuation (or more) of deviant behavior attends discussion of other living situations.

To be sure, a number of groups have specialized interests in homes. Architects write about the ways that design affects living. City planners discuss the environments around homes and the effects of various "mixes" of different kinds of people and different kinds of buildings. Specialists in child care, responding to the breakdown of nuclear families, discuss the varieties of groups or foster homes most helpful for children cast adrift, and deplore the inadequacy of public services for such children (Eisenberg, 1965; Governor's Commission, 1973). And sociologists like Goffman (1961) have described the devastating effects that living in total institutions such as mental hospitals have on residents. Claiming that much of the deviant behavior seen there is generated by the place itself, they have called for a change in policy. And mental health and youth corrections planners, smarting from such criticism and promising to save the state money, have lately given verbal and some administrative commitment to the idea of moving people from such institutions back to ones thought more conducive to full living (Ohlin et al., 1974). And the way that *that* movement has gone has led to fear and anger in the neighborhoods involved and to new concerns (the "back wards in the streets") among professionals in the field (McGrath, 1974; Rabkin, 1974).

Are these special issues arising out of special circumstances? I suggest that they are not. I argue here that these problems are part of a larger, undeveloped subject, that of the relationships between where people live and how they live and grow. I will develop this argument from a point of view derived from clinical work. Clinicians are inclined to appreciate the issues involved in residence because the overrepresentation of homeless people in all patient populations forces clinicians willy-nilly to deal daily with the problems ("disposition problems") of where people are to live. A clinical perspective, that of the interaction between people's needs at each stage of life and the ability of the environment to meet these needs, offers a useful framework in which to organize thoughts about residence.

Two reasons for looking into the relationships between residence and development can be mentioned at the outset. First, the subject of residence has been, in this century, as indicated above, relatively neglected in our discussions of what affects growth and health. The neglect has been both conceptual, when we think of what holds our society together, and programmatic, as we skimp on allocating resources to institutions we would like to think do not exist (or exist only for deviants).

Second, of the many variables that shape our growing up and sustain our health, the institutions around us, like our homes, lend themselves to intervention more readily than do the more personal aspects of our lives, like attitudes, feelings, and relationships. Without proposing new social interventions, I advocate that we consider the interactions of social structure and development, and so examine which parts of our social system promote growth and which retard it. Such an examination must include both those features of society, which arise by design or avowed public policy, and those that seem "just to happen," by lack of such attention—or the appearance of such lack.

I have come to see certain existing institutions as "of a kind," and to group them together under the heading "middlehomes." In this chapter I will discuss the clinical-developmental point of view on residence; offer definitions of different kinds of homes, including middlehomes; discuss different kinds of middlehomes; show how middlehomes have become a conspicuous (if little recognized) feature of the social landscape; present vignettes of predicaments in which middlehomes matter; and, finally, discuss implications of this subject for clinical training and public policy.

DEVELOPMENTAL NEEDS AND HOMES

From the point of view of human development, the purpose of homes is to meet people's needs or to offer a setting conducive to the meeting of those needs. "Needs" are understood in three ways. First are the universal *survival needs* for shelter, clothing, and food. While the practical task of organizing resources in such a way as to provide these necessities for everyone seems to remain beyond the capacity of many societies, such needs are easily understood and present little conceptual problem.

At the other extreme are *idiosyncratic needs* arising out of illness or distorted emotional growth—everything we usually consider as relating to medical and psychological treatment. These also are easily understood.

The third category, *developmental* needs, lies midway between the general and the particular, and is the most complex. These needs arise because of an individual's point in development. Every parent is more or less aware of the needs of a child at any given stage of development, as are good teachers with regard to their pupils. In clinical work, of course, some assessment (often unspecified) of such needs lies under all our best efforts. Because they are so often unstated and because they lie at the heart of what I want to say about middlehomes, however, developmental needs warrants some special emphasis.

The conceptual framework I am using here comes most immediately from Erikson (1963, 1976). Development is seen as a sequence of stages. In each stage, through the related processes of growth, neurological maturation, and psychosocial development, the individual possesses new capacities, which may be translated into new motor, linguistic, and cognitive abilities, ways of feeling, and, consequently, social experiences. To be fully "worked into" the existing personality, such capacities need, and ideally call forth from the environment, such input that the individual assimilates what is new, and keeps growing despite change. The variety of inputs needed at different ages has been described, for different capacities and from different points of view, as Piagetian aliment or the combination of emotional relationships that Winnicott (1965) called the "facilitating environment." In addition to specific capacities, in each stage the person must build on what accrued in earlier stages and reconcile his growing inner sense of identity with the psychosocial possibilities available in the world outside.

The view of development shares with earlier psychoanalytic theory, from which it arose, an appreciation of crucial early affective encounters between the infant and young child and the environment, and of the relatively permanent psychic structures laid down in early childhood. It differs or goes beyond that theory in several ways: in focusing on other capacities as well as affective ones and therefore seeing libidinal development as a part, not the whole, of early experience; in postulating the *mutuality* with the environment, and not simply the vicissitudes of drives, is the "goal" of early interactions; and in contending that development continues beyond latency and adolescence, that the work of development at each stage of life is the integration of the personality's inner capacities with outer possibilities, and that the outcome of development can be seen as a series of inner senses, like a sense of basic trust and a sense of autonomy, related to practical abilities, cognitive skills, and identities, as well as to emotional evolution and interpersonal relating.

For this discussion, several points in this interactional model are relevant. First, neither the model of the individual evolving in isolation nor that of the environment acting on a blank slate accounts adequately for development. Both act on each other, both need each other, both are developing, at different points in the life cycle. From this point of view, a term like the "facilitating environment" seems more appropriate than a more passive-sounding phrase like "average-expectable environment."

The issue in the developmental study of residence is now definable: What kinds of homes, for what kinds of people, at what stages and with what specific needs, are facilitating environments? One thing is clear: since there is no age without developmental tasks, and no people without developmental needs, no home that is purely custodial can be adequate.

As an illustration of this point, it is worth recalling some examples of homes that have not met people's developmental needs. Large infant asylums were prevalent until Spitz (1946), Bowlby (1952), and Provence and Lipton (1962) demonstrated the need of infants for individual, personal care. Jails and state hospitals, with lasting labels to offer, continue to be the only refuge available for many confused adolescents, despite the irrelevance of therapy or actual harm thus done to many adolescents, who need to experiment with various identities without being confirmed in a negative way (Erikson, 1968). And old-age homes often try to maintain a kind of aseptic neatness by throwing out or putting away the cluttery life souvenirs of their residents, in spite of the residents' developmental needs, specific to old age, of maintaining their personal integrity in the face of deteriorating alertness and memory, and of "making sense of life" as they approach its end (Erikson, 1963; Curtin, 1972).

It goes without saying that any list of developmental needs is not meant to be taken as dogma, or as the latest bit of revealed truth, but as an approximate formulation, the best we can do at any given time, of what human development is about. As such, any list is influenced by contemporary ideas about human nature, the nature of childhood, and the nature of differences among people (Aries, 1965; Rothman, 1971).

HOMES: OWN HOMES, MIDDLEHOMES, HOMES OF DISASTER

If homes are "meant" to meet people's needs, they can be classified according to where and with whom needs are being met.

First is the "own home," the home where one's biological parents care for one, or where one cares for one's own children. This term overlaps with the terms "primary home" and "home of origin or procreation."

Social reformers and sociologists have drawn attention to a group of "homes" located at the other end of the spectrum, both in size and in degree of relatedness. These are the large-scale, primarily custodial institutions to which the word "home" can be applied only with difficulty or with irony, but where, nonetheless, society strives to meet the needs of many people not otherwise cared for. Goffman (1961) used the term "total institution" to emphasize the extent to which such institutions control every aspect of their inmates' lives. Alongside that term I would set the term "home of disaster": most total institutions are homes of disaster both because people generally arrive there through some "disaster" (either a mishap in their own lives or in the ability of more desirable homes to care for them) and because the institution's response to people's needs is often disastrous. Homes of disaster comprise most prisons, traditional mental hospitals, most chronic medical hospitals, and such places as large orphanages and "training schools" for delinquent juveniles.

A third class of homes, for which the name "middlehomes" seems useful, lies between the "own homes" and the "homes of disaster." It can be argued that they exist not just in response to exceptional or special circumstances, but as a regular and predictable and *necessary* feature of modern society.

As the name suggests, a middlehome lies in between, both sociologically and emotionally. In a middlehome, from a sociological point of view, people's ties are less bureaucratically determined than in a home of disaster, but less shaped by kinship of other "personal" relationships than in a home of origin or procreation. Emotionally, relationships in middlehomes are neither as diffuse as in large institutions nor as charged with feeling as in one's "own home." Indeed, the degree of emotional intensity or diffuseness predictable in middlehomes of certain structure (or, put differently, the degree to which a middlehome evokes the emotional atmosphere of the "own

home") may be a deciding factor in determining where some people
with certain needs have the best chance of continued growth.

We define these three groups of homes according to who lives
where, and who is meeting whose needs. Many needs, developmental
and other, are met by institutions somewhere "in the middle" where
people do not reside, or live the full day. Day hospitals, boys' clubs,
many schools, and day care centers are examples. These might be
called "part-middlehomes," but a more useful name would be
"dayhomes." This name suggests both the fact that people spend the
daytime there and the fact that needs are being met there, as in
24-hour homes.

The characteristics of the several kinds of homes can be represented as follows:

	Scale	Relationships of residents	How well needs tend to be met	Services may be supplemented by:
Primary home	Small	Biological	Variable	Often by dayhomes
Middle home	Small to intermediate	Not biological, but often "as good as kin"	Variable	Often by dayhomes
Home of disaster	Large	Primarily bureaucratic	Poorly	Usually nothing; "total institution"

TYPES OF MIDDLEHOMES

"Middlehome" is an inclusive term. The following dimensions
identify different types.

1. The first dimension is presence or absence of *therapeutic intent.*
One group of middlehomes, exemplified by boarding schools and
most summer camps, may be called the *growth-may-proceed* type.
Those sharing its services are assumed to be more disposed to grow
than to stay put or to regress. In Anna Freud's terms, the forces for
growth outweigh the forces for regression. It follows that meeting
the developmental needs of each member of the home will be enough
to let him or her grow. Such fostering of growth, of course, is usually
quite un-self-conscious. Human development assumes that people
generally, to the extent that their needs have been met historically
and in the present, will do without planning what is "right" for the
development of those around them. This holds for infants, toddlers,
preschoolers, school-age children, teenagers, young adults, parent-
householders, and older people. Reciprocity and mutuality are

involved in this shared fostering of each other by each generation: many of the infant's behaviors activate feelings in the parents and elicit parenting behaviors in them that are "just what is needed" by the baby (and by his parents). "The family brings up the baby by being brought up by him" (Erikson, 1963). The interchange will occur to best advantage where the wider social network supports materially and emotionally each person's responses to those around him.

Winnicott's argument (1965) that a normally endowed infant could expect to thrive in the growth-fostering environment he called "facilitating" can be extended to all ages and all developmental stages. The first type of middlehome is one that provides such an environment for each member.

The second type takes on an additional task: *supplementing* the experience of children (and adults) with environmentally slowed development and *correcting* developmental deviations. An example is a residential treatment center for children. This kind of middlehome is intended to provide the kind of experience thought of in psychotherapy as a "corrective emotional experience." It undertakes to offer that kind of experience, to try to undo or make up for earlier experience, for people with lags or deviations in intellectual, physical, or social growth, as well as emotional development. The residential treatment center has an explicit "therapeutic" or "corrective" mandate, whereas the boarding school wishes only to provide a facilitating environment.

2. Another dimension of middlehomes is the *length of time* one spends in one, which may vary depending on the purpose of the middlehome and on the stage of life of its members. Children and adolescents stay in adoptive, foster, or group homes for the period of *dependency;* runaway youths may "crash" in a hostel or shelter for the duration of a *crisis;* young people may live in a boarding school, boot camp, or college dormitory for as long as is required for a given piece of *training or education;* and patients or ex-patients stay in a concept house (drug addiction rehabilitation center), residential treatment center, some halfway houses, or convalescent home for a period of *treatment, rehabilitation, or recovery.* The ultimate length of stay applies in some communes, monasteries, nursing homes, halfway houses (as for some formerly hospitalized mentally retarded adults who continue to be dependent for many day-to-day services), and old-age homes, where some members will stay as long as they live.

3. The efforts of many groups, governmental and voluntary, to provide shelter and other services for alienated and runaway youths during and since the 1960s have made clear the importance, especially for this group, of such dimensions of middlehomes as the

degree of *structure*, real and symbolic cultural *identifications* (especially when they relate to government and other established agencies), presence or absence of an *ideology*, any obligatory *labels* attached to residence there (especially labels related to patienthood), and the stability or transience of *emotional ties*. For many de facto emancipated runaways, the only acceptable shelter has been one that eschewed official trappings, advertised its involvement in the "counterculture," and offered its residents considerable latitude of behavior (within broad limits) and an emotional atmosphere where one could "keep one's distance." All of these features can be related to the developmental issues of adolescence, especially when inherited institutions appear to have lost their integrity.

The challenge of providing some kind of service to such youths was initially recognized and met only by voluntary groups; some state and federal mental health and public welfare agencies have recently begun to channel limited financial support, but not government structure, to such services.

4. Another dimension is degree of *"family-ness."* An example of clinical decision-making in child care may illustrate the usefulness of understanding the various types of middlehomes in clinical terms. Some emotionally troubled children living outside, but still emotionally tied to, primary families are unable to tolerate living situations that stir up family-like feelings. They may thrive in group homes or other institutions, but in foster homes, which seem to raise the hope and dash it simultaneously that the fantasied "ideal parents" are at hand, their behavioral symptoms recur. For some of these children, in adolescence, a series of state hospital admissions, punctuated by repeated failed attempts to find a "better" out-of-hospital placement (from which, time after time, the child runs back to the hospital), speaks to the comparative safety such children may feel in a place with more structure and less personal, more diffuse relationships where the staff change every eight hours and no one is called "mother."

The astute clinician or caseworker is guided in making recommendations for such children and adolescents by considerations of just such matches between the needs of the child and their predictable interaction with one or another kind of home.

HISTORICAL BACKGROUND: HOW HAVE MIDDLEHOMES ARISEN?

Middlehomes appeared during the transition from traditional to modern societies, and now constitute a regular and necessary, if underrecognized, part of modern society.

Among the reasons for their appearance is the increase in the numbers of people living outside primary homes. Demography accounts for some of the increase through increased numbers of out-of-family births and orphans. But if there are more people in these groups, their lives have surely been complicated by redefinitions of the family and the family's role that have occurred at the same time. The nuclear family has become both the modal and the normative living unit, while the extended family is seen as educationally or economically obsolete, personally old-fashioned or irrelevant. Since the extended family specialized in personal services and in geographical contiguity and in women who fulfilled themselves primarily within the home, several kinds of marginal family members previously included *in* both family and home are now defined *out:* the cousin's illegitimate daughter, the child with Down's Syndrome, the retarded uncle, or the senile grandparent.

Rothman (1971) has written of some of the ideological reasons for this change, notably the belief of people in the United States in the early nineteenth century that deviance was an affront to their claims to being the Elect of Columbia. These attitudes have grown narrower as social class pretensions have been added to the earlier ideological ones. Put simply, the modern nuclear family has less room in it than larger families in traditional communities had. There are more primary-home orphans.

As much as social change has altered family life and produced more primary-home orphans among the dominant classes of the industrialized West, at least some family structure has remained. In societies shattered by war and not rebuilt, or in the underclass in industrialized societies where dislocation from county to city occurs along with chronic unemployment and possible social and ethnic discrimination, whole sections of society have seemed to consist mostly of primary-home orphans. The family-less state in which children grow up in such conditions in Latin America, North America, and Asia has been portrayed on film and in print (Lewis, 1965; Wolff, 1970). The need for middlehomes in these areas is a small part of the need for social reorganization on a larger scale.

On their own in such areas, children may establish bootstrap middlehomes, families of a sort, in deserted apartments (Brown, 1973). Energetic societal efforts to cope with large numbers of family-less children have occurred, especially in the aftermath of war and revolution (Makarenko, 1951).

Even where society is not so shattered, families' capacity for a certain kind of caring has declined. Women work outside the home. Grandparents live far away. First parents, finding themselves facing their offspring with little exposure to and less experience with child rearing, feel a special kind of anxiety and may wish they were back at more familiar work. For all of these reasons, people feel more ready to turn those in their care over to surrogate care givers. Dayhomes such as day care centers come into vogue. In other families, frustrated parents encourage, allow, or reluctantly resign themselves to their children's "running away" to join a kind of floating urban world of adolescents and preadolescents seeking (with or without societal sanction or support) new kinds of middlehomes.

There are educational, ideological, and recreational reasons for concentrating people, especially young people, together outside of primary homes. Such motives account for middlehomes ranging from the British public school to the boarding schools of revolutionary Cuba, in which rural youths live in the mansions of the dispossessed rich. Also included in this group are summer camps and college dormitories, which we might call middlehomes of special opportunity.

Modern society seems to bring with it a new kind of consciousness in which one does not feel the same person in all one's relationships. In contrast to the presumed simplicity of personality in homogeneous societies where one related to all one's acquaintances in the same way and thought of oneself the same way at home, at work, and at play, several contemporary observers, from various points of view (Berger et al., 1973; Trilling, 1972), describe a plastic personal quality or multifaceted identity as a quality of modern man and woman. Whatever its other implications, this feature of modernity certainly creates new developmental needs: How can one learn so many social roles, so much sensitivity and ability to modulate one's behavior (and self-concept) with the situation? Frequently, such learning requires living, during the developing years, in more places than the primary home. Many middlehomes and dayhomes have arisen and others have been populated, in response to this need. Schools (day and boarding), camps, and other kinds of outings away from home come to mind.

Other middlehomes have arisen in flight from this complex, highly differentiated world. Witness the homogeneous contemporary communities where people can "once again" feel whole and the same in all relationships. Against the background of modern society, such communes, monasteries, and treatment communities look like the simple, undifferentiated traditional societies of the past.

Another variety of respite, for those with fewer resources (or less luck in finding facilities to match their resources), is the kind of shelter to which alcoholics and other family-less adults may drift. Many of these are homes of disaster in both the senses mentioned earlier.

Finally, given the growing disparity between unmet needs (some traditional, some new) on the one hand, and the diminishing ability of traditional homes to meet these needs on the other, modernizing societies first tried to cope by building what became the homes of disaster: asylums, prisons, orphanages, poorhouses. Their size was large; their inmates' status very low; and the terms of residence or commitment long. In our terms, their most striking feature was their failure to meet more than custodial needs. Rothman (1971) spells out the course of their decline and gives plausible reasons for it.

In the last two decades, many inside and outside the professions that arose to oversee these institutions have concluded that such large-scale chronic care facilities do more harm than good. Eisenberg (1973) has described this enlightened movement as the rediscovery of moral treatment. At present in the fields of mental health, mental retardation, penology, and youth "corrections," workers in this movement are closing the homes of disaster and moving their inmates back into smaller institutions more like primary homes and more adequate to meet the needs of those who have long been incarcerated. These smaller institutions are, of course, middlehomes.

In one sense, the closing of the homes of disaster has created another important reason for middlehomes. In another sense, deinstitutionalization has only unmasked a long standing need that the homes of disaster obscured.

This historical review is intended to make only one point, which should not be lost in the discussion of deinstitutionalization: that even if halfway houses seem to have arisen as a (sometimes belated) complement to the current phasing out of the big training schools and state hospitals (for motives that mix humanism with governmental thrift), other middlehomes, the bulk of middlehomes, are not just a part of this administrative movement but are a part, an inevitable part, of modern society.

The neglect of this thrust in our society, the refusal to see middlehomes as meeting a general, not just a current need, is a story in itself.

CLINICAL VIGNETTES

A baby is born prematurely to an unmarried adolescent. The mother gives up the child at birth. The infant's first weeks are spent near death's door, with respiratory problems, which eventually resolve, and a tragic loss of part of one limb as a complication of one of the therapies. The baby would have been "placed" routinely for adoption, but his severe course, with the "possibility of brain damage, which cannot be ruled out" and his new deformity make him "difficult to place," both because many prospective adoptive parents now demur, and because the agency is reluctant to "let him out for adoption" until some long period of observation will, supposedly, give firm answers to all the questions about his eventual capacities. He stays in the nursery months longer than medically indicated, the nursery becoming his first middlehome. This long stay is not ideal for the infant—both because of the risk of hospital-acquired infection and because it deprives him of the chance to begin to know, as early as possible, his eventual adoptive parents. A placement "in between" the acute-care nursery and an adoptive home might be found, but plans get bogged down in the confusion over his "suitability for adoption." Finally, a professional family, wise to the ways of agencies, delighted with the baby's development, but adamant that his coming to live with them not be delayed past the period when an infant first "locks onto" his parents, forces the issue and prevails upon the agency to let them adopt the child without further delay.

An early adolescent is brought repeatedly to a hospital emergency ward because he's "out of his mind," "out of control," "doing it again," and so on. The offensive behaviors include taunting and then threatening to whip a girl at school, and having a confrontation with, then running from, a female teacher, but mostly heated arguments and fist fights at home, sometimes with his mother, sometimes with an older sister. Once or twice, he uses a knife threateningly, but no one is hurt.

Interviewed, the boy is at first sullen, then a little more talkative, but completely "sane" at all times. A father in prison for murder, a mother trying to cope with (which to her means control) a large family in his absence, and this boy's arrival at the threshold of a pubertal manhood that no one in this family is quite sure can be handled (by any man, much less by him) complete the picture behind this boy's panicky outbursts. It is clear, in particular, that the mother and her female relatives are unconsciously fomenting and secretly enjoying the exciting tantrums they complain of so dramatically. But they seem unable to stop the cycle. Rejecting the idea of going to the police (too frank a confirmation of the family's worst identity), they request that the boy be "put away" as "mental," though he is anything but "insane." Frantic calls around town to find a relative, friend, or halfway house where the boy can stay a while so that both sides can cool off are unsuccessful. The mother finally gets her conscious wish: this nonpsychotic, frightened boy is indeed "put away" for a hospital stay that will change nothing in the long run and that immediately offers a painful label, "mental patient," to a boy who needs much less of this, but also much more, of a different kind of institution: something "in between." Nor have we even begun to consider what alternative living arrangements for the parents—in between home and hospital for the exhausted mother and between home and distant prison for the convicted father—might have better served this family's needs.

A father of two sustains severe brain injuries in an auto accident. Unsure who he is, unable to remember much of what has recently happened, and easily irritated by situations he used to take in stride, he bounces around for a while between the acute hospital where he was treated after the accident and a rehabilitation hospital that sends him out when a medical complication arises, and is not able to "readmit" him without a lengthy repeat screening procedure. At home, he rapidly becomes overly suspicious and mentally disorganized. He eventually ends up on the psychiatric ward of the hospital where he was first treated, to rebuild slowly his personality as he recovers whatever part of his neurological loss may come back. In this supportive, low-pressure world, he copes well, but misses the chance to continue whatever fathering or work he is able to perform; at home, he goes to pieces. He needs a home somewhere in between these two.

A 78-year-old woman is brought to the hospital, white as a sheet and gasping for breath, in a repeat of her arrival there, nine months before, the time of her last hospitalization. Living alone in a single room on a diet of tea and cookies and refusing or forgetting to take the pills that the visiting nurse tries to remind her of, she has again managed to become so depleted of iron and vitamins that a severe anemia has put her marginal heart into congestive failure and swollen her lungs with fluid. Intensive medical work for a few hours and then careful management over several days are successful but leave the staff with what they call a "disposition problem." She wants to go back to her single room in the heart of a decayed neighborhood once proudly "lace-curtain" Irish, where she has lived since she was a girl, even as she watched in recent years her "own kind" flee to the suburbs and blacks and Puerto Ricans move in. But there she will again miss the social network that a generation ago might have sustained an elderly woman living all alone. In her isolation, even with the support of the visiting nurse, she will again sip tea and nibble cookies until she is again anemic and is again rushed, breathless, to the hospital. But the nursing home the staff would send her to, in their long debates over "what to do with her" once she is physically well, would be far away. And besides, she points out, she is not sick. What kind of home, or network of support in her own place, can we find for her, in between?

Workers in social welfare or child guardianship could document problems of this kind greater in number and complexity than these examples, from the medical setting where I have found them. Such problems are hardly unique to medicine. But from the medical context, we can make several observations about middlehomes. First, the problem brought in as "medical" or "psychiatric" is often simply a search for a middlehome, or a *better* middlehome. The medical setting is an important portal of entry (or of transfer) for many who cannot live in primary homes. Second, when middlehomes fail, our "medical" facilities are often called upon to fill a gap and serve as a temporary middlehome, or else to put the pieces together again for people who suffer, like the old woman mentioned above, a loss of care because their living place is not a good home. Third, a surprisingly large amount of "medical" time and talent is devoted to solving, or trying to solve, middlehome problems. Many hospital residents spend hours each week with the medical social worker, and more hours on the phone, trying to solve the clinical dilemmas for which they have only the name "disposition problems." Disposition of the patients becomes the physician's problem, because the patients have nowhere to go, even though the physician lacks the training or ancillary back-up, and the profession lacks a conceptual framework to manage such problems.

MIDDLEHOMES (AND DAYHOMES): WHY THE SILENT PARTNER IN THE HEALTH SYSTEM?

Compared to the large amounts of literature on the modern hospital and on outpatient practice, very little work has been done to describe, to conceptualize, to make and test hypotheses about, and to plan programs for this other buttress to people's health, middlehomes and dayhomes.

Sociology has said little more than medicine. Both theory of socialization and social control and empirical studies of societies leave unexamined the large range of living places "in between" the well-described primary homes and homes of disaster. Among community studies, for example, Lynd and Lynd (1956) assume that residence in one's "own family" is not only the norm and the mode in Middletown, but a near universal statistical reality. Middlehomes are reflected only in one footnote on adoption and on one page on the county home.

Such a blind spot in sociology may be related to the neglect of developmental models, in particular the kind of interactional developmental model presented here. Without that, sociology has relied on models of social role learning in which the individual's contribution is not emphasized. Only among some anthropologists with a psychoanalytical orientation has a developmental framework been widely used in which children and their shifting developmental needs are prominent. The sociology of the changing developmental needs of adults receives attention in another chapter (see chapter 11).

It is true that some middlehomes, especially halfway houses for discharged mental patients, are currently in vogue. Governments are eager to favor the development of halfway houses, particularly if they will save money over the expensive state hospitals and prevent more scandals in which poor community planning leads to "back wards in the streets" among discharged patients. Financial support is as yet still meager. It is one thing to run after a galloping social problem with an imaginative solution and quite another to plan comprehensively for a comprehensive social need. The latter has not been done. Why not?

I can point to three partial answers. One is the ambivalence for everything collective or altruistic that seems a part of the American ideology of every-man-for-himself. Americans often act as if they thought that self-reliance and freedom of choice would be jeopardized by an acknowledgment that there are things we must do for each other and many people who cannot do everything for themselves. Among all the kinds of dependence and neediness in human society, we single out one kind, economic needs, to be called "dependency," and use that in a pejorative sense. In the 1920s, in Middletown, Lynd and Lynd wrote, "The working philosophy toward helping the 'dependent,' tends to be: people in actual need must be helped, because you wouldn't let a dog starve, but we must not make it too easy for them, and by all means let's get the unpleasant business over with and out of sight as soon as possible." (Lynd and Lynd, 1956).

The same wish seems to shape our current ignoring of problems, especially when they imply a need for social services for the reasons Gunnar Myrdal (1968) had in mind when he said that all ignorance is opportunistic.

Ignoring our collective problems, and our collective and altruistic efforts to deal with them, is an unfortunate habit, because we thereby conceal much that we do that is cooperative or group-minded. While we concentrate on our "individualism," the slogans blind us to parts of ourselves and our neighbors that do not seem to fit the conventional wisdom. We find ourselves in a vicious circle: believing that efforts-in-common are not our way; then, failing to recognize such efforts when they occur, we become less likely to work cooperatively. Our impulses to be diligent in the service of others, or in company with others, may atrophy as they receive little conscious and public encouragement (Eisenberg, 1972).

Another reason is the strength of feelings aroused in all of us by consideration of such issues as parenting, the family, and homes. It is hard to review neutrally the historical changes that led to the appearance of middlehomes; this may be the most affectively charged aspect of modernization, touching such issues as the effect of slum life on children, epidemic runaways, women's work and child care. Social policy planning, however, requires suspension of judgment on the *processes* by which people have come to live in middlehomes, in order that one can recognize the *fact* that they do, and plan accordingly. Separate attention to the ways that the family has become less of a home is appropriate and may in itself form the basis for other policy. But wishing people were not homeless, or planning family-supportive systems that, had they existed, might have kept them "at home," does nothing for those presently afloat. And to hope that people with problems, if no planning is done, will just disappear (a hope expressed by many confronting runaway teenagers in the sixties) is both vain and cruel. On a national level, the veto of the Child Development Bill of 1972, justified with the rhetoric of preserving the family, ignored the reality of where children are actually spending the day. That rhetoric, like all ignorance, served the interests of those in power and retarded the interests of the disenfranchised: middlehome populations, more often than not, include the dispossessed and the disenfranchised.

Two other reasons for our lack of either a middlehomes concept or a middlehomes policy concern medicine more particularly. One is the tendency to speak of the "health system" as if it began and ended with the efforts of doctors and other health personnel. The social, cultural, and environmental aspects of health, quite unplanned or at least not part of the "health maintenance" program, but nonetheless important to health (Mechanic, 1972; Townsend, 1974), are harder to keep in view, especially when looking from inside the hospital. There is irony as well as myopia in this situation, because of the huge amount of doctors' time that ends up being spent, for example, on middlehome problems. What I propose is that we as doctors acknowledge this part of our work, think about it systematically, and begin to include it openly in our training and practice.

Community psychiatry is the one area of medicine that has recognized and attempted to foster, with regard to mental health, "all the other" health-sustaining aspects of community life (Kaplan, 1974). Here I would expand that view (1) to insist that such supports, including middlehomes and dayhomes, are essential for all forms of the health of a society, not just sanity and psychological well-being, and (2) to attempt to bring them, conceptually, into medicine.

The other reason has to do with the conceptual framework with which physicians view events. Most of medicine and psychiatry focuses on the individual patient or potential patient, in whom disease is conceptualized as the faulty development or current malfunction of an anatomic organ whose normal function we believe we understand. Even psychiatrists, refusing to despair at having no dissectable diseased organ to grapple with, have fastened with a vengeance on a physicalistic mythology, imagining hydraulic fluid flowing among the (postulated) organs and positing a "stable character structure" and "psychic institutions."

In the midst of this, we all, physicians of body and mind alike, come to grips only reluctantly and fleetingly with two other views of life: first, we hesitate to gain an understanding of the ever flowing world of relationships among individuals and identities-through-doing-and-knowing that shape our lives and those of our patients (Minuchin, 1974); second, we neglect developmental medicine in our thinking even when we recognize it in practice. Heraclitus' dictum, "A man never steps into the same river twice; the second time, both the man and the river have changed," is quoted more often by classicists than by physicians. It reflects both the existential balance-of-relationships view, and also the progressive-through-time view of life. These notions have a hard time with our medicine, derived as it is from the fixed sections of the pathologists, the stable if changing internal milieu of the physiologists, and the points of fixation of the psychoanalysts. But they are essential to understanding people's changing developmental needs, and the middlehomes, which are meant to ease those interactions, provide resilience to the person during times of change, and respond imaginatively to the demands of each season of life.

WHY A NEW CONCEPT?

I hope that this discussion will bear fruit in three areas: health care and health planning; social theory and planning; and the ways we think about psychological development and society.

First, in the area of health, an appreciation of middlehomes supplements current notions of how people's health is maintained. If useful, this concept should be worked into medical curricula and into the conceptual models physicians use to think about disease, just as in other eras aspects of life not at first thought relevant to health and disease (like the quality of the water or the amount of dust in the air) were described, recognized as relevant, conceptualized, and integrated into medical thinking and practice. Research could then begin to answer the questions as yet not even asked, about what kinds of homes will be most helpful, for what kinds of people, with which kinds of problems, at which ages, in order to flesh out empirically the impressionistic bones of this subject. Then, an understanding of what middlehomes are and of how they function, and of how residence affects health, would enable clinicians to approach "placement" problems with a clearer notion of what the issues are and of what best match between patient's needs and middlehomes assets may be sought.

Second, in the area of social theory, a conceptual understanding of the function of middlehomes in modern society is long overdue not simply for heuristic purposes, but because all efforts at social planning depend on an awareness of how society works and of what current social needs are. No one can do justice to any segment of society without knowing about it, and, in fact, society has hardly done justice to middlehomes and the related dayhomes, as anyone familiar with the financial situations of most of the institutions discussed in this chapter can attest. Yet, more than financial rewards are at stake: general recognition would greatly boost the morale of those who work in middlehomes and dayhomes, who presently have to live with the fact that they work in a kind of orphan-area, for which there seems to be no place in the national view of the way things are.

Third, with regard to psychological development: our child welfare, foster home, adolescent shelter, and old peoples' home systems remain in a state of moral and financial penury partly because of the lack of a unified theory of what milieu settings contribute to personal growth, and partly because of failure to make use of comprehensive theories that already exist. A definition of middle-homes' contribution to the development of people's adult strengths is a necessary step to remedy that lack. The benefits will accrue on two levels: more attention will be paid, and maybe even more money, when advocates of boys' clubs, or of better day care, or of decent halfway houses, for example, present their case; and also, in the fields of psychiatry and social work, a new tool will be available with which to think about the meaning for a given person, say, on leaving a psychiatric hospital, of going to his or her primary home or going to one of a variety of middlehomes.

THE SOCIAL ECOLOGY OF GENEROSITY

A review such as this one of the range of institutions that support people's growing up and thriving, and that enhance their ability to help others likewise to grow and to thrive, may serve as a reminder that our ability to respond to the needs of others depends on two things: our experience of generosity when young, and our sense of the kinds of moral and material supports around us right now. Human generosity is a delicate growth in need of cultivation at all ages. At some point, society will recognize that cultivation to be one of its major tasks (Titmuss, 1972).

Such an awareness—and a knowledge of human development in general—imposes on those who share it a social and political responsibility, especially with regard to children. For we can afford neither the wishful thinking that deprivation does not matter because "children bounce back," since we know that beyond a point some of the effects of deprivation are irreversible; nor the therapeutic nihilism that remedial efforts are not worth trying once "damage has been done," since our incomplete knowledge of the point of irreversibility obliges us to give every child the benefit of remedial services (Eisenberg, 1975).

Such a responsibility obliges us to pay close attention to those living outside of primary homes, in the middlehomes and the homes of disaster, since they, by definition, are not having their needs met by primary homes and since the meeting of people's needs in middlehomes and homes of disaster is both more conspicuous and a more a public concern than is the case with those "still at home" who remain the private responsibilities of their families.

A survey of such institutions does not allay one's concerns. The problems include not only inadequate social and financial support, but, according to one's social and ethnic background and wealth, great variation in access to and quality of facilities and services. This maldistribution holds whether we speak of foster care, boarding schools, convalescent homes, or old-age homes. Existing middlehomes, in short, are allocated according to the concepts of the market economy.

In the largest sense, the question raised by this chapter is whether we are going to continue to regard the meeting of such basic human needs as we have discussed in this chapter—people's residential needs in a developmental sense—as a private matter, with people purchasing the goods according to their means, and with society providing, where conscience leads and resources allow, varying degrees of inadequate services and facilities for those who cannot afford to buy their own. The other proposition, that shelter, in particular developmentally adequate shelter, be recognized as a human right to be provided by society at large (along with the other acknowledged developmental necessities like clean air, and water, food, schooling and medical care) seems more in keeping with our knowledge of human development and with our best sense of our obligations to each other and to the health and strength of coming generations.

REFERENCES

Aries, P. 1965. Centuries of Childhood: A Social History of Family Life. New York: Knopf.

Berger, P., B. Berger, and H. Kellner. 1973. The Homeless Mind: Modernization and Consciousness. New York: Vintage.

Bowlby, J. 1952. Maternal Care and Mental Health. Geneva: World Health Organization.

Brown, C. 1973. The Group. New York Times Magazine, December 16, pp. 22 et seq.

Curtin, S. R. 1972. Nobody Ever Died of Old Age. Boston: Little, Brown.

Eisenberg, L. 1965. Deprivation and foster care. Journal of the American Academy of Child Psychiatry 4:243-248.

———. 1972. The human nature of human nature. Science 176:123-128.

———. 1973. Psychiatric intervention. Scientific American 229:116-127.

———. 1975. Primary prevention and early detection in mental illness. Bulletin of the New York Academy of Medicine 51:118-129.

Erikson, E. H. 1963. Childhood and Society. 2nd ed. New York: Norton.

———. 1968. Identity: Youth and Crisis. New York. Norton.

———. 1976. Reflections of Dr. Borg's life cycle. Daedalus Spring:1-28.

Goffman, E. 1961. Asylums: Essays on the Social Situation of Mental Patients and Other Inmates. Garden City, N.Y.: Anchor.

Governor's Commission on Adoption and Foster Care. 1973. Report to Governor Sargent. Boston: Governor's Commission on Adoption and Foster Care.

Kanter, R. M. 1972. Commitment and Community. Cambridge, Mass.: Harvard University Press.

———. 1973. Communes: Creating and Managing the Collective Life. New York: Harper & Row.

Kaplan, G. 1974. Support Systems and Community Mental Health: Lectures on Conceptual Development. New York: Behavioral.

Lewis, O. 1965. La Vida: A Puerto Rican Family in the Culture of Poverty—San Juan and New York. New York: Random House.

Lynd, R. S., and H. M. Lynd. 1956. Middletown: A Study in American Culture. New York: Harcourt, Brace, & World.

Makarenko, A. S. 1951. The Road to Life. Moscow: Foreign Language Publishing House.

McGrath, S. D. 1974. Community treatment—a broken promise? Schizophrenia Bulletin, Fall (10):4-5.

Mechanic, D. 1972. Social-psychologic factors affecting the presentation of bodily complaints. New England Journal of Medicine 286:1132-1139.

Minuchin, S. 1974. Families and Family Therapy. Cambridge, Mass.: Harvard University Press.

Myrdal, G. 1972. Asian Drama: An Inquiry into the Poverty of Nations. New York: Random House.

Ohlin, L., R. B. Coates, and A. D. Miller. 1974. Radical correctional reform: a case study of the Massachusetts youth correctional system. Harvard Educational Review 44:74-111.

Provence, S., and R. Lipton. 1962. Infants in Institutions: A Comparison of Their Development with Family Infants. Report of a Five-Year Research Study. New York: International Universities Press.

Rabkin, J. 1974. Public attitudes toward mental illness: a review of the literature. Schizophrenia Bulletin, Fall(10):9-33.

Rothman, D. J. 1971. The Discovery of the Asylum: Social Order and Disorder in the New Republic. Boston: Little, Brown.

Spitz, R. 1946. Anaclitic depression. Psychoanalytic Study of the Child 2:313-342.

Titmuss, R. M. 1972. The Gift Relationship: From Human Blood to Social Policy. New York: Random House.

Townsend, P. 1974. Inequality and the health service. Lancet i:1179-1190.

Trilling, L. 1972. Sincerity and Authenticity. Cambridge, Massachusetts: Harvard University Press.

Winnicott, D. W. 1965. The Maturational Processes and the Facilitating Environment: Studies in the Theory of Emotional Development. New York: International Universities Press.

Wolff, P. H. 1970. An Evil Hour (film). Boston: Committee of Responsibility.

CHAPTER 11

REVEREND CALDWELL
A Life History in the
Civil Rights Movement

William R. Beardslee, M.D.

Reverend Caldwell is one of a group of civil rights workers who has remained active from the early 1960s until the present, working to realize the goals of the Civil Rights Movement. This chapter is his own description of how he survived in the movement, of what he sees as having kept him going.

The piece is one of a series[1] describing civil rights workers' firsthand accounts of how the workers were able to survive the pressures of the movement. The aim of the series is to develop an understanding of how the workers say they were able to survive; this is both a first step for understanding how they were able to survive, and a crucial part of a full understanding of how they were able to survive.

I became interested in what I think is an unusual psychological strength under pressure through my own work in the Civil Rights Movement in the 1960s. The larger clinical issue of how people cope successfully with severe emotional stress, be they patients, or families of patients, or whatever, has been of great interest to me throughout my training. Reverend Caldwell's history, and the other histories in the series, are relevant to the larger clinical issues in that they provide examples of successful coping.

I chose to approach the question of coping in the movement by obtaining firsthand histories after reviewing the literature about the movement. Although there is much valuable writing about the

[1] Beardslee, William R. 1977. *The Way Out Must Lead In, Life Histories in the Civil Rights Movement*, Atlanta: Center for Research in Social Change, Emory University.

movement, from a variety of perspectives, there is no in-depth, well worked out psychological study. There are no straightforward, standardized psychological tests that are directly applicable. There are numerous analyses of the movement, with many different kinds of explanations offered. In reviewing the literature, I was most impressed with the firsthand accounts, either told exclusively by the participants or mediated through a sympathetic listener. Of the latter, the books of Robert Coles (1967, 1971) have influenced me a great deal. I came to do the work as I did because of my attraction to the firsthand account, and because of an underlying impression from my own experience in the movement and from my subsequent clinical work. This impression was that the people who had endured such stress had had to develop an unusual degree of self-perception in order to survive. I felt that these people who had seen so much change and who had changed so much themselves must have thought about their pasts and about their needs and about what kept them going.

My method was to interview Reverend Caldwell and the others in depth about their life histories, their current situations, and their own perceptions of what has kept them working.

In trying to characterize the life histories, I asked the people about their early lives, then briefly about their initial involvement in the movement and the reasons for it, then the questions central to the inquiry: what kept them going over time; what did they see as the source of their strength; how did they deal with hard times in the movement, such as the deaths of close friends. I concentrated on the self-perception of the people, what their own explanations of themselves were. I asked in detail about the role of an ideology in their lives, whether it was a religious faith, nonviolent philosophy, or a political credo. I tried to get a sense of the progression of each person's life. I paid particular attention to the period after 1967, as it was a watershed point in the movement both in terms of change in ideology and in that many people left the movement at that time. I asked more or less the same questions of each of the people, although the order varied and the questions were general and open-ended. Each person was allowed to develop the answers to the extent that he or she saw fit.

In the reporting, I tried to be as true to the sense of the words as possible. I did not retell the history in my own words, although I edited and reorganized it somewhat. Where it seemed relevant, I included a brief description of the person's current setting. This is especially important in Reverend Caldwell's situation, as his story is so closely bound to a particular piece of land.

I have not elaborated conclusions beyond what the people themselves conclude about themselves, as this is primarily an attempt to look at the quality of self-understanding that has developed in conjunction with the work in civil rights.

Thus, Reverend Caldwell emphasizes his early experiences with his grandmother as formative. In his movement experience, he talks about the power and support of the group, music's important function in relation to group cohesion and his own faith, troubled as that is. These then are his own conclusions, which are, I believe, quite valid.

"I do have hope, although it's a very troubled hope. I think the biggest thing we've got going for us is the fact that we have a group and it's working amid all the failures. It's working as the source of comfort and support for us. It encourages me that there's a possibility to hope to connect this piece of land we have up with other pieces of land that other people own and finally bring about a strength and a togetherness that can't be broken. I haven't given up the idea of changing this damnable monster that we have.

"A crisis came in many young guys' lives in the movement when they felt that all that they had done was in vain. They felt white folk were going to be in charge, and they saw what they had done going down the stream. My analysis of it is that they weren't able to regroup and devise new ways of living at that point. I advised them to find a way to take care of themselves while there was still a chance. That's what we're trying to do here."

Reverend Caldwell spoke to me in rapid-fire bursts, his head bobbing up and down as he emphasized a point, or illustrated another. He is a tall, well-muscled man. We met on the huge tract of farmland that occupies all of his attention at present. The land is communally owned by the movement group in the area. As we talked, we drove along the boundaries of the land. It is rich, flat farmland, dark soil in long, regular rows, with patches of red clay and white clay, and occasionally broken with thickets of brush, groves of fruit trees, and ponds. Reverend Caldwell spoke with great pride of the land and the farm equipment. He knew every acre well.

He is the acknowledged leader of the Civil Rights Movement in the area. In the course of his twelve years of work there, he has organized the community in a variety of efforts, from challenging public accommodations, to voter registration, to school desegregation, and finally to acquiring the land.

The land is communally owned, any decisions about it are made by the movement community as a group. In the early days of the movement, both here and in many other places, the workers lived on a subsistence wage and pooled what money there was for the whole group's needs. Reverend Caldwell, his family, and his co-workers still live this way. His wife is also a movement worker. They have two young children.

The group includes many workers who have been there for a number of years. In the troubled times of the late sixties, Reverend Caldwell remained committed to the possibilities of blacks and whites working together, when so many turned away from those possibilities. The project that he leads now, as then, has both blacks and whites working on it.

He himself is caught up in the vision of what the farm could be, and he thinks entirely in terms of how to keep it going. As an example, when we talked of health care needs, his interests were in how a clinic could be used as an organizing tool in getting support for the larger farm project.

In the course of our talking, we visited the farm manager's office, where there is also a market and a store. It was the middle of winter, and the reverend and the manager talked at length about what cash crops—that is, truck-farming vegetables—to plant in the spring, what quantities, which to experiment with and which to plant in bulk, which seeds to buy and how much they would cost. They talked about marketing, whether they would have the transportation needed or would have to rent some, how to load the vegetables, which markets to deliver to, how to display and label the items once delivered, and how much they could expect to make.

They talked of plans to develop the store and the market. The manager emphasized that the many people who work on the farm spend their earnings in the town, and thus the money is lost. He wants the money to be spent in the community and said, "I want that dollar to touch as many hands as possible."

What was striking throughout my visit was the dependence of the success of the whole undertaking on such things as the shrewdness and the timing of the marketing, not just on people's faith and work. Financial solvency is all the more important in light of the lack of it in the first few years of the farm's operations.

Reverend Caldwell described the struggle to raise the money to buy the land. Some of the money came from private sources, some from foundations, and some from commercial loans. He spoke of the continued struggle to keep the farm going. He is embattled, accountable to outside sources for funds and to the black community, and under pressure from both. The farm has by no means earned money up to its full capacity. There are complaints of mismanagement in agricultural technique. There is by no means unqualified support from the black community. There have been complaints about working conditions. To compound the problem, Reverend Caldwell led the movement in the area for years before the land was acquired. He led the effort to acquire the land. Thus, people have very high expectations of him, both in the community and in the outside organizations.

In talking of how he had come to the position he now holds, he spoke first about his grandmother.

"I've always said if the Lord called me, He called me through the mouth of my grandmother. I really believe that she had the greatest influence on my leaning toward the ministry, and I know that she influenced my going to church.

"I could talk all day about my grandmother. She was a human being. She had her faults, but she had an inside beauty. She was a mixture of Indian and white folk that brought out the American best. She was a beautiful woman, light-skinned with straight hair, the rest of her characteristics were Negroid.

"A the age of 70, she could still jump in the air and kick her heels twice. That always amazed all the children. Also, she would play with us, she'd get down on the floor and play with us. Grandma just had ways, I guess, that everybody wanted to mimic. It wasn't what she did so much outside. It was the inside that made you respond to her.

"We grew up poor, in a rough neighborhood, and yet we weren't rough people. My grandma wasn't rough, as such, but she wouldn't take no stuff from nobody.

"I remember, also, my momma. Since we were poor, we didn't have the things that we needed. I felt ashamed a lot of times at school about what I had to wear and the fact that I didn't have enough money to pay for lunch. But somehow my momma overlooked all of that and kept pushing me. She didn't try to get away from her responsibilities as a mother as many young girls do these days, and I appreciate her for that.

"It took me a long time to understand the way my mother acted. That's something I've thought about for a long time and have finally worked out in my mind through introspection, rethinking, looking, searching, reading. I'm trying to understand this. I remember that my mother was quite young, and she and I sort of grew up together.

"I remember one time when my mother refused to eat when we were eating. I had a notion that she wasn't eating at all, so I made up my mind to watch her that whole night to see if, in fact, she ate. She went to bed and didn't eat at all. The next day I demanded that she eat. I told her that I knew she hadn't eaten. So she did eat that time. That's the one thing I remember that really started me thinking about being responsible about things at home.

"For some reason, I was very visionary as a child. I guess I'd say that there were many times that I was just able to see further as a child than my parents, elderly people, other adults around me. If there's anything that I believe would be a gift that's mine, it would be the gift of insight and sensitivity to people and some funny kind of ESP.

"As a child, I used my imagination either to ward off, as it were, the bad spirits, or bring good spirits to my aid. Practically speaking, I entertained myself. When I was scolded or made to stay in or beaten, I would say I was going to be something. I wasn't going to be here. It wasn't going to be like this always.

"That was one way I dealt with bringing the spirits; another was the fact that I saw things in the future and people were scared. I just found out recently that my immediate family was afraid of me, of things I would say about people who would die or not die, things like that. I don't know what it is. Sometimes there's some experience of my life in which I feel like I've been there before or have seen the experience before, or can say what's going to happen. It frightens me, too, sometimes. When I was younger, it didn't frighten me. I'd just come out and say it. It might be that we would be riding up a hill and I could tell a car was coming before we saw it. It might be that someone would start talking or thinking and I'd say exactly what that other person was already thinking or saying. That sort of thing is what I call ESP.

"I come out of a basic Baptist background and a strict Fundamentalist understanding of the Scriptures. I built a church at the age of about 8 or 9 with my group. It was rectangular in structure, set at about one-sixth, and it hung over at the edges about a foot. That was the chapel part. The congregational part was the flat top." The reverend paused and then said, "The whole thing was later converted to a tank," and he laughed.

"There were a lot of other things we did as children. We made some inventions, whistles, for example. We all did them together, the whole gang. It was a group that went places together and stayed together. I started talking about that because it reminds me that it may have some connection with my feeling about how we operate on the farm now, that good experience that I had in my childhood, working with a small group, making decisions together not exactly as we do now but, you know, I'm stretching the point, but there might be some connection. I'm just thinking it out.

"I was a member of the Police Boys' Club and I was superintendent of my Sunday School. I was teaching the Bible there at the Sunday School. I was convincing enough to adults to allow me to supervise them. I was exercising my mind in the Bible class very strongly. I was outspoken among adults, one or two of whom I really respected for wisdom; not for their actions, but for their wisdom." He laughed.

"The Police Boys' Club allowed me not to be afraid of policemen. I learned boxing as a child and so I wasn't afraid to fight. I grew up in a rough neighborhood where I was beaten up a lot, but people knew that if they beat me they'd have to keep on beating me. I was a small boy, but they knew that if they ever beat me, boy, they'd have me on their hands for a long time. I'd be throwing rocks from around the corners at them, and fighting back. I wouldn't give up. I'd keep fighting till I won.

"I remember this one man who said he was helping me. He was a teacher. I wasn't a hard person. I was soft, tender-hearted, and he saw weakness in that, so he really stomped me around. He hit me. He cussed me every day, actually cussed me out. He'd throw something down on the floor and make me pick it up. He pulled a real Simon Legree, saying he was trying to help me to make me strong, you know. That was strength, but I had already fashioned a kind of strength about myself, not one that I had determined to be strength, but that was in fact strength. My strength was my stick-to-itness. So that was my growing up.

"Before the sit-ins in Greensboro I got interested in sit-ins through a fellow, a good friend of mine named Howard. For some reason, he came up with the idea of going to churches to see if they really believed what they were talking about. This was 1954 or 1955. He came to see if I would help him test the churches in the town where I grew up. It might be interesting to tell you that that town is the only city that, for instance, the first and only city in this country where the City Council has come out against South Africa. I mean against the banks supporting apartheid. They have a majority black council down there.

"Anyway he came to me with the idea, and we talked about it, and we executed it by going to various churches. It was the white churches, on Sundays, and we were turned away from some. One church let us in and sat us right in the front. I thought that they were trying to embarrass us, putting us up front. We got some threats. But we kept going. The point is that it was significant because it was before Greensboro. I did it and forgot it, no big thing. Nobody went to jail.

"In my time I've worked just about every work that a child could work and I worked many, many jobs that any man, a black man, would have to work to exist. I've done everything from shining shoes to waiting tables, dishwashing or being a bus boy, or doing cafeteria work, or working for a furniture company . . . everything.

"But the greater part of my life was spent in school. I had a rough time in college. I had to work, earning money almost full-time at times, and in my last year of college I did work full-time at two jobs. One job I was working was in the cafeteria, and I spent two hours every meal; that's six hours. Then I was working at night as an orderly in the college grill—you know, a bar-type place where you come in and buy a hamburger—eleven to seven shift. I was making pretty good grades, too.

"I used to write essays as part of my class work. There was one teacher who wouldn't accept that I had written them. She wouldn't give me credit for what I wrote. I remember one thing that I wrote that I've analyzed several times. I described a man who was thirsty. I don't remember the whole story now, but anyhow this man got thirsty doing something in the desert and he had a delusory vision of water and found himself swimming in the mud and the mud dried on him and the ants came. I would use my imagination, you know."

He narrated very simply the way he had joined the movement and did not elaborate on it.

"At college, another friend, Frank, came to me and talked about these demonstrations. Then the SCLC [Southern Christian Leadership Conference] made a call for kids who were doing demonstrations to come to North Carolina, Greensboro. We had a meeting in Charlotte. That's where SNCC [Student Nonviolent Coordinating Committee] got started. I thought it was a good idea to go and find out what other guys were thinking about and what they were doing, and I thought why shouldn't we get together on these things? Somebody else had organized it, and I went and listened. I didn't have much to say, but I said a few things and became a part of it. I went back to school and then left to work with SNCC and was sent to this area.

"When we first came here, we decided to go to Rock Hill because some kids at Rock Hill were demonstrating and were doing what we had talked about doing, refusing bond. We thought we should go in there and refuse bond also to show people in the country, to ask the people in the country, to come and fill that jail.

"There were four of us. We went to participate with those thirteen kids who were in jail there, and we went to jail in the same way. That was a big experience there. I learned a lot about nonviolence, really, about nonviolent action."

The reverend talked in detail about the transformation that took place in him because of that and other jailings.

"I think in going to jail I found out about as much about the church as I did about myself. My understanding of the church started to change in jail. I was looking at things probably in a different way than most of the young guys there, since I was both fighting being a minister and at the same time knowing that I had to be a minister. I was looking for peace. The inward calling, at times, was greater than the call my grandma put on me, because it had started internalizing itself and being more a part of me than my grandma. My grandma had died and I was still alive. Being in jail, the experience of Paul and Silas and all those guys that I knew about became more real, and so Christianity became more real itself. That's why that experience had greater meaning to me.

"Actually loving your neighbor and doing unto others became real to me only in the movement. Before, it was just conceptual, and going to church on Sunday, and loving, you know, because it's wrong to hate, and feeling guilty if you hate because of the wrong. Whereas in the movement, I moved from loving as a doctrine to loving as a discipline, to loving as a way of life, to now loving and hating as a healthy way of life."

After his initial involvement, he stayed in the one area in which he works now. He has seen all the phases of the movement from the vantage point of his one area. We talked first about the general problems of being in the movement for a long time.

"A problem in the movement was that we had to act. We couldn't say, 'Well, we're going to stop our actions on the grounds of not enough information to come to a conclusion.' That's what we accused others of doing. We couldn't do that. We did not have the choice not to act.

"We wanted to destroy an evil society. The problem was, if we destroy, on what are we going to build? We have to think about all this the whole time that we're working, with every little problem that we solve. What are we doing when we help a union develop? Are we really helping the cause that we propose, or hurting it? If we get a union involved, we know that the national officers are fat, sometimes corrupt, and that they make deals with the corporations that we're fighting. We know all these things, and we have to wonder whether we're really helping our cause or hurting it. So, out of the old society, we are taking some things to build the new. There's a problem in that, and we have to deal with that general problem and come to a satisfying or unsatisfying solution and act.

"A particular problem we faced here was that this is a place where the heat of battle between black and white wasn't buffered by the Mississippi image, but it was buffered by the image of a good state, a border state. The whole state is buffered by the image. People don't believe that things that happened here can happen, while they believe it about Mississippi.

"So it was difficult for us to get the kind of pressure of conscience from the nation. Dr. King did come. Then he left. Then we were in the same situation. We didn't ever get the resources the other places got again during the movement and after the movement. You don't see a lot of development down here, and that's the cause of it; that's the reason. Everything we got, we got it inch by inch by inch. It was hard in Mississippi, but then, after the explosions, after those three guys died, things began to ease up and the people in Mississippi got more resources than we got here. People don't understand that. As a result, it just has taken us longer to develop what we had to develop, but I don't . . . let's see what I want to say . . . we suffered for it, but I wouldn't say that I'd rather have it that way.

"Progress is misleading. I could say that our progress has been like a ring in our noses. Progress has been a stumbling block for us as organizers, because the people became satisfied and aren't willing to take the steps that need to be made. After all the fuss about public accommodations, it doesn't encourage me to see that we're going in all those same places, spending all our money, and coming out as poor or poorer for it.

"All kinds of bad things happened in the movement. On top of all the problems, there was the ordinary selfish greediness of individuals no matter who they were. If we couldn't comprehend either all of it or some of it or enough to deal with it as it touched us, then we'd be overwhelmed by everything. We'd start overeacting to things.

"Then, too, after you start batting your head up against a wall, trying to break the wall, or trying to get leverage to move the wall and make it more comfortable in your box, then you either fall back on your history and be swayed or cajoled or be praised by it or if it is not there to be affirmed in the historical past, then you have to grab hold of the present moment, or you've got to have a vision. When people had a vision, they were able to be stabilized in the present situation.

"In many people's lives in the movement, there came a time when support was needed, and in some cases there was no support. To be more specific, you see . . . what I'm trying to say is that if, while a person was trying to understand himself, maybe he went to his childhood and saw what out of his childhood he had to take to make himself strong enough to deal with what this and that influence were doing to him. He needed somebody to help him put it together. He was not getting any reinforcement from the predominant society and perhaps at that time was at odds with his girlfriend or his wife, so he was dealing with not getting any support there, either. Also, a person in the movement during those times was most likely a young person just out of adolescence, suffering from the wounds that adolescence leaves, and then all these other things were thrust upon him at once. Maybe also he was kicked out of the movement or something in the movement was not going fast enough for him or his livelihood was threatened. Whatever the reason was, the point is that he had a crisis because he didn't have the resources or the reassurance that he needed, and if he was not able to deal with that particular crisis, it had a domino effect and shattered his image of himself. Many people left the movement because of that.

"What happened to me, I didn't lose hope and I kept a group. I always told everybody else to do that. You can't make it in this kind of thing by yourself. You have to have something to reassure you. Not only that. You have to have something to keep you straight as far as not giving in to the rewards of this society.

"The songs that we sang had more influence than anything else in enabling us to endure what the white people put on us to endure without our going berserk.

" 'Dark Song,' and 'Freedom, Oh Freedom,' 'Let us Break Bread Together,' those were the songs we used to sing all the time before we met at meetings. 'We Shall Overcome' we would sing at the end of meetings. That was mostly sung in large groups where we wanted people to leave with the marching spirit and a sense of accomplishment. This song operated on me as well as them.

"Music is an opiate, a good opiate. Music does tend to bring together the spirit. Music is what kept the slaves together, enabling them to endure the lash. While we're sitting down here, our spirit is separate, you might say. When music moves, we move to the same spirit. So, in that sense, we feel that our spirit is moving together. We look at one another and communicate.

"Music can tell you what has gone on and what can go on. Music carries a depth charge with it. It can set off what we all know is there, the explosion that causes us to sing, 'God damn it, I ain't going to do it no more.' It's the rebel in us. It linked us with our past; it gave us a bridge from which to move during our present, and it hooked us onto the future. It gave us through another aspect, its creative aspect, a way to say where we were going. "I'm going to tear down your wall. I'm going to do this or I'm going to do the other." We all composed verses and songs. That music is something."

We concluded by talking about the reverend's personal position, not about the movement in general.

"I don't think my vision has changed a lot over the course of time. I had been talking black before Black Power . . . I had praised Garvey; at one point, I'd praised Malcolm X. I could see Malcolm coming into our camp, finally understanding that color is not the enemy; racism is. I think he saw that and he would have been a great resource for us . . . A racist is a racist. There ain't no color to a racist; that's what I'm saying. Any man can be . . . any man who uses race to his personal or group advantage is a racist.

"As for other hard times, I wouldn't want to say all the effects King's death, or Malcolm's, or other things had on me. Some could be described; some couldn't be described, and some I wouldn't want to describe. My direction was clear; it wasn't changed. My vision was a paradoxical vision. King's dream was part of my dream . . . but I also understood and had the nightmares that Malcolm had and the nightmares that Stokeley Carmichael, Rap Brown, and others had. To keep health, I have to be able to wake up out of my nightmare and have as much of the dream as I can and still be sensitive to reality.

"I've always felt that I'm a potential fanatic. If I were to stop believing that we could change things and there will be a better day . . . for me it would be the same as dying, and I fear my dying would not be easy on white people. I mean, Rap Brown, what he said about violence was nothing compared to what I would do. If he said to kill ten, I'd say ten thousand. I'd say that, after all that's been done here. But for now I keep on believing.

"I haven't even given up the philosophy of nonviolence, the strategy of nonviolence. I participated in it just a month ago. We were successful in getting the school board to allow certain changes in the educational process, getting teachers' jobs back, getting kids back in school, all that sort of thing. We operate in an environment now where one is to be ashamed of being nonviolent, you see, in our culture, I mean among those who were in the movement and call each other black.

"There weren't that many people that ever believed in nonviolence. People never believed in nonviolence as a goal or as more than a strategy. I never believed in nonviolence as apart from Christianity. I just incorporated Christianity, my understanding of Christianity, into nonviolence, what I learned from other people. I haven't really studied nonviolence on my own enough. I've read a few books but not really gotten down into it. I never really needed to. I taught it to other, younger people who probably feel it stronger than I do, but I had something stronger than it before I got into it. What I was into was the part of religion that says not to do this or not to do the other thing and not to let no man mistreat you as a human being and that you'd be willing to die for things. I've had all that in my whole life as a Christian, not in my life as a theoretician of nonviolence. I don't see any distinction there. See, if somebody asked me if I believed in nonviolence, I'd say yes, but I'd know immediately that they don't understand what I'm talking about.

"I'm in a flux about nonviolence and Christianity now. I'm reading Bonhoeffer and Tillich and the German school in general. On the other hand, I'm accepting the world of materialism and what is and where our people are as opposed to where they say they are, you know, how they act as opposed to how they say they understand love."

The reverend returned, finally, to a characteristic of himself that he had described earlier, and that sustains him now. "Stick-to-itness is what got me through the hard times in the movement, and also the hope that you can change some—if you stick to it."

REFERENCES

Coles, Robert. 1967. Children of Crisis, Vol. 1: A Study of Courage and Fear. Boston: Atlantic-Little, Brown.

Coles, Robert, 1971. Children of Crisis, Vol. 2: Migrants, Mountaineers, and Sharecroppers. Boston: Atlantic-Little, Brown.

Name Index

Subject Index